Home Care Therapy:
Quality, Documentation, and Reimbursement

A Handbook for Physical Therapists, Speech-Language Pathologists, and Occupational Therapists

Tina M. Marrelli, MSN, MA, BSN, RNC

Home Care and Hospice Consultant
Marrelli and Associates, Inc.
Boca Grande, Florida

Linda H. Krulish, MHS, PT

President, Home Therapy Services
Powell, Ohio

Marrelli and Associates, Inc.
Boca Grande, Florida

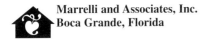

Marrelli and Associates, Inc.
Boca Grande, Florida

Printing in the United States of America
Cover design by Joann Schissel
Technical assistance by David F. Davis

Marrelli and Associates, Inc.
P.O. Box 629
Boca Grande, Florida 33921
(941) 697-2900, (800) 993-6397, FAX (941) 697-2901
E-mail: news@marrelli.com
Web Site: http://www.marrelli.com

Library of Congress Catalog Card Number 99-94255
International Standard Book Number 0-9647801-2-7

ACKNOWLEDGEMENTS

Heartfelt and special thanks to Lynda S. Hilliard, Sandy Martin Whittier, and Carroll Tollner Fernstrom for their thoughtful input and (re)reviews (and answering questions too numerous to remember). And, as always, I could not have done it at all (or at least not within this millennium) without the humor and help of Buddy and Bill Glass.

Tina M. Marrelli

A sincere thanks to the home care therapists, nurses, managers, and patients who have contributed to this work through example, contribution, and thoughtful review. Special thanks to the world's most supportive family...my sweetheart Bob and the little ones - Amanda, Noah, Holly, and Logan.

Linda H. Krulish

REVIEWERS

Gloria Bartholomew Nelson, MS, CCC, SP
Director, Gloria Bartholomew Nelson Associates
The Nelson Center
Annandale, Virginia

Margaret N. Carr, PT, MBA
Editor of the *Community Home Health Quarterly Report*
of the American Physical Therapy Association
Carr Consultants
Niles, Illinois

Kathryn S. Crisler, MS, RN
Assistant Director
Center for Health Services and Policy Research
University of Colorado Health Sciences Center
Denver, Colorado

Carroll Tollner Fernstrom, OTR/L
Licensed Occupational Therapist and Consultant
Professional Occupational Therapy Services
Richmond, Virginia

Mary M. Friedman, MS, RN, CRNI
Principal & Home Care Consultant Home Health Systems
Nurse Surveyor, Joint Commission on Accreditation
    of Healthcare Organizations
Marietta, Georgia

Deborah H. Heatherly, BSN, MA
Manager of Home Care Sales Operations
Hill-Rom
Charleston, South Carolina

Lynda S. Hilliard, RN, MBA, CNAA
Director of Quality Management, Education, and Compliance
VNA and Hospice of Northern California
Emeryville, California

Sandra G. Marody, PT
Physical Therapist
Wetzel County Hospital
New Martinsville, West Virginia

Rebecca A. Robinson - Brown, OTR/L
President
Robinson - Brown & Associates
Columbus, Ohio

Sandra M. Whittier, MSN, BSN, RNC
Clinical Coordinator Nursing and Rehabilitation
Home Health and Hospice Care Network
Whidden Hospital
Swampscott, Massachusetts

Carolyn (Sue) Wilkie, RN
Medicare Provider Consultant
Provider Education
Wellmark, Inc.
Des Moines, Iowa

Darlene Boenig Zakrajsek, MS, PT
Director of Rehabilitation Services
Meridia Home Health
Mayfield Village, Ohio

Preface

Providing skillful and compassionate care in the home setting brings its own challenges to all care team members. The rehabilitation team, usually thought of as being comprised of speech-language pathologists (SLP), physical therapists (PT), and occupational therapists (OT), and their specialized assistants, have never been as important as they are today in the emerging new vision of health care. This vision continually seeks a balance between cost, value and quality. These priorities of improved quality (e.g., evidence-based care, OASIS, expected and demonstrated improved outcomes) and increased cost-effectiveness and efficiencies has only heightened the importance of the therapy team members and their unique services and skills.

The effectiveness of the entire patient care team, as well as an understanding of the important roles and contributions of the rehabilitation team, is key to improved patient outcomes. This book, truly interdisciplinary, is the first of its kind in home care, and is authored by a nurse and a therapist. The book seeks to pull together the varying glossaries and therapy practices in home care, to work toward the standardization of care and practice. Our hope is that we contribute to improving home care services generally and therapy services specifically in the individual care provided daily to patients in communities everywhere.

Tina M. Marrelli and Linda H. Krulish

As we go to press...

The OASIS requirements have been revised and readers are encouraged to keep apprised of regulatory changes related to OASIS.

CONTENTS

Guidelines for Use

The goal of this book is to provide information and resources to enhance the coordination, appropriate utilization and quality of the therapy provided to patients in their homes. The book provides a comprehensive discussion of home care issues, including reimbursement and regulatory updates, and provides a common framework from which readers can work as the roles of therapists and other rehabilitation team members in home care continues its evolution. Because "home care" can mean so many different kinds of care provided in the home, we have strived for consistency throughout the text. With this in mind, be aware that the order of the rehabilitation therapists, physical therapists, speech-language pathologists, and occupational therapists as presented on the cover are reflected in the *Home Health Agency Manual*, also called the *HHA Manual* (HCFA Publication - 11). This is the Medicare manual that defines the specific coverage and other issues related to Medicare home care practice. As Medicare has set many of the standards for home care, we present this information in the same order as Section 204 of the *HHA Manual* thus being consistent with that Medicare publication.

Part One of the book includes an overview of home care, dividing pertinent issues into four topic areas or "domains." They are:
1) Domain One - The Reimbursement and Payer Domain;
2) Domain Two - Customer Service and Quality Imperatives;
3) Domain Three - The Patient's Home as Environment of Care; and
4) Domain Four - Patient Care Planning and Related Processes.

Domain One contains information about the Medicare home care benefit and tips and tools to improve documentation skills and clarify issues related to the Medicare home health benefit, including the definition and determination of the patient's homebound status.

Domain Two describes customer service and quality issues and provides valuable information for managers and visiting clinicians in assessing and improving care and operations through customer service and competency assessment initiatives.

Domain Three provides practical insights into the unique issues and considerations created by the patient's home as the site for care delivery and that environment's impact on achieving desired outcomes.

Domain Four addresses issues revolving around care planning and the care cycle. This section provides essential information describing the specific covered services of each discipline with an emphasis on the therapist's case manager role, care coordination, and "therapy only" case considerations.

Part Two addresses two specialty practices in therapy, pediatrics and home hospice care, and these chapters contain useful forms, tips, and tables for practice. The first chapter in Part Two, "Pediatrics and Therapy: Making A Difference in Young Lives" provides an overview of the care provided to children with special needs. The next section, "Hospice and the Therapist: Efforts Directed Toward Comfort and Safety" addresses the special role of hospice care as our health system seeks to improve care at end-of-life. This section provides readers with a review of this important segment of health care and where therapists and others can make an important difference in the quality of life of patients and their loved ones.

Part Three presents in detail the unique and specialized roles of the physical therapist, speech-language pathologist, and occupational therapist in home care. In addition to describing the general role of each discipline, this section provides narrative information that more fully defines the areas of assessment and interventions utilized by each of the therapy disciplines. The information presented in this section is excerpted from publications of each of the national therapy associations, and represents a broad scope of clinical practice. Additionally, standards of practice and guidelines for care provision are also included along with a listing of additional resources and contact information for each of the national therapy associations. By presenting this information, all members of the home care team can further understand the unique roles of the rehabilitation team members and in this way perhaps be more effective in the early identification of patients needing a referral to a(nother) specialized service or intervention. Because excerpts from the national therapy associations have been reprinted with permission in this section, these references are listed as footnotes.

Part Four provides a comprehensive overview of the assessment process with an emphasis that assessment or evaluation serves as the foundation for all care planning and outcome achievement. The characteristics of what comprises an effective therapy assessment, additional responsibilities related to the admission process, and correct completion of the Health Care Financing Administration (HCFA) Form 485 are outlined in this section. Readers may refer to this section for valuable information about the Medicare requirements. This section also addresses the role of therapy providers and the requirements of a patient health status assessment with the defined components that comprise this holistic assessment.

Part Five is devoted to providing an overview of the Outcome and Assessment Information Set (OASIS) and related issues, including the role of OASIS in the larger purviews of outcomes-based quality improvement (OBQI) and prospective payment system (PPS) rate determinations.

Specific information related to the scope and specificity of the OASIS data set, the discipline-neutrality of the data elements, the development of OASIS - integrated tools, and data competency — are also presented. Sample competency tools are integrated into this section as well as a discussion related to the assessment of therapy staff's knowledge in required areas. A sample therapy tool that has integrated the required data set and is completed based on a patient case scenario provides practical visualization and application of the comprehensive assessment and the OASIS concepts addressed.

Part Six focuses on function. This part presents interdisciplinary therapy "care guides" related to a variety of functional limitations experienced by a wide range of patients receiving home care therapy services. At the start of this section a broadly constructed general care guide summary is introduced. This is intended to increase the awareness of the range of rehabilitation roles and activities in home care, and to facilitate an interdisciplinary approach to identification and management of the unique and comprehensive needs of the individual home care patient. Following the general care guide are eighteen specific care guides, which are listed alphabetically and presented in a functional manner. These specific care guides are presented in alphabetical order for easy retrieval of needed information and are intended to cue particular areas for assessment, interventions, and goals that together may improve patient performance.

The intent of these specific care guides is that the reader may readily identify patient rehabilitation needs and thus more comprehensively plan, individualize, and document patient care. Each of these care guides is defined by a specific performance area, such as "ambulation" and is divided into four standardized areas for easy identification of needed information. There is also the corresponding OASIS component(s) identified, where applicable.

The standard areas addressed in each specific care guide are:
1) Identified/Assessed Problems/Restricted Performance Areas,
2) Safety Checklist,
3) Actions/Interventions/Activities and
4) Specific Functional Goals.

#1 and #2 are listed alphabetically and may be used by all team members to more fully identify individual patient problems and safety and environmental challenges while parts #3 and #4 identify interventions and goals specifically indicated for the home care PT, SLP, and OT and are categorized in that manner and order for easy review of the information.

These care guides are not intended to be an exhaustive list of all the possible functional limitations that may be identified in the home care patient, nor do the proposed interventions and goals represent the boundaries of all available care options or opportunities.

It is important to note that the care guides are organized using the disablement model focusing on the functional impact of the patient's condition, as opposed to the medical model which organizes patients solely on the basis of the medical diagnosis. The premise on which the care guides are based includes an assumption that treatment plans and interventions are based on the individual patient and their unique medical, co-morbidity, rehabilitative, social, and discharge planning needs. Therefore the interventions, goals, and outcome measures outlined in the care guides may not be appropriate for every patient with a given functional limitation. The intent is to encourage investment in the patient assessment to determine not only the patient's functional limitations, but any other identified factors which should be considered in the care plan development to maximize outcomes through the achievement of optimal function or the attainment of the patient's highest possible functional capacity. As many clinicians are very familiar with the classification of patient populations by diagnosis, it is important that the reader review the introduction in this section, as it provides a conceptual description of the disablement model necessary to cost effectively utilize the therapy care guides. Included are examples of how to transition from a medical model (diagnosis) to a disablement model (impairment/functional limitation).

Part Seven contains equipment considerations that are referred to throughout the text and information about performing a comprehensive wheelchair assessment. Following this information is a home safety program.

Part Eight addresses aspects of human resource management such as competency tools and position descriptions for PTs, SLPs, and OTs in home care therapy.

Part Nine contains two of the most important parts of the *HHA Manual* (HCFA Publication - 11.) These are the "Coverage of Services" Section for Therapists and the "Correct Completion of the HCFA Form 485" and are printed here in their entirety. *It is important to note that Medicare makes Manual and policy changes and all clinicians and managers are encouraged to review new materials and information as it becomes available.*

Part Ten lists useful resources. This section includes a comprehensive list of abbreviations and a glossary of home care therapy terms. Licensing board information for PT, SLP, and OT by state is listed with addresses and phone numbers. Finally, there is an extensive Directory of Resources which lists educational and practice resources for clinicians.

About the Authors

Linda H. Krulish, MHS, PT is the owner of Home Therapy Services in Columbus Ohio, which provides direct patient care and consulting services to the home care industry. Linda H. Krulish received a Bachelor of Science in Physical Therapy in 1987 and completed a Master in Health Sciences in 1991, both from the Medical University of South Carolina. Ms. Krulish has served in home care organization management roles, including those as director of business development and specialty program development. Ms. Krulish provides presentations for organizations and associations on various topics related to the provision of therapy services in the home, is active in the American Physical Therapy Association (APTA), and serves as an officer in the Community Home Health Section. Ms. Krulish developed the *Home Therapy OASIS Assessment Forms* in 1999. She is an advocate for improving the quality and cost-effectiveness of home care services through enhancing outcomes of the interdisciplinary team. Therapy-specific questions can be directed to Ms. Krulish at (614) 250-5438 or via e-mail at linda.krulish@oasisanswers.com.

Tina M. Marrelli, MSN, MA, RN, C is the editor and publisher of *Home Care Nurse News*. Ms. Marrelli is also the author of the "Little Red Book", the *Handbook of Home Health Standards* and *Documentation Guidelines for Reimbursement* (third edition, Mosby, 1998), the *Hospice and Palliative Care Handbook: Quality, Compliance, and Reimbursement* (Mosby, 1999), *Mosby's Home Care and Hospice Drug Handbook* (1999), the *Nurse Manager's Survival Guide: Practical Answers to Everyday Problems* (second edition, Mosby, 1997), the *Nursing Documentation Handbook* (Mosby, 1996), and the *Handbook of Home Health Orientation* (Mosby, 1998). Ms. Marrelli is the co-author of *Home Health Aide: Guidelines for Care* (Marrelli, 1996), *Home Care and Clinical Paths: Effective Care Planning Across the Continuum* (Mosby, 1997), *Home Health Aide: Guidelines for Care Instructor Manual* (Marrelli, 1997) and the *Manual of Home Health Practice: Guidance for Effective Clinical Operations* (Mosby, 1998). Ms. Marrelli is also the editor of *Home Care Provider* (Mosby).

Ms. Marrelli received a Bachelor's degree in Nursing from Duke University School of Nursing and has directed various home care and hospice programs. In 1984 she received a Master of Arts in Management and Supervision, Health Care Administration and in 1996 she received a Master in Nursing.

Ms. Marrelli worked at the Health Care Financing Administration (HCFA) for 4 years in the areas of home care and hospice policy and operations, where she received the Bureau Director's Citation. She is a member of Sigma Theta Tau, is certified by the American Nurses Association (ANA) credentialing center as a home health nurse, and serves as a member of the National Hospice Organization's (NHO) Standards and Accreditation Committee. Ms. Marrelli was the 1998 recipient of the Arizona Association for Home Care's prestigious "Genie Eide Award" which recognizes dedication and contributions to the home care industry.

Correspondence, including feedback, recommendations, suggestions or additional information may be directed to her at the following address: Marrelli and Associates, Inc., P.O. Box 629, Boca Grande, FL 33921-0629. She can also be reached by calling (941) 697-2900, (800) 993-6397 or via the web site at www.marrelli.com or by e-mail news@marrelli.com.

PART ONE
Home Care: An Introduction

Home care can be defined in many ways. By varying definitions and the services provided, home care can encompass home infusion services, medical equipment services, home health care, private duty services, hospice and the traditional Medicare program or medically-directed care model. Clearly, it is the provision of the health care services at the patient and family's home that makes it truly a unique setting and practice. In some ways, home care is the antitheses of the care provided in an inpatient setting. Examples are numerous; in the hospital, patients are directed or told what to wear (a hospital gown), the hours (e.g., visiting hours) and the ages of visitors (e.g., no children under age ___), and other requirements and rules. At some level the hospital setting was designed around the provider physician's and hospital staff's needs; not the patient and family needs. As the entire health care system goes through a re-design for the new vision of health care, home will continue to be the setting of choice for many patients and their loved ones. In the home the patient truly is the focus of care and care planning processes revolve around the patient and caregiver's needs.

Home Care: A Working Definition

There are many models and definitions of home care. For our purposes there is an appropriate definition of home care put forth by the United States (U.S.) Public Health Service that is both holistic and interdisciplinary. This definition states that: "Home health care is that component of a continuum of comprehensive health care whereby health services are provided to individuals and families in their places of residence for the purpose of promoting, maintaining or restoring health, or maximizing the level of independence, while minimizing the effects of disability and illness, including terminal illness. Services appropriate to the needs of the individual patient and family are planned, coordinated, and made available by providers organized for the delivery of home care through the use of employed staff, contractual arrangements, or a combination of the two patterns." (United States Public Health Service, Department of Health and Human Services, 1980). In this way home care organizations provide skillful and valuable services, particularly rehabilitation services to patients in their homes.

Other services may vary depending on the organization and the payer, but generally always provide nursing and home health aide services, which have been the two services most frequently used and needed by patients. Other services that organizations may provide include social work, respiratory therapy, dietitian or nutritional services, massage therapy, chaplaincy, and homemaker services. Home health aides, besides being well-loved and valued by patients and families (and team members!), have historically provided the largest number of visits and been the largest number of full-time equivalent employees in home care. Figure 1-1 displays the "Average Number of FTE Employees Per Agency, By Size of Agency" and Figure 1-2 displays the "Average Number of FTE Employees Per Home Care Agency."

FIGURE 1-1

FTE JOB TITLE/POSITION	1–100 Visits/Week	101–300 Visits/Week	301–500 Visits/Week	501+ Visits/Week	Overall Average
Registered Nurse	4.64	9.50	10.61	29.76	**14.99**
Licensed Practical Nurse	2.08	2.39	3.54	3.51	**2.88**
Home Health Aide	8.16	10.22	10.81	36.90	**18.07**
Homemaker	0.88	1.14	1.07	2.14	**1.39**
Occupational Therapist	0.03	0.50	0.55	1.11	**0.61**
Physical Therapist	0.36	1.26	1.13	4.72	**2.13**
Respiratory Therapist	0.08	0.14	0.09	0.09	**0.11**
Speech Pathologist	0.01	0.30	0.41	0.58	**0.36**
Case Manager/Care Coordinator	0.67	1.03	1.19	2.96	**1.58**
Secretarial/Clerical	1.37	3.62	2.11	8.90	**4.57**
Sales/Marketing	0.25	0.45	0.47	0.56	**0.45**
Administrative	1.43	2.18	3.97	4.23	**2.98**
All Other*	1.06	0.97	1.57	6.36	**2.73**
TOTAL**	**21.03**	**33.70**	**37.53**	**101.83**	**52.83**

Table title: AVERAGE NUMBER OF FTE EMPLOYEES PER AGENCY, BY SIZE OF AGENCY

* "Other" includes medical social workers, pharmacists, accounting staff, dietitians and quality assurance staff.
** Column totals represent the average of each facility's total full-time-equivalent employees.

FIGURE 1-2

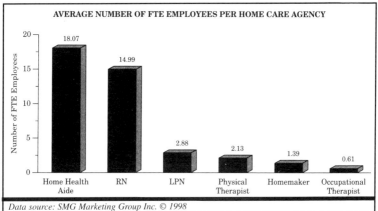

Data source: SMG Marketing Group Inc. © 1998

Figures 1-1 and 1-2. Reprinted with permission from Hoechst Marion Roussel Managed Care Digest Series™, **Institutional Digest,** *1998, p. 39.*

Whatever the specific definition of home care or the services your organization provides, one main tenet remains. We are all striving to provide patients and their families with patient-centered care. The term "patient-centered care" was designed to improve care processes. It is important to note that patient-centered care is not used only as a cost control or an effort to downsize. Other components include that care is customer-service oriented, that the patient and care provider decide upon and agree on the goals and outcomes, and that the care processes and interventions are based on clinically-sound data or research. The best models of home care operations today use patient-centered care and realize that to be successful, it requires ongoing staff education and training.

The Big Picture: Four Domains

Home care is complex as there are many types and components. There are four main areas or "domains" that comprise home care. They are: 1) the Reimbursement and Payer Domain, 2) the Customer Service and Quality Imperatives, 3) The Patient's Environment of Care (Why Home Care Is So Unique!) and 4) Patient Care Planning and Processes. These four domains can be seen visually as shown in Figure 1-3.

FIGURE 1-3   The Big Picture: The Four Domains

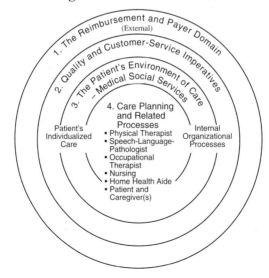

This can also be seen as the four areas that efficient therapists or nurses must have a working knowledge of to be successful in this specialty area and positively impact patient outcomes. This section addresses these four areas and the therapist's roles in meeting these myriad requirements, oftentimes all at once. The information is organized in a manner that moves from the larger external environment down to the main focus of this text - the actual care processes in home care that support quality patient care from holistic rehabilitative and interdisciplinary perspectives.

Domain One: The Reimbursement and Payer Domain

Medicare has set many of the standards for home care. Because of this, all clinicians need a working baseline of knowledge related to how patients qualify for Medicare coverage, the rules related to the specific services, and other information that can assist the clinician, the organization and patients and their families when addressing Medicare questions. There are six services that can be covered or are coverable by the Medicare home health benefit when the patient meets certain defined requirements called "Medicare qualifying criteria." Homebound and other qualifying criteria are discussed later in this section. The six Medicare coverable services are: 1) Nursing, 2) Physical Therapy (PT), 3) Speech-Language Pathology (SLP) services (also called speech therapy), 4) Occupational Therapy (OT), 5) Home Health Aide (HHA) services and 6) Medical Social Services (MSS). Please note that the "Coverage of Services" section of the *HHA Manual* (HCFA Pub.-11) relating to therapy is located in Part Nine for review of specific examples of covered care with numerous patient examples for the Medicare therapy services. The six services listed here are in the same order as listed in the Medicare Manual. *Readers are strongly encouraged to review this material and know these rules and the specific language for an understanding of Medicare home care.*

Medicare: An Update

Medicare is the U.S.'s national medical health insurance program for (primarily) the elderly. It is the largest medical insurance program in the world, and covers or provides medical insurance benefits for approximately 39 million patients, who are called Medicare beneficiaries. This Medicare beneficiary population is comprised primarily of three groups: 1) those patients over age 65, 2) the disabled population (regardless of age), and 3) those patients with End-Stage Renal Disease (ESRD). The Health Care Financing Administration (HCFA) is a component of Health and Human Services (HHS), under the responsibility of the Secretary of HHS, who administers the Medicare and Medicaid programs. Medicare generally, and Medicare home care specifically are going through turbulent changes. Medicare is the largest payer of home care services. Throughout the 1980's and early 1990's expenditures for and utilization of home care services increased significantly. Many reasons were attributed to these unprecedented increases, including an increase in the number of patients using home care and the number of services or visits per patient. Other factors were also clearly at work including improved technology, the aging population, and the decreased lengths of stays in hospitals fueling the need for alternative care sites, particularly home care. At the same time, HCFA data showed no end in site to the escalating costs that had (at least) three separate, identified components:

1) more Medicare patients receiving home care,

2) more services provided per patient, and

3) more (higher) costs reimbursed to provider organizations, e.g., the home health agencies (HHA), per patient. At the same time, HCFA found there was wide variation by state for the number of visits provided for Medicare patients served.

Specific state rules also vary widely related to home care practice. Some states have licensure for home care, some have certificate of need (CON) processes or related regulatory legislation that many believe controls growth and the number of provider organizations, while other states have neither. At the same time, hospitals and nursing homes are shortening stays which many believe increases the need for home care services and home care has historically been the "safety net" for many patients.

Clearly the comparisons could not be "apples to apples", but the data shows at some level that in health care it can be said that "geography is destiny." This means the more supply you have in a given geographic territory, such as home care agencies or orthopedic surgeons, the more home care services or hip replacements may be provided in that area.

Home Health Care: Last Vestige of Cost-Based Reimbursement

Still another reason for the unparalleled growth in home care was attributed to the actual reimbursement structure, called cost-based reimbursement. This payment methodology generally does not support the most effective use of limited resources (e.g. Medicare dollars, number of visits, etc.) Most therapists and nurses are very aware of the hospitals' entry into the world of prospective payment or a prospective payment system (PPS) through the implementation of the diagnoses-related groups (DRGs) in the early 1980's. All other Medicare reimbursed programs are currently already reimbursed through PPS or a managed care program, including hospice and skilled nursing facilities (SNFs) or nursing homes. In fact, Medicare-certified hospices have been reimbursed on a prospective system with four levels of care since its inception in the 1980s. Hospitals went from cost-based to a PPS as noted above and that change has significantly decreased the length of stays for hospitalizations as well as the number of hospitals and the number of available acute care beds in communities. Hospitals are still trying to decrease their lengths of stay and manage their "empty beds" to stay effective and viable for the future. Yet numerous reports say that we still have too many acute care beds in many parts of the country. SNFs or Medicare - reimbursed nursing homes went to a PPS mechanism in 1998.

Home care is currently in the throes of an interim payment system or IPS, which is the period of initial reimbursement cuts and data collection prior to the implementation of the PPS. Mandated by the Balanced Budget Act (BBA) of 1997, the home care industry has suffered devastating cuts in reimbursement and many home care organizations across the country have been forced to close their doors. The PPS will be supported by the data collected from a standardized data set, similar to the tool and reporting mechanisms that the SNFs went through in the past few years.

OASIS: Home Care's Newest Regulatory Requirement

The standardized data set is called the Outcome and Assessment Information Set (OASIS) and is the name of the mandated set of data elements (called "Moos") with the thought of HCFA collecting the data and attributing costs to functional statuses, thus changing significantly and forever the structure of home care reimbursement. In addition, the OASIS data set provides a basis for standardization for the entire team as it is discipline-neutral and should contribute to more standardized documentation in assessments, and other documentation. It may also assist with a common glossary among providers such as those terms used in care coordination communication.

The OASIS, which is a component of the Medicare Conditions of Participation (COPs) for home care, is a major factor in the operations and final structure of the home care industry. The data collected will assist the HCFA in determining specific payment rates for home care organizations, based on the patients' functional problems and numerous other factors. OASIS measures patient changes or outcomes between (at least) two points in time, such as on admission and discharge, and its collection is discussed in-depth in Part Four and Part Five, the "Assessment" and "OASIS" sections of this text.

Whatever the final form of PPS in home care, the future of home care depends on our understanding the implications and nuances of PPS on our practices and organizations. The incentives have changed and are being realigned with those of other payers and managed care entities. Whatever the model and final structure of the PPS, we know that we must identify ways to care for patients at home in a less costly and more effective manner. This means moving from more visits to less visits, redesigning the organization to reduce costs, and supporting decreased lengths of stay. Other changes will involve improving patient education, increasing the quality of the care provided, identifying alternative methods to case manage more effectively (e.g, telephonic home care), and placing more emphasis on supporting patient and family responsibility, self-care, and achieving health maintenance. At the same time, we must achieve desired patient outcomes and increase efficiencies operationally and clinically as we will have increased admissions and discharges. We saw this change occur (which continues to be the standard) since the inception of the DRGs in hospitals. Simply put, we will have more activity related to admissions and discharges with a shortened time span in which to provide needed patient services. We must truly think "out of the box" and pilot creative and innovative ideas to get to the achievement of pre-determined outcomes while staying within the confines of limited resource utilization. Like the hospitals with the emergence of the PPS DRG system, we will see heightened respect and use of tools such as clinical paths and standardized, evidence-based protocols.

Medicare: Undergoing Significant Change

It is important to remember that Medicare was signed into law and opera-tionalized in the mid 1960's, almost forty years ago. Clearly that was a very different time, when we did not have the technology and life span changes that have significantly changed the frameworks of both the Medicare patient popula-tion and the health care environment. At the same time, the patient population has significantly increased and changed. Medicare was created as a medical model, an intervention-focused program. Now, with the aging of the population and the increased life span for many patients, health care needs are primarily focused on chronic care conditions of our growing elderly population. These chronic care conditions includes diabetes, chronic lung and heart problems and many others.

At some point in our practice lifetimes, the Medicare program may become a prevention-focused model or program, but this kind of cataclysmic change may take years to design. "How things have always been" is not a good reason to continue an old structure that no longer meets the needs of the intended bene-ficiaries. In fact, the changes have started and in the Balanced Budget Act (BBA) of 1997 some new and very prevention-focused services were signed into law. These include: annual screening of mammograms for all Medicare enrolled women over age 40 (with no part B deductible), pap smears, colorectal screen-ing exams for Medicare patients aged 50 and over and for all Medicare patients at risk for colorectal cancer, and diabetes outpatient self-management training and education for all Medicare patients with diabetes. Other prevention and health-maintenance focused new covered services include procedures to measure bone mass, bone loss or bone quality for women at clinical risk for osteoporosis or for others at risk for losing bone mass. Also signed into law was Medicare coverage for influenza, pneumococcal and Hepatitis B vaccines.

Medicare Part A

The Medicare program is divided into two parts - Medicare Part A and Medicare Part B. This section explains the differences between these components of Medicare. Medicare Part A programs include hospital, home care, nursing home, and hospice insurance. Medicare Part A programs pay at 100% - this means (at this time) there is no co-payment for Medicare Part A services, such as home care patients. It is important to note that Part A in some instances has deductibles, such as the deductible for hospitalization.

Part A programs are also unique in that they have Conditions of Participation (COPs). The Medicare COPs spell out the specific conditions and requirements that must be achieved and maintained by organizations to receive Medicare reimbursement for Medicare patients who are provided care. Examples of home care COPs include those addressing patient rights and responsibilities, comprehensive assessments including OASIS, compliance with federal, state, local laws and accepted professional standards and principles including specific therapy and nursing practice acts. Other COPs address coordination of patient care, spelling out what constitutes nursing and therapy services, clinical documentation and protection of record requirements and other components that support quality patient care.

Part A organizations, such as home care and hospice organizations go through a certification process, also known as state surveys. Prior to becoming Medicare-certified and at regular intervals throughout the organization's existence the state survey agencies, for example, the Ohio Department of Health, visits on-site to the organization and surveys Medicare-certified home care and hospice organizations in Ohio. The HCFA contracts with the state health agencies to provide this survey and certification service. The certification and state survey process is comprised of record reviews, staff and patient interviews and other methods to demonstrate adherence to and achievement of the Medicare COPs.

Part A claims are paid by insurance companies that contract with the HCFA and are called intermediaries. All home care and hospice claims are paid by one of five specialized intermediaries, called the Regional Home Health Intermediaries (RHHIs). The five are divided into geographic areas and Figure 1-4 shows the RHHIs with their specific areas of responsibility, listed alphabetically by state. The five RHHIs have responsibilities related to their paying only

Figure 1-4   State Assignments to Regional Home Health Intermediaries (RHHIs)

RHHIs	STATES
Associated Hospital Services of Maine www.bluecares.com/plans/bcbs-maine.htm.	Connecticut, Maine, Massachusetts, New Hampshire, Rhode Island, Vermont
Blue Cross and Blue Shield of Wisconsin www.bcbsuw.org.	Michigan, Minnesota, New Jersey, New York, Puerto Rico, Virgin Islands, Wisconsin
Blue Cross and Blue Shield of South Carolina (Palmetto) www.pgba.com	Alabama, Arkansas, Florida, Georgia, Illinois, Indiana, Kentucky, Louisiana, Mississippi, New Mexico, North Carolina, Ohio, Oklahoma, South Carolina, Tennessee, Texas
Wellmark, formerly known as IASD Health Services Corp. www.wellmarkbcbs.com	Colorado, Delaware, District of Columbia, Iowa, Kansas, Maryland, Missouri, Montana, Nebraska, North Dakota, Pennsylvania, South Dakota, Utah, Virginia, West Virginia, Wyoming
Blue Cross of California www.bluecrossca.com	Alaska, Arizona, California, Hawaii, Idaho, Nevada, Oregon, Washington

for covered Medicare claims. An indepth discussion of documentation follows later in this section, but it is important to note that the RHHIs look to the clinical documentation to assist in supporting covered care, such as the patient's homebound status and the need for skilled care. *The RHHI and other Medicare contractors, can only pay for covered care. The clinical documentation contains the important information to help support Medicare coverage.*

The RHHIs do not formulate the regulations and many of the mandated requirements; these are found in the Social Security Act, the Balanced Budget Act (BBA) of 1997, the *Home Health Agency Manual -HCFA Pub.-11*, the Medicare COPs and state laws, such as nurse and therapist practice acts, Federal laws or requirements like the OSHA standards, or those promulgated by the Centers for Disease Control and Prevention (CDC) on infection control and others.

Medicare Part B

The other part of Medicare is Medicare Part B. Medicare Part B covers physician services, ambulance transportation, home medical equipment (HME), (also called durable medical equipment or DME), and outpatient services. *Not all patients have Medicare B because it is a voluntary program and the Medicare beneficiaries must pay a monthly premium for this Part B coverage.* In addition, Part B has a patient co-pay component. For example, with the use of DME, the patient pays a 20% copayment on all covered items. DME claims are paid for by carriers called the Durable Medical Equipment Carriers (DMERCs) who have the responsibility from HCFA for the processing and adjudication of those specialized claims. Figure 1-5 lists their four geographic areas organized alphabetically by state.

Medicare Changes Pursuant to the BBA of 1997

The BBA of 1997 revised the Part A home health benefit to provide that home health visits that are not a part of the first 100 visits following a patient's "qualifying" stay in a hospital or skilled nursing facility are now considered Part B home health services. For Medicare patients who are enrolled in both Parts A and B, Part A finances post-institutional home health services furnished during a home health spell of illness for up to 100 visits. After the individual exhausts the 100 visits of Part A post-institutional home care, Part B finances the balance of the home health spell of illness. The HCFA's common working file (CWF) system is responsible for the tracking of this information.

Figure 1-5   State Assignments of the Durable Medical Equipment Regional Carriers (DMERCS)

	DMERC	STATES
Region A:	United HealthCare P.O. Box 6800 Wilkes-Barre, PA 18773 (717) 735-9445 www.medicare-link.com	Connecticut, Delaware, Maine, Massachusetts, New Hampshire, New Jersey, New York, Pennsylvania, Rhode Island and Vermont
Region B:	AdminaStar Federal Inc. P.O. Box 7078 Indianapolis, IN 46207 (317) 577-5722 www.astarfederal.com	District of Columbia, Illinois, Indiana, Maryland, Michigan, Minnesota, Ohio, Virginia, West Virginia and Wisconsin
Region C:	Palmetto Government Benefits Administrators Medicare DMERC Operations P.O. Box 100141 Columbia, SC 29202 (803) 691-4300 www.pgba.com	Alabama, Arkansas, Colorado, Florida, Georgia, Kentucky, Louisiana, Mississippi, New Mexico, North Carolina, Oklahoma, Puerto Rico, South Carolina, Tennessee, Texas and the Virgin Islands
Region D:	CIGNA Medicare P.O. Box 690 Nashville, TN 37202 (615) 251-8182 www.cignamedicare.com	Alaska, Arizona, California, Guam/American, Hawaii, Idaho, Iowa, Kansas, the Mariana Islands, Missouri, Montana, Nebraska, Nevada, North Dakota, Oregon, South Dakota, Utah, Washington and Wyoming

Medicare Risk and Health Maintenance Organization (HMO) Programs

No doubt you have cared for patients who signed up for an alternative to the Medicare fee-for-service home care program so they would receive "free" medication and other services (currently) not covered under their regular, traditional fee-for-service Medicare coverage. Approximately 17% of Medicare beneficiaries are in some kind of managed care plan, such as a health maintenance organization (HMO). It is expected that by 2005, approximately 30% of all Medicare beneficiaries will be enrolled in Medicare + Choice plans, a new government initiative that began in 1998. These new programs, have the goal of encouraging Medicare beneficiaries into various insurance products and programs. Unfortunately, at the same time, in certain parts of the country, some HMOs have stopped serving some Medicare beneficiaries in certain (mostly rural) geographic areas of the country. At the same time, HMO and other insurance programs vary widely in structure, organization, services offered, benefit packages, clinical practices and protocols, and payment policies. These problems of access, cost, and quality are the three primary challenges facing our health care system today.

Compliance: Everyone's Role

No discussion of Medicare would be complete without addressing compliance issues. All Medicare providers (organizations and their team members) have an obligation to conform and "comply" with the rules and requirements of the Medicare program. Simply put, all team members must have a working knowledge of the Medicare rules and comply with the rules related to the law, coverage and documentation. Unfortunately, stories about unscrupulous providers and evidence of fraud and overutilization have made newspaper or headline news in certain parts of the country. Every time this happens, the entire industry suffers reputation erosion. In fact, there are some fundamental steps that can assist organizations in their quest for quality and compliance.

Strategies for Organizations to Ensure Ongoing Compliance

• **Make sure that agency staff know the "rules" related to Medicare.** This includes the *Home Health Agency Manual* Coverage of Services section, the definition of homebound status, the 15 covered nursing services, covered therapy services, and covered aide services (personal care and activity of daily living assistance, etc.); accurate HCFA Form 485 and OASIS completion responsibilities; compliance related to physician orders (e.g., state licensure and other requirements); and documentation requirements generally, and the specific ones at your individual organization related to accuracy, completeness and timelines for submission.

- **Perform comprehensive audits** that encompass the span of care activities from admission through discharge. Typical review questions include: Does the patient meet Medicare and the organization's admission policies and criteria? Are physician orders timely? Are all business practices and billing processes supportive of, and in compliance with Medicare and other requirements?

- **Standardize care and operational processes** and strive to decrease the risk caused by varying or different systems, methods, and operations, whenever possible.

- **Provide patient education handouts** and tools at admission to assist in identifying that the patient (still) meets Medicare criteria (e.g., homebound, skilled care, etc.) and establishes mutually-agreed-upon goals with projected timelines for achievement.

- **Verify and document that there are doctor orders** prior to the provision of care and that the physician orders cover the projected frequency and duration during the certification periods.

- **Validate that the physician orders are countersigned** and dated by the physician prior to billing for the provided care.

- **Use checklists for clinical record reviews** and other methods to monitor for compliance on an ongoing basis.

- **Develop mechanisms to verify that patients are provided care as ordered** and that the written documentation and related components of care planning (how we obtain verbal orders, evidence of care coordination, conformance with the ordered care, etc.) support Medicare and other requirements.

- **Perform unannounced or random supervisory visits.** This is a way to support compliance - a kind of ongoing mini "mock survey" related to the most important components of compliance.

- **Promote an awareness among agency staff that the federal government has made controlling health care fraud and abuse second only to fighting violent crime** on its law enforcement agenda. Readers are referred to the *Office of Inspector General's Compliance Program Guidance*, a 65-page document, which can be accessed free from the OIG website at http://www.dhhs.gov/progorg/oig/modcomp/hha.pdf. It is imperative that we know and adhere to the rules as this is the basis for everyone's important role in maintaining compliance.

Documentation to Support Covered Care

The RHHI is only responsible for paying for care that is covered under the Medicare home care program guidelines. The RHHIs make these decisions, or adjudicate the claims and make payment determinations based on a careful review of the patient's clinical record. This section seeks to address the major components of documentation requirements for Medicare and other third party payers.

Because Medicare is a medical insurance program, there must be justification in the clinical notes supporting medical necessity for the care and for the level or intensity (frequency and duration) of the care. The "law requires that payment be made only if a physician certifies the need for services and establishes a plan of care. The Secretary [of Health and Human Services] is responsible for ensuring that the claimed services are covered by Medicare, including whether they are `reasonable and necessary'." (Section 203.1 of the Coverage of Services section of the *HHA Manual* (HCFA Pub.-11.) *It is the responsibility of all clinicians to provide this clinical documentation that identifies their role in all components of the provision of home care, including assessment information, care planning, intervention, communications and care coordination, and evaluation.* Thus the burden is on the clinicians to document the care, provide the rationale for care, and to support covered care throughout the patient's stay in home care.

Medicare Requirements for Home Care

There are certain requirements or "qualifying" criteria that the patient must meet to be covered for home care services by Medicare. The patient must meet all of these requirements:

1) The home health agency is Medicare-certified;
2) The patient is homebound as defined by Medicare;
3) The patient is an eligible Medicare beneficiary;
4) The services are coverable as defined in the HHA Manual - (HCFA Pub.-11) and meet the specific coverage rules related to the six services of nursing, physical therapy (PT), occupational therapy (OT), speech-language pathology (ST or SLP), medical social services (MSS) and/or home health aide (HHA) services;
5) The services are medically reasonable and necessary based on the patient's unique condition; and
6) A physician certifies and provides oversight of the patient's plan of care.

Homebound: A Major Qualifying Criteria

Patients in home care must be homebound as defined by Medicare. When performing your initial assessment the clinician must identify the functional criteria that supports the homebound status. The following is an example of the functional detail that assists in identifying key criteria related to documentation to support homebound status. The referral from the physician reads: "PT and OT assessment for patient with chronic obstructive pulmonary disease (COPD) with decreased strength and level of activity post-hospital discharge. Please evaluate for therapy services".

Homebound: Patient Example - Mrs. Smith

After you knock and wait for a few minutes, the door is finally opened and an elderly, **frail**, ninety-pound, 79-year-old woman **using a quad cane** s-l-o-w-l-y opens the door to welcome and let you in. (You called this morning to set up this initial assessment visit so she has been expecting you.) You immediately notice **she can hardly talk**, due to being **so short of breath** and is **using every accessory muscle** you can see around the collar of her worn sweater just to breathe. You also scan the room and get an immediate picture - you see a **hospital bed, bedside commode** and an **oxygen tank** in the living room. This lady and her home is the classic Medicare home care patient. She states **the only time she leaves the house is for her monthly physician visit** which **takes exhaustive effort on her part**. She says it takes until the next day just to recuperate from the activity. She does receive **maximum assistance from her two daughters** who **drive her to the doctor's office**. In fact, she tells you that her daughters are going to ask the doctor at the next scheduled visit if there is anyway he could start making home visits.

Every patient is different and it may be a group of assessed findings that makes a particular patient homebound. To help clarify homebound status, and because it is prudent to get in the habit of referring to the *HHA Manual* (HCFA Pub. 11) whenever a question arises related to homebound, readers are encouraged to review the homebound part of the *HHA Manual* (HCFA Pub -11), and the six examples which follow in Box 1-1 and are reprinted in their entirety.

Box 1-1 Homebound

"204.1 Confined to the Home.-

A. Patient Confined to the Home.-In order for a patient to be eligible to receive covered home health services under both Part A and Part B, the law requires that a physician certify in all cases that the patient is confined to his/her home. An individual does not have to be bedridden to be considered as confined to the home. However, the condition of these patients should be such that there exists a normal inability to leave home and, consequently, leaving home would require a considerable and taxing effort. If the patient does in fact leave the home, the patient may nevertheless be considered homebound if the absences from the home are infrequent or for periods of relatively short duration, or are attributable to the need to receive medical treatment. Absences attributable to the need to receive medical treatment include attendance at adult day care centers to receive medical care, ongoing receipt of outpatient kidney dialysis, and the receipt of outpatient chemotherapy or radiation therapy. It is expected that in most instances, absences from the home that occur will be for the purpose of receiving medical treatment. However, occasional absences from the home for non-medical purposes, e.g., an occasional trip to the barber, a walk around the block or a drive, would not necessitate a finding that the patient is not home-bound if the absences from the home are undertaken on an infrequent basis or are of relatively short duration and do not indicate that the patient has the capacity to obtain the health care provided outside rather than in the home.

Generally speaking, a patient will be considered to be homebound if he/she has a condition due to an illness or injury that restricts his/her ability to leave his/her place of residence except with the aid of supportive devices such as crutches, canes, wheelchairs, and walkers, the use of special transportation, or the assistance of another person or if leaving home is medically contraindicated. Some examples of homebound patients that illustrate the factors used to determine whether a homebound condition exists would be: (1) a patient paralyzed from a stroke who is confined to a wheelchair or requires the aid of crutches in order to walk; (2) a patient who is blind or senile and requires the assistance of another person to leave his/her residence; (3) a patient who has lost the use of his/her upper extremities and, therefore, is unable to open doors, use handrails on stairways, etc., and requires the assistance of another individual to leave his/her residence; (4) a patient who has just returned from a hospital stay involving surgery suffering from resultant weakness and pain and, therefore, his/her actions may be restricted by his/her physician to certain specified and limited activities such as getting out of bed only for a specified period of time, walking stairs only once a day, etc.; (5) a patient with arteriosclerotic heart disease of such severity that he/she must avoid all stress and physical activity; and (6) a patient with a psychiatric problem if the illness if manifested in part by a refusal to leave home or is of such a nature that it would not be considered safe to leave home unattended, even if he/she has no physical limitations.

The aged person who does not often travel from home because of feebleness and insecurity brought on by advanced age would not be considered confined to the home for purposes of receiving home health services unless he/she meets one of the above conditions. A patient who requires skilled care must also be determined to be confined to the home in order for home health services to be covered.

Although a patient must be confined to the home to be eligible for covered home health services, some services cannot be provided at the patient's residence because equipment is required that cannot be made available there. If the services required by a patient involve the use of such equipment, the HHA may make arrangements with a hospital, skilled nursing facility, or a rehabilitation center to provide these services on an outpatient basis. However, even in these situations, for the services to be covered as home health services, the patient must be considered confined to his/her home; and to receive such outpatient services a homebound patient will generally require the use of supportive devices, special transportation, or the assistance of another person to travel to the appropriate facility.

If a question is raised as to whether a patient is confined to the home, the HHA will be asked to furnish the intermediary with the information necessary to establish that the patient is homebound as defined above."

Source: *Home Health Agency Manual* - (HCFA Pub. 11)

Homebound status is an essential qualifying requirement or criteria that must be met for Medicare coverage. The patient is either homebound and the plan of care is initiated or the patient is identified as not being homebound or confined to the home as defined by Medicare and therefore cannot be admitted to the organization's home care program under the Medicare benefit. For all these reasons, it is crucial that all therapists, nurses, and other team members receive an orientation to the homebound criteria and the specific documentation and other requirements related to homebound status necessary for the employing or contracting organization. If the patient is not homebound and therefore does not qualify for coverage under the Medicare program, another payer source may be available for coverage of the home health services. The clinical record of Medicare patients must show the patient's homebound status. Examples of documentation could include:

- Mrs. Smith is short of breath from rising from the chair, takes two steps and stands for a minute to catch a breath,
- Mrs. Smith's gait is unsteady, she hangs onto chairs for support, and uses a cane to walk in her home, and
- Mrs. Smith is currently unable to walk down her stairway to exit her home without the assistance of another person.

The importance of homebound and the documentation of homebound lends itself to a discussion about home care documentation and the significance of that documentation. The following information lists some of the roles of effective documentation.

Roles of Effective Documentation

1. Reflects the care provided to a specific home care patient.
2. Provides the basis for coverage and reimbursement.

3. Protects the clinician and the organization from alleged practice or fraud complaints.
4. Provides the organization with information for benchmarking or data collection.
5. Supports the tenets of quality care and recognizes that quality is in the details (e.g., completion, accuracy, adherence to organizational timelines, and other standards).
6. Validates the standardization of care and care practices.
7. Acts as the basis for reviews related to quality of care, reimbursement, and documentation.

Documentation: An Overview

In documenting to support covered care by any insurer, it is important that basic requirements be met regarding all clinical notes for any patient. The following are some of these requirements:

1) Documentation be written at the time the care is provided (e.g., in home care, usually in the patient's home unless there are safety concerns for the clinician)
2) Ink must be used and the documented information is clear and legible (if the insurers cannot read it they certainly won't pay for it!)
3) Products that cover-up or white-out entries are not to be used on documentation notes or anywhere else in the clinical record.
4) If an error does occur, that the clinician follows the organization's policies or accepted standards related to correction. Oftentimes it may be that a single line is written through the entry, it is marked and signed with initials, and the date noted. Document any addendum also within accepted standards and per organizational policies.
5) Notes should be objective and reflect the specific care provided, particularly the reason for the visit, the interventions provided, and the patient's response to the interventions (e.g., exercise regimen, teaching, etc.)
6) The patient's name and other identifying information required by the organization is complete, accurate, with the date and time of the visit noted (arriving and leaving).
7) The patient's history and physical exam be included in the clinical records or notes.
8) X-ray reports and other information or findings supporting medical necessity and the patient's unique medical condition that require skilled therapy assessment/evaluation, intervention, and care be clearly documented.

9)   There are specific orders for the therapy, including the projected frequency, duration and specific modalities for intervention to support positive patient outcomes.

10) Overall, that the documentation accurately reflects the condition of the patient. Always write notes knowing you may have to prove why you saw the patient and think: "Would I authorize payment or reimbursement with this submitted note?"

The Important Role of Documentation: A Checklist Approach

1.   Is the patient's homebound status stated in clear, concise, specific and measurable terms? (e.g., supported in notes by diagnosis, safety precautions, functional problems, symptoms and medical condition(s))

2.   Are all physician orders obtained prior to care and services being provided?

3.   Does the therapy baseline assessment/evaluation and other documentation state why the referral was made, the patient's functional or mobility changes/problems, medical history including current status and specifically what the loss due to the illness or injury was (e.g., amputation, cognitive/perceptual changes, dysphagia, etc.), and the interventions and plans for the care? Are goals for the plan clearly stated with functional implications identified?

4.   Are the agreed-upon goals identified specific enough? Are they measurable, where possible, and do they state what needs to be accomplished/completed in a given period of care?

5.   Does the HCFA Form 485 contain all the pertinent information, such as ICD-9 codes, medications, and others related to the patient's condition?

6.   Are the OASIS items completed in a timely and accurate manner?

7.   Are there orders for all the therapy interventions or changes to the plan of care related to therapy services?

8.   Do the skilled therapy visit notes and re-evaluations use the same objective measurement tools as those of the initial assessment/evaluation to demonstrate and measure the patient's progress (or lack of progress) toward achievement of the stated goals? Is the level of participation/involvement of the patient and family clearly stated in the documentation?

9.   Does the therapy documentation state how or why home health aide services are needed (or not needed) for this specific patient?

10. Is there care coordination and communication documented for the therapy team members including those with nurses, physician(s), social workers, therapists' assistants and others involved in the patient's care?

11. Does my documentation reflect or support the need for (an)other team members? (e.g., interdisciplinary referral to nursing, aide, PT, SLP, OT, SW).

The Care Process: Assessment and Documentation

The assessment, evaluation and re-evaluation visits are comprised of many components which assists in eliciting needed information to determine the patient's needs for the plan of care. Whatever the format of the assessment form, the patient's medical/surgical history should be noted in relation to this admission or referral for care. This information includes the date(s) of the onset or exacerbation of the illness and injury, any safety factors that place the patient at risk, the patient's functional capacity and status prior to the current condition or state, any history of prior treatment/intervention and outcomes (e.g., other joint replacements, exacerbation with surgery dates), and the patient's status on discharge from the hospital and the reason therapy is needed or initiated.

The establishment of measurable goals at the onset of care is one of the therapist's most important responsibilities. This process is dependent upon the comprehensive assessment, a thoughtful analysis of all the data and consideration of the patient/family/caregiver's goals. This includes: what do they hope to achieve as a result of the therapy and what are the expected specific functional outcomes? Checklists or narrative forms should assist the therapist in describing any test or baseline results or findings in specific and quantifiable language. Whatever the format, the therapist must document any functional capacity deficits. Always address safety considerations (e.g., history of falls, throw rugs, judgment skills, swallowing problems, s/p fracture, etc), range of motion (ROM) and activities of daily living (ADL) capacity, mobility and strength problems and identified precautions. In addition, being aware of the patient's pre-existing function is most important in the development of a realistic plan.

The Care Process: Intervention and Documentation

Many therapy documentation forms or tools are comprised of a blend of checklist and narrative information. Whatever the format, the RHHI must be able to identify the covered skilled care provided by the therapist on each visit. As noted in the "Coverage of Services" sections of the *HHA Manual* (HCFA Pub.-11), therapy interventions may include assessment, therapeutic exercises, gait training and others. It is important to remember that the patient's condition usually also contributes to that patient receiving covered and appropriate therapy services. Documentation should clearly illustrate an accurate reflection of the patient's conditions and health status, including functional limitations. The need for therapy services is contingent upon the patient's unique problems and as such, must be documented explicitly. With this in mind, the documentation should also reflect that the (Medicare) patient is homebound and the specific reasons requiring the initial and ongoing skilled services of the therapist(s). Homebound status should be addressed and clearly documented by all team members. All instructions and teaching that is provided by the home care clinician to the patient/caregiver or family must be documented. Documentation must state the specific task (e.g., gait training) or information taught (e.g., therapeutic exercises), the patient's response to the treatment or instruction, and the evaluation of that teaching (such as an accurate return demonstration by the patient's caregiver, etc). It is also important to demonstrate progress toward goals in the clinical notes or to provide an explanation of why if there is minimal or no progress.

Our roles as educators are more important than ever. Teaching skills and activities that support patient adherence or compliance have never been as important than in the current health environment. *Teaching and education directed toward patient self-care and health maintenance will only be more important as the health care vision of the future changes from an acute intervention-focus to that of a health maintenance or disease management model.* With this in mind, efforts directed toward education of patients and caregivers must be valued for their significance related to the patient stability and overall health. At some level, home care is based on instructing patients, caregivers and family members, when available. The use of the words "instructed" and "educated" (or other interventions/actions accomplished) must be clearly noted in the clinical notes, visit records or other documentation.

Documentation Problems: Common Reasons for Payment Denials

Denials are always a traumatic experience for the therapist who provided the care, the patient who receives the denial notice, and the home care organization who must follow-up with a labor-intensive and time-consuming (read:costly) process to try and recoup the money lost for a visit and care they thought was covered. Home care services are now under an intense level of scrutiny, which has not been experienced since the mid-late 1980's, prior to the landmark Duggan vs. Bowen lawsuit. Some of the increased medical or "focused" reviews are triggered by excessive utilization. This means that services are provided in excess (either dollars per patient or amount of services provided per patient) of what the RHHI has deemed acceptable. When the RHHIs ask for more information, hopefully the clinician has provided the organization with the documentation that supports the need for the treatment from a medical necessity perspective (e.g., related to the extent of the patient's illness, loss, or injury).

The *Medicare Manual* states in Section 203.1: "Use of Utilization Screens and 'Rules of Thumb'. Medicare recognizes that determinations of whether home health services are reasonable and necessary must be based on the assessment of each beneficiary's individual care needs. Therefore, denial of services based on numerical screens, diagnostic screens, diagnosis or specific treatment norms is not appropriate." [*Home Health Agency Manual* (HCFA Pub-11).] The care provider or therapist must present the documentation that supports the need for the patient's level of care that is initiated during the assessment and supported throughout the care processes.

Some medical reviews are random and others are based on screening for outliers or patterns of aberrancy as compared to other organizations. As you review this list, you will see that many are documentation problems and speak to the need for the documentation to be timely, clear, and support why the skills of the therapist are needed, based on the patient's unique medical problems. The lists are divided by the reason for the denial. Keep these in mind as you comprehensively document your patient's care. Strive to document correctly and thoroughly on every visit, ask yourself - "does this visit or other note support coverage?"

General Medical Review Problems (Or What to Avoid)

- No doctor's orders
- PT, OT and/or SLP not [medically] reasonable and necessary
- Missing/incorrect documentation
- No valid certification or recertification of the plan of care

Specific Therapy Problems

- Poor assessment, lacking prior level of patient function
- Lack of documented objective goals with functional measurements
- Use of "check box" forms without enough [narrative] unique patient information
- No orders, poorly written orders, or incorrectly written orders
- The record does not support the need for the specialized skills of the therapist
- No clear reason for the therapy referral (and no diagnosis or problem that supports therapy)
- Frequency does not appear to be appropriate or correlated with the documented functional needs
- From the records, the therapy does not appear to be reasonable and necessary
- Repetitive and unclear notes of routine services that do not support medical

necessity and the need for the therapist
- Lack of knowledge about Medicare coverage criteria (e.g., homebound, covered therapy services or other care)
- Poor documentation of the therapy assistant maintaining communication and care coordination with the therapist. The documentation must show effective, up-to-date interactions and communications between the assistant and the therapist.

Summary

Home care generally and Medicare specifically are going through tumultuous times. Whatever the final structure of PPS, we must work together to hold costs within defined rates and limits for survival. At the same time, we are held accountable for numerous aspects of care and successful operations. We must determine ways to provide needed patient care within the confines of the changing reimbursement and practice environments.

Domain Two: The Customer Service and Quality Imperatives

We all remember that President Clinton's proposed Health Security Act was initiated to address three major problems with the U.S. health care system. They are: access, cost, and quality. The continuing problem of cost escalation of health care services is frequently in our newspaper headlines or the television news and provides grist for the political mill. It is no secret that the U.S. spends more than any other country in the world on health care, yet some countries have better infant morbidity and mortality rates. At the same time, patients, the consumers of care want value for their hard-earned dollars regardless if their health insurance programs pay or reimburse for it. At the same time, many people want more health insurance coverage, but do not want to pay more for these added benefits. We have numerous external factors that demand quality and mandate movement toward measurable outcomes related to the provision of health care. Some of these factors include accreditation bodies such as the Joint Commission on Accreditation of Healthcare Organizations (JCAHO), the Commission on Accreditation of Rehabilitation Facilities (CARF), Community Health Accreditation Program (CHAP) and others; utilization review entities, case management firms and others.

We also have emerging and growing patient populations in home care that are demanding more of the already limited financial resources - four of these patient populations are: 1) the elderly - who were brought up on the Medicare program years ago with its paternalistic ("we'll do everything for you and patients had little input") and intervention-focused medical model; 2) the infants or neonates - the neonatal intensive care units (NICU) graduates who with technology are growing or sick at home and may need care for some years; 3) the baby boomers (the authors included) - the largest cohort yet who are (appropriately) concerned about the country's limited resources related to Medicare funding long-term (or when we all need it in the coming decades) and 4) the head injury or shock trauma patients who after their severe injuries or losses usually need rehabilitation or other services, for the rest of their lives post severe injury. They may need services such as hyperalimentation or a home therapy program. All of these factors in our external environment demonstrate that the cost/quality equation is becoming harder to balance for the clinicians, the organizations serving patient consumers and the insurance payers.

At the same time, most patients and families do not know their specific insurance coverage for home care until they need it and they oftentimes are frustrated with the limits of their home care coverage. For example, not too many years ago a patient may have had therapy for six months, this same patient with a similar stroke three years later might receive less services, in terms of length of service and in authorized visits. This can be very confusing to consumers of care and their families as they perhaps have the perception that home care therapy services would be provided on a long term basis. This is a major change and a difficult learning curve for clinicians and patients and their families.

Quality 101: An Overview

Quality, the buzzword that emerged in the 80's, is an important concept that is here to stay in health care and has become a cornerstone for effective organizations and their team members. The basic premise of quality in home care is that the right clinicians provide the right intervention(s) for the right patient and at the right time. This means striving to "do it right the first time." Having the "right clinicians" starts with hiring skilled clinicians, with defined performance expectations clearly specified in job or position descriptions (see Part Eight for examples of position descriptions). Competence or competency assessment is a long-term quality process comprised of initially assessing the knowledge and skills of the clinical team members and then on an on-going basis, reassessing that those skills are up-to-date, maintained, and are appropriate to the types of patients being seen and treatments provided. In this way patients and their families are assured that competent clinicians knowledgeable in their area of expertise, will contribute to the achievement of patient outcomes in a safe and standardized manner. This process of continually reviewing clinical team members' knowledge and skills is key to the provision of the best home care.

Competency Assessment: Foundation for Excellence

Competency assessment refers to the process that an organization has in place to assess, maintain, and improve the competence of all care and services provided by clinical team members. This means that nurses, therapists, and others are clinically competent and up-to-date in their skills, knowledge, and problem-solving or critical thinking abilities. Organizations usually develop and implement a process for assessing the competence for all care staff who see patients in the home. Readers are referred to Part Eight for competence assessment tools. This includes both employees and any contracted staff, including therapy team members. Usually another therapist or a peer of the same discipline performs some of these competency assessment activities.

Components observed or queried may include infection control, equipment use, communication skills, home visit activities and many other aspects of home care practice. Many times clinical documentation review is a key component of competency assessment activities. This process would verify compliance with Medicare rules, and other payer and organizational requirements as well as determine whether the clinicians have an understanding of paperwork and regulatory requirements. This usually includes reviewing for homebound status information, what the skilled therapy interventions were every visit, phone communications with the physician, nurse, and other disciplines involved with the patient demonstrating care coordination and other components of a clinical record review for compliance. There may also be a written test process.

Most organizations seek to assess competence on low-volume, high-risk skills. For nurses this may be tracheostomy, peripherally-inserted central catheter (PICC) lines, pediatric or other specialty patients. For therapists, this may be removal of staples, medication management, or other areas defined by the organization. Annually, the competence data should be analyzed to identify learning needs for team members. The results of this learning needs assessment then become the identified topics for continuing educational sessions and through these recurring processes the quality cycle continues.

"Right interventions" refers to the fact that the team members have a standardized method of performing job functions, as mandated by the organization's policies and procedures. An example could be that at XYZ Home Care, all clinicians follow a standardized format for the assessment visit of all patients. This could include the forms, the order in which information is explained to the patient and family (e.g., consent, bill of rights, advanced directives, etc.), the standardized explanation of homebound given on admission, the explanations related to the on-call systems, how complaints would be handled and many other components of the initial assessment. In this way, through standardization and incorporation of identified best practices, the managers (and the consumer and community) know that all patients get XYZ's special brand of home care, regardless of the individual team member providing the care.

It is easy to see that education and quality go hand-in-hand. This is why in many organizations education is part of the quality division. Learning needs assessment should be conducted with all field staff as needed and an educational calendar for inservices planned at least yearly. For example, infection control is an important component of quality in home care and hospice organizations. The following information Figure 1-6, is entitled "Home Care Bag Contents by Discipline" and lists specific bag content by clinician. This information identifies the infection control and other supplies needed for clinicians in the provision of patient care, by specialty.

Other educational topics that are usually helpful because of our changing environment include improving or updating assessment skills (e.g., physical, interviewing techniques, etc.), medication updates, ethical decision-making, and care coordination. Up-to-date drug, documentation and care planning, and other resource texts should be readily available (e.g., in visit bags) to staff as resources to help assure safe, standardized and effective patient care. Cross training and interdisciplinary orientation and ongoing educational efforts can also contribute

Figure 1-6   HOME CARE BAG CONTENTS BY DISCIPLINE

PT	OT	ST

Newspaper
Agency designated
  antimicrobial skin cleanser
Cal Stat®
Paper towels
Plastic aprons
Disposable gloves
Disposable gown
Disposable mask
CPR MicroShield
Protective eyewear
Stethoscope
Sphygmomanometer
Thermometer/covers
Alcohol wipes
Biowipes
Asepti-Chlor™ towelette
Gait belt
Goniometer
Shoe covers
	Newspaper
	Agency designated
	  antimicrobial skin cleanser
	Cal Stat®
	Paper towels
	Plastic aprons
	Disposable gloves
	Disposable gown
	Disposable mask
	CPR MicroShield
	Protective eyewear
	Stethoscope
	Sphygmomanometer
	Thermometer/covers
	Alcohol wipes
	Biowipes
	Asepti-Chlor™ towelette
	Gait belt
	Goniometer
	Shoe covers
		Newspaper
		Agency designated
		  antimicrobial skin cleanser
		Cal Stat®
		Paper towels
		Plastic aprons
		Disposable gloves
		Disposable gown
		Disposable mask
		CPR MicroShield
		Protective eyewear
		Stethoscope
		Sphygmomanometer
		Thermometer/covers
		Alcohol wipes
		Biowipes
		Asepti-Chlor™ towelette
		Laryngeal mirror
		Thick-it samples
		Make-up mirror
		Flashlight/penlight
		Gait belt
		Lemon glycerine swabs
		Shoe covers

Figure 1-6 HOME CARE BAG CONTENTS BY DISCIPLINE
(cont'd)

MEDICAL SOCIAL WORKER	DIETITIAN	HOME CARE AIDE

Newspaper
Agency designated
  antimicrobial skin cleanser
Cal Stat®
Paper towels
Plastic aprons
Disposable gloves
Disposable gown
Disposable mask
CPR MicroShield
Asepti-Chlor™ towelette
Protective eyewear
Shoe covers
	Newspaper
	Agency designated
	  antimicrobial skin cleanser
	Cal Stat®
	Paper towels
	Plastic aprons
	Disposable gloves
	Disposable gown
	Disposable mask
	Protective eyewear
	CPR MicroShield
	Alcohol wipes
	Biowipes
	Food models
	Plastic plate
	Asepti-Chlor™ towelette
	Shoe covers
		Newspaper
		Agency designated
		  antimicrobial skin cleanser
		Cal Stat®
		Paper towels
		Plastic aprons
		Disposable gloves
		Disposable gown
		Disposable mask
		CPR MicroShield
		Protective eyewear
		Stethoscope
		Sphygmomanometer
		Thermometer/covers
		Alcohol wipes
		Biowipes
		Asepti-Chlor™ towelette
		Hair dryer
		Shoe covers

Figure 1-6   HOME CARE BAG CONTENTS BY DISCIPLINE (cont'd)

RN/LPN Standard Care	RN IV Therapy	RN Enterostomal Therapy
Newspaper	Newspaper	Newspaper
Agency designated antimicrobial skin cleanser	Agency designated antimicrobial skin cleanser	Agency designated antimicrobial skin cleanser
Cal Stat®	Cal Stat®	Cal Stat®
Paper towels	Paper towels	Paper towels
Plastic aprons	Plastic aprons	Plastic aprons
Disposable gloves	Disposable gloves	Disposable gloves
Disposable gown	Disposable gown	Disposable gown
Disposable masks	Disposable masks	Disposable masks
CPR MicroShield	CPR MicroShield	CPR MicroShield
Protective eyewear	Protective eyewear	Protective eyewear
Stethoscope	Stethoscope	Stethoscope
Sphygmomanometer	Sphygmomanometer	Sphygmomanometer
Thermometer/covers	Thermometer/covers	Thermometer/covers
Plastic Ziploc bags	Plastic Ziploc bags	Plastic Ziploc bags
Plastic Biohazard specimen bags	Plastic Biohazard specimen bags	Plastic Biohazard specimen bags
Sharps container	Sharps container	Sharps container
Blood drawing kit	Blood drawing kit	Blood drawing kit
Syringes and needles	Syringes and needles	Syringes and needles
Insulin syringes	Insulin syringes	Insulin syringes
Dressings	Dressings	Dressings
Culture tube	Culture tubes	Culture tubes
Sterile urine spec. cup	Sterile urine spec. cup	Sterile urine spec. cup
Sterile gloves	Sterile gloves	Sterile gloves
Sterile instrument set	Sterile instrument set	Sterile instrument set
Tape	Tape	Tape
Betadine wipes	Betadine wipes	Betadine wipes
Accu-Chek Advantage and supplies	Accu-Chek Advantage and supplies	Accu-Chek Advantage and supplies
Sterile applicators	Sterile applicators	Sterile applicators
Sterile tongue blades	Sterile tongue blades	Sterile tongue blades
Moni-Chlor™ towelettes	Moni-Chlor™ towelettes	Moni-Chlor™ towelettes
Asepti-Chlor™ towelette	Asepti-Chlor™ towelette	Asepti-Chlor™ towelette
Staple removal kit	Staple removal kit	Staple removal kit
Paper tape measure	Paper tape measure	Paper tape measure
Surgi lube	Surgi lube	Surgi lube
Skin prep	Skin prep	Skin prep
Telfa pad	Telfa pad	Telfa pad
Steri-strips	Steri-strips	Steri-strips
Shoe covers	IV start kit	S/H powder
Flashlight	Central dressing kit	S/H paste
	IV angio caths	Curved scissors
	Needleless connectors	Duoderm
	Shoe covers	Stoma measuring guide
	Flashlight	Shoe covers
		Flashlight

Figure 1-6   HOME CARE BAG CONTENTS BY DISCIPLINE (cont'd)

RN Diabetes Education	RN Maternity Services	RN Mental Health Services
Newspaper	Newspaper	Newspaper
Agency designated	Agency designated	Agency designated
antimicrobial skin cleanser	antimicrobial skin cleanser	antimicrobial skin cleanser
Cal Stat®	Cal Stat®	Cal Stat®
Paper towels	Paper towels	Paper towels
Plastic aprons	Plastic aprons	Plastic aprons
Disposable gloves	Disposable gloves	Disposable gloves
Disposable gown	Disposable gown	Disposable gown
Disposable masks	Disposable masks	Disposable masks
CPR MicroShield	RESUSCI® patient face shield	CPR MicroShield
Protective eyewear	Protective eyewear	Protective eyewear
Stethoscope	Stethoscope - Adult/Infant	Stethoscope
Sphygmomanometer	Sphygmomanometer	Sphygmomanometer
Thermometer/covers	Thermometer/covers	Thermometer/covers
Plastic Ziploc bags	Plastic Biohazard specimen bags	Plastic Biohazard specimen bags
Plastic Biohazard specimen bags	Sharps container	Plastic Ziploc bags
Sharps container	Blood drawing kit	Sharps container
Blood drawing kit	Syringes	Blood drawing kit
Syringes and needles	Dressings	Syringes and needles
Insulin syringes	Culture tube	Insulin syringes
Dressings	Sterile urine spec. cup	Dressings
Culture tubes	Sterile gloves	Culture tubes
Sterile urine spec. cup	Sterile instrument set	Sterile urine spec. cup
Sterile gloves	Tape	Sterile instrument set
Sterile instrument set	Urine specimen bags (Infant)	Moni-Chlor™ towelettes
Tape	Cord clamps	Asepti-Chlor™ towelette
Betadine wipes	Clamp remover	Staple removal kit
Accu-Chek Advantage	Pen light	Paper tape measure
and supplies	Asepti-Chlor™ towelette	Surgi lube
Sterile applicators	Steri-strips	Skin prep
Sterile tongue blades	Biowipes	Telfa pad
Moni-Chlor™ towelettes	Paper tape measures	Steri-strips
Asepti-Chlor™ towelette	Surgi lube	Flashlight
Staple removal kit	Staple removal kit	Accu-Chek Advantage
Paper tape measure	Shoe covers	and supplies
Surgi lube		Sterile applicators
Skin prep		Sterile tongue blades
Telfa pad		Shoe covers
Steri-strips		
Glucose tablets		
Shoe covers		
Flashlight		

Reprinted with permission from Meridia Home Care Services, Mayfield Village, Ohio, 1999.

to improved team work, standardized care, and effective operations.

The best organizations truly walk the talk of quality. These are organizations where "questioning why" is seen as a good thing, where the culture is that "no one is as smart as all of us," and there is true team work where staff members work with each other as part of a cohesive team which revolves around patient needs. Performance improvement (PI), which is the hallmark of quality initiatives, is key to survival in the health vision of the future. There is a saying "if you cannot measure it, you cannot manage it." With this in mind, organizations set performance expectations and monitor performance based on the data collected.

Data Management: Increasing Focus

Organizations must more effectively manage their data. The OASIS has brought home care up-to-date with other health entities such as hospitals which must track the results of their care and interventions on patients. For quality and survival the following is the utilization data that most organizations track: the average visits and length of stay (LOS) by diagnoses or major diagnostic category (or at least the top 5 diagnoses); the average visits and LOS by payer (such as Medicare, Champus, etc.); the average visit and time utilized per visit by each discipline; the percentage of patients admitted to home care from an inpatient setting; rehospitalization rates from home care, emergency room visits; and numbers or rates of discharges due to hospitalization.

Other measures of quality control include customer service and satisfaction survey feedback, infection control information, measuring the turn-around times for HCFA 485 forms and other physician orders, outcome reports that demonstrate appropriate visit and other resource utilization. Some of this data can then also be used as marketing material for managed care entities who are result (read: data) oriented, and many others. Whatever the information collected, the data is systematically aggregated and analyzed; the results are then summarized and activities planned to further improve the performance of that particular process with the goal of improved performance. Organizations and clinicians must continually seek new ways to think about how to provide quality services and seek opportunities to streamline or redesign activities to support the best work of any home care organization. The goal is for patients to have achieved agreed-upon predetermined outcomes that were attributable to the interventions of the clinician and provided in an equal partnership with the patient. Only through this mechanism can the value of home care be successfully demonstrated. The other hallmark that supports quality and survival in this competitive and changing environment is customer service.

Customer Service

Effective customer service is the cornerstone of quality. Customer service is a skill that too often has not been stressed and valued enough in the health care environment generally. And, unfortunately, in some instances it has been completely forgotten. Many customers or consumers of health care accepted less than perfect or merely adequate customer service, attributing it to the way the health care industry has operated. Clinicians may sometimes think of customer service only in relation to the patient and family satisfaction survey or a form that may be sent out after discharge or at other times, depending on the organization. It is most important to think of quality (way) beyond the confines of patient satisfaction.

The patient's perception of care or satisfaction has emerged as a necessary monitor in this world of increased competition. All clinicians know that "bedside" manners are very important to patients and their families. In the past, good bedside manners were thought to be "enough" to define effective customer service.

The home as a health care setting has introduced a whole new aspect to the traditional meaning of bedside manners. One measure of customer service attributes is the use of customer service satisfaction evaluation tools or survey forms. The external environment, including increased competition and regulatory entities, has brought the concept of customer service to a new and important level. An example of a satisfaction questionnaire that outlines itemized areas for feedback follows for review in Figure 1-7. In some cases, organizations may lose sight that home care is a service industry. With home care's direct patient and family contact, one of the most important ingredients for success is the human element.

It goes without saying that all team members should treat every phone call or encounter positively, always keeping in mind that the party is a customer. Of course, all tasks need to be prioritized, but from a customer service perspective some activities are to be valued more than others. For example, because home care services are heavily reliant on phones, this may be an opportunity for improved customer service. Remember if you are a referral source or a family member, you provided their first impression of home care. Numerous studies have shown how much first impressions count - they are very difficult to change once an assessment has been made by the customer or consumer.

One way to know how your organization is perceived is to call your organization (or the on-call system) to get an idea of the impression the customer gets. Is the name of the organization and the person answering clear as an objective listener? How does the person sound? Phones should always be answered timely and per policies as implemented to meet customer service goals. For example, many organizations have a standard of three rings maximum prior to

Figure 1-7

SATISFACTION QUESTIONNAIRE

DATE ____ / ____ / ____

Thank you for allowing us to provide care for you or your family member. We are interested in your ideas or opinions about our care/services. Please take a moment to answer the following questions. Additional comments are welcome and can be recorded on the back of this form. If you need assistance in completing this form, please feel free to contact our office.

For questions 1 - 10, please circle the appropriate number that best describes your opinion.
1-Strongly Agree   2-Agree   3-Disagree   4-Strongly Disagree   5-No Opinion or Not Applicable

1. I was satisfied with the care provided by the:					
a. Nurse(s)	1	2	3	4	5
b. Physical Therapist	1	2	3	4	5
c. Occupational Therapist	1	2	3	4	5
d. Speech/Language Pathologist	1	2	3	4	5
e. Medical Social Worker	1	2	3	4	5
f. Home Health Aide(s)	1	2	3	4	5
2. I was involved in decision-making regarding my plan of care.	1	2	3	4	5
3. My opinions were considered in the planning for discharge.	1	2	3	4	5
4. Staff treated me, my family, my home and belongings with respect.	1	2	3	4	5
5. Staff explained my conditions, rights and responsibilities, and other procedures related to the care I received.	1	2	3	4	5
6. The staff generally arrived as scheduled.	1	2	3	4	5
7. I was able to reach my nurse/therapist promptly and my phone calls were returned.	1	2	3	4	5
8. When I called the agency, office staff were courteous and available and directed my call correctly.	1	2	3	4	5
9. I would use this agency again.	1	2	3	4	5
10. I would recommend this agency to friends and relatives.	1	2	3	4	5

11. Suggestions for improvements/additional comments:

12. What most impressed me about the agency's care/service was:

Thank you for your valuable feedback. This confidential information will be used only in efforts to improve care/service.

Sincerely,

_____
Organization Director or Administrator Signature

I ☐ would/☐ would not like to discuss my responses further.

Please return the completed questionnaire in the enclosed, self-addressed, stamped envelope.

_____   ____ / ____ / ____
Optional Signature of Person Completing Form   *Date*

SATISFACTION QUESTIONNAIRE

Reprinted with permission from Briggs Health Care Products, Des Moines, Iowa, 1999.

answering, while others have a policy that calls are always returned (e.g., within a one - hour maximum) when following up on phone mail messages.

The level of customer service that an organization provides on a daily basis can make the difference in the reputation and long-term survival of the organization. The goal of the organization and its team members is to meet the specific home health care needs of the public. Being on-time for scheduled appointments and calling ahead if you are running late or ahead of schedule supports positive customer service feelings and is valued by many patients. Be aware of the crucial role we have as visiting clinicians in facilitating the achievement of the organization's customer service goals.

Who is the Customer?

The term customer itself raises many questions. Who are your customers? Which customers are more or most important when compared to others? There are several levels of customers in any home care or hospice organization. There are the external customers, comprised of patients, their families, and companies connected with patients, such as hospital referral sources, referring physicians, managed care company nurses, and others. Equally important are the internal customers: the home care and hospice team members, including clinical, managerial and administrative, billing and others who work together to create an effective team. How positively and collaboratively the whole team works together and communicates is a measure of customer service. In fact, many organizations value and heavily weigh customer service from a performance evaluation perspective. In larger organizations, where there are other offices or local offices and corporate headquarters, these entities and the team members are also customers of the organization. Members of alliances, networks, systems and other relationships of which the organization is a part are customers too.

Any successful organization will attribute part of their achievement to knowing and listening to their customers and responding to them appropriately. It goes without saying that it is almost always easier to prevent customer-service problems than to try to solve them once a problem has occurred with a patient or family. If a problem occurs, be proactive in addressing the dilemma, rather than reactive. Strive to correct the error and move on. See if that problem is a one-time problem or if the system needs to be reviewed to prevent similar problems in the future. Clinicians and organizations are judged on how well the last patient (or the most vocal patient!) was served. People who believe and act as if they are there to truly serve the community make the difference between mediocre organizations and great ones.

Like never before, there is a need and urgency to go beyond the one-to-one contact level with the patient and family. Thus documenting all contact, whether it is in person, on the phone, or in a written note, is necessary to reflect this level of comprehensive, quality care. The level must be holistic, across the entire organization, and encompass all team members.

Summary

Customer service, respect for patient rights, and quality go hand-in-hand in organizations seeking to provide effective care for patients. The care and other components in the organization that support the clinical operations have opportunities to continually improve. This cycle of quality must be a hallmark of every home care and hospice organization. Specific areas are chosen for improvement and data measured, collected and analyzed. The results are distributed, studied, and educational and other efforts are directed toward ongoing improvement. This cycle is the force which drives the achievement of both customer service and quality imperatives.

Domain Three: The Patient's Environment of Care: Home (Or The Reason Home Care is So Unique)

In a nutshell, the patient's home and environment is why homecare is so different from other care settings. We are guests in the patient and family's personal space and it is the opposite of the relationship and power base often seen in the hospital or in the outpatient setting. In the patient's home, clinicians are immediately exposed to relevant data related to the patient's unique environment.

The therapist's observational and assessment/evaluation skills are key to the early identification of potential safety problems or looming hazards identified in the patient's home environment. A home safety assessment is a part of the mandated comprehensive assessment in home care. Some of the more common safety hazards include ferocious or unusual pets (or unsanitary pet care), uneven steps or side walks, lack of maintenance on floor boards or porches, throw rugs, space heaters and other hazards. Rug edges which pose a safety threat or may slide, can cause risk of falls. Other hazards include cluttered hallways, decreased patient judgement, telephone cords, blaring televisions, inadequate lighting, excessive smoke, and numerous others.

Patient Example: The Setting Negatively Impacting Care Goals

As a neophyte home care nurse I will never forget walking into an elderly woman's **townhouse** in Baltimore and seeing **a hole in the middle of the living room floor** about the size of her couch. After a tactful comment about it on the initial assessment visit, she remarked "honey, it's been there for a good many years and **my dogs (all four)** know to walk around it now." She also commented that it was **going to get fixed by her nephew, but he had recently died** in a car accident and could we help her? Having been sent out to assess her **hypertension and new medications**, I knew she would also need PT and OT for her **new CVA** as I could see her **gait problem** and **difficulty with transfers.** I had visions of the aide having her practice with her walker and some dire consequences occurring (ie., they both disappear through the hole in the floor) during the exercise regimen.

The rest of the story is that we had a care conference immediately and the social worker, physician, and the team worked together and the floor was fixed through community assistance. Without intervention, this patient's plan of care could not have been implemented nor goals achieved. Many environmental problems are not that bad, though many are worse, and part of our role is identifying what we can and cannot do related to the patient's environment. Readers are referred to Figure 1-8 "Home Environment Safety Evaluation" for review. In Part Seven, "Optimizing Home Safety", there is equipment assessment information as well as a comprehensive home safety program.

Figure 1-8

HOME ENVIRONMENT SAFETY EVALUATION

Check Yes, No or N/A (Not Applicable) for each of the following items. For all "No" responses identify, in the space provided, item number, action plan to correct the problem and document the date the patient/client was instructed.

		YES	NO	N/A
1.	There is a working telephone and emergency numbers are accessible.			
2.	Electrical cords and outlets appear to be in good repair in the patient/client area (i.e., cords not frayed, outlets not overloaded, etc.).			
3.	There are functional smoke alarm(s).			
4.	Fire extinguisher is available and accessible.			
5.	Access to outside exits is free of obstruction.			
6.	Alternate exits are accessible in case of fire.			
7.	Walking pathways are level, uncluttered and have non-skid surfaces.			
8.	Stairs are in good repair, well lit, uncluttered and have non-skid surfaces. Handrails are present and secure.			
9.	Lighting is adequate for safe ambulation and ADL.			
10.	Temperature and ventilation are adequate.			
11.	Medicines and poisonous/toxic substances are clearly labeled and placed where client can reach, if needed, yet not within reach of children.			
12.	Bathroom is safe for the provision of care (i.e., raised toilet seat, tub seat, grab bar, non-skid surface in tub, etc.).			
13.	Kitchen is safe for the provision of care (i.e., working appliances, hygienic area for food prep, etc.).			
14.	Environment is safe for effective oxygen use.			
15.	Overall environment is adequately sanitary for the provision of care.			
16.	Other			

FOR ALL ITEMS CHECKED "NO" ABOVE, SPECIFY ACTION PLAN AND DOCUMENT DATE PATIENT/CLIENT WAS INSTRUCTED

ITEM NO.	DATE INSTRUCTED	TEACHING MATERIALS PROVIDED	REVIEWED	ACTION PLAN

CHECK ANY OF THE FOLLOWING THAT NEED TO BE OBTAINED

☐ Raised toilet seat	☐ Plug covers	☐ Wheelchair	☐ Other_____
☐ Tub seat	☐ Cabinet latches	☐ Lifeline or other PERS	☐ Other_____
☐ Grab bar	☐ Window locks	☐ Car seat	☐ Other_____
☐ Non-skid surface (bath)	☐ Ipecac syrup	☐ Seat/bed cushion	☐ Other_____
☐ Infant tub	☐ Smoke alarm	☐ First aid kit	☐ Other_____

Emergency preparedness plan discussed with/provided to patient/client?   ☐ Yes   ☐ No, explain:_____

SIGNATURE OF PERSON COMPLETING EVALUATION _____ DATE __/__/__

CARE MANAGER SIGNATURE/TITLE _____ DATE __/__/__

PART 1 — Clinical Record	PART 2 — Patient/Client	PART 3 — Care Manager

PATIENT/CLIENT NAME - Last, First, Middle Initial   ID#

Form 3542/3P   © 1994 Briggs Corporation, Des Moines, IA 50306
R595   To order, phone 1-800-247-2343 PRINTED IN U.S.A.

HOME ENVIRONMENT SAFETY EVALUATION

Reprinted with permission from Briggs Health Care Products, Des Moines, Iowa, 1999.

Environmental Safety Considerations: Identifying At-Risk Patients

High-risk home care patients such as the patient example above, may have one or numerous environmental factors contributing to their inability to achieve established goals. Though not every one of these factors, taken alone, may trigger the need for intervention by a medical social worker for assessment, taken together the clinician may see a trend that may need to be evaluated to ensure the patient's long-term safety. Factors which may be high-risk indicators relative to the patient's home safety status include the following:

- The patients' age (e.g., the frail elderly)
- The patient who lives alone
- The caregiver's age and ability, capability, and willingness to care for the patient
- The patient (or caregiver) not answering the phone or door
- Incontinence problems or complaints (including odors)
- Impaired ability or inability to perform ADLs
- Lack of the basic requirements or inadequate requirements for safety and health (e.g., food or refrigeration availability/capability, safe municipal or other water for drinking and hygiene needs, heat, protection from the natural environmental elements, etc.)
- Abusive environments where either the patient is abusive to the caregiver or the caregiver is abusive to the patient
- Problematic social interactions (e.g., no or poor relations with others, loner, hermit-like, geographically or socially isolated, "fires" the aides or others, refuses family help, etc.)
- Lack of appropriate equipment and the home's limited adaptability to such equipment (bathtub upstairs with no railing on stairs)
- Physical structure of the home is of concern (patient uses a wood stove for heat in the winter and now needs oxygen therapy)
- Financial limitations
- Poor understanding, confusion, sundowning, inappropriate affect, paranoia, perceptual, judgment impairment, cognitive or psychological problems
- Patient/caregiver not following safety precautions
- Depression or grief symptomatology (tearful, crying, sad, history of loss - Note: the average Medicare home patient is an elderly widow)
- Poor appetite or nutritional status
- Multiple pathologies or co-morbidities (e.g., CHF, COPD, Cancers, etc.)
- Medically noncompliant
- Hygiene concerns from pets or infestations such as fleas, lice, worms, or inappropriate defecation
- Language barriers or difficulty in accessing assistance

- Multiple emergency room visits or hospital admissions
- History of falls or fracture (e.g., hip, wrist, etc.) due to falls
- Little or no financial resources
- Physical and geographical location (e.g., patient lives where there are few or no community resources, etc.)
- Substance abuse
- Inability to perform community skills such as banking, shopping, acquiring prescriptions, laundry, etc.
- Other factors

Medical Social Services: Important Role

Environmental problems as listed above should start us asking these questions: 1) What impact are the environmental problems having on the patient's health status? and 2) does this patient need medical social work intervention? Safety considerations may help make the determination or trigger the mechanism for an evaluation by the organization's medical social worker (MSW). It is important to note that Medicare calls social work service "medical social services (MSS)." This is because it highlights that Medicare is a medical insurance program and all care and services are directed toward the improvement or resolution of medical problems, illnesses, or injuries.

A medical social worker referral is appropriate when there are one or more factors impeding the implementation and effective actualization or operationalization of the plan of care. Often, psychosocial or environmental factors are involved including the following:

- Patients cannot afford their ordered medications,
- Patients cannot afford ordered food supplements needed to maintain weight or optimize nutritional status
- Patients are tearful since their spouses or friends deaths and state they "don't want to do anything"
- There are concerns about mental capacity, or signs of abuse, neglect, or financial exploitation
- Patients needs a personal emergency response system as they have had falls and are at risk for more
- Other examples may be where the patient needs sterile dressings or infusion services per the plan of care and the patient does not have a refrigerator or other supports or structures that are needed to facilitate maintenance of minimal infection control or safety standards.

According to Medicare, "medical social services which are provided by a qualified medical social worker or a social worker assistant under the supervision of a qualified medical social worker may be covered as home health services where the beneficiary meets the qualifying criteria and the services of these professionals are necessary to resolve social or emotional problems which are or are expected to be an impediment to the effective treatment of the beneficiary's medical condition or his or her rate of recovery and the plan of care indicates how the services which are required necessitate the skills of a qualified social worker or a social work assistant under the supervision of a qualified social worker to be performed safely and effectively." (*HHA Manual* (HCFA Pub-11, 206.3).

Services of the Medical Social Worker

- Assessment of the social and emotional factors related to the beneficiary's need for care, response to treatment and adjustment to care
- Assessment of the relationship of the beneficiary's medical and nursing requirements to the individual's home situation, financial resources and availability of community resources
- Appropriate action to obtain community resources to assist in resolving the beneficiary's problem. (Note: Medicare does not cover the services of a medical social worker to complete or assist in the completion of an application for Medicaid because Federal regulations require the State to provide assistance in completing the application to anyone who chooses to apply for Medicaid).
- Counseling services which are required by the beneficiary and
- Services provided on a short-term basis to a patient's family or caregiver to remove a clear and direct impediment to the effective treatment of the patient's medical condition or his/her rate of recovery.

Medical social worker services, like home health aide services, cannot "stand-alone." This means that the services they provide must be under the umbrella (or in conjunction with) qualifying services such as nursing, PT or SLP services It is important to note that OT also addresses significant safety concerns, usually related to ADLs. Though the OT cannot initiate home care services, OT can continue to provide services after the other qualifying "stand-alone" services of either nursing, PT or SLP have opened the case.

For clarification purposes, the OT can remain providing visits, even after all other qualifying service(s) have stopped their visits. In this way the OT can remain throughout care and continue to intervene and reassess for progress up until the patient's discharge. The patient's important ADL and other functional problems or concerns are then addressed and undergo re-evaluation by the OT, throughout the duration of the patient's home care services. Medical social work services, like the aide services, can continue in conjunction with OT services.

Summary

The patient's home environment, when looked at from a holistic perspective often makes the difference between a patient being able to remain at home while receiving health care services or having to find alternate housing situations, such as assisted living facilities or nursing homes. The MSW is a very important team member. Though their services are multifaceted and based on each patient's individual needs, the MSW provides services that support the maximization of patient health and function through the identification of financial or community access barriers and challenges with interventions directed toward referral and linkage to appropriate resources. The MSW also is key in the facilitation of patient/family/caregiver responses to care interventions through counseling and family support.

Therapy and all other home care team members use all of their creative skills to develop a net for some of these at-risk patients, particularly elders who want to remain in their own homes. The assessment of the information gathered by all team members and referrals made to the social worker can oftentimes assist in putting together a plan that assists patients to remain safely in their home environments.

Domain Four: Patient Care Planning and Related Processes

The formation of the care plan is the essential component that creates the route or road map for the team and patient to follow to achieve desired outcomes. Once the assessment or evaluation has been performed, thoughtful analysis of all the data occurs, the goals are identified, and the patient's care plan is established with direction from the doctor and input from the patient/caregivers and other involved team members. Readers are referred to Part Four the "Assessment" section, for indepth information about the comprehensive assessment and Part Five for review of the OASIS data set, and associated tools and forms.

Because care planning and related patient and family needs are directed from the assessed and reassessed findings, the services involved are based on the patient's specific pathology requiring intervention and other problems specific to their needs. It is this vision of where the patient can/will be upon discharge that creates the path to meeting rehabilitation goals that all team members, including the most important member, the patient, help support.

Therapy team members are highly valued for their contributions to functional improvements experienced by patients. These can include such gains or improvements as improved gait, independence or improved ability to perform self-care activities, weight stabilization, improved social interactions, safe oral eating, improved mental attitude, increased stamina, increased bladder control and function, improved communication and numerous others. **These functional improvements oftentimes make the difference between patients staying at home or being institutionalized.** This is particularly poignant when we realize that there are estimated to be one-third of Americans age 65 or older either disabled or with at least one chronic illness and these numbers are estimated to grow significantly over the next 20 years.

Skilled Therapy: The Basic Rules

For therapy services to be covered by Medicare, the service may be reasonable when:

1) Generally, that there is an expectation that the patient's condition will improve and in a reasonable or predictable period of time and that the therapy services are reasonable and necessary to restore the function lost, due to the illness or injury. An example is the new patient after a recent cerebral vascular accident (CVA) (the illness/injury) who needs intervention and a home exercise regimen implemented related to right-sided paresis and receptive aphasia (the functions lost due to the illness/injury). This means that the patient has an illness or injury where the therapist(s) can either:

a) assist the patient toward functional improvement from a rehabilitation perspective (the above example) or

b) help assure safety for those patients that have limited rehabilitation potential or an overall poor prognosis by fully establishing an effective home program to maintain their status and/or prevent further deterioration of the condition. An example is the hospice home care patient with a pathological fracture who refuses surgery and needs instruction in an effective program to enable the patient to remain safely at home and prevent further injury or complications. This safety-focused program will also assist the other team members, such as the caregivers, family, nurses, and aides, in providing safe care for this at-risk patient in such activities as turning, positioning, and supporting effective pain management.

2) The service is complex and requires the specialized skills [of the therapist] and services for safe and effective treatment. Home care therapy patients are those patients who have had a recent episode or deterioration of their status resulting in a loss of functional ability from a neurological, orthopedic, cardiac, pulmonary or other system problem. Remember that therapy team members can only provide these important rehabilitation services because of their specialized education and experience. Medicare and other payers pay for therapists' and nurses' higher level skills such as those required for instructing the patient, beyond simply the "tasks" that may be associated with a particular activity.

3) The services that therapy (and other services) provide are reasonable for each specific patient's individual illness and injury and the services provided are consistent with the patient's illness/injury and are within accepted standards of practice. Teaching exercises, techniques, and precautions (such as those for hip precautions after hip replacement surgery) must be based on the patient's illness or injury.

4) The patient's unique findings and medical complications which require the specialized skills of the therapist are clearly documented in the clinical documentation. This includes the OASIS data elements, the discipline-specific assessment forms, visit notes, communication notes, care conference or coordination meeting notes, and others.

Coverage Versus Scope of Practice Dilemma

For all services, it is important to note that there is sometimes a gap between what services can be provided under a therapist's professional scope of practice and what is coverable or payable by insurance payers, such as Medicare. An example could be hearing aid training or the teaching of sign language for speech-language pathologists. Though these are very important for the patient from a communication perspective, they are generally not covered by Medicare. Readers are encouraged to check with their managers for clarity in specific coverage and other requirements.

Physical Therapy Services In Home Care

Physical therapy (PT) services are provided by a qualified licensed physical therapist (PT). There are also physical therapist assistants (PTA) who work under the direction of the PT in certain states, based on licensure and/or state practice acts. These roles are defined by state law and practice standards. The following are the acceptable or coverable services provided by the PT in home care according to the Medicare *HHA Manual* (HCFA - Pub.11).

1. **Assessment** - The skills of a PT to assess a patient's rehabilitation needs and potential or to develop and/or implement a PT program are covered when they are reasonable and necessary because of the patient's condition. Skilled rehabilitation services concurrent with the management of a patient's care plan include objective tests and measurements such as, but not limited to, range of motion, strength, balance coordination, endurance, or functional ability.
2. **Therapeutic Exercises** - Therapeutic exercises which must be performed by or under the supervision of the qualified PT to ensure the safety of the patient and effectiveness of the treatment, due either to the type of exercise employed or to the condition of the patient, constitute skilled PT.
3. **Gait Training** - Gait evaluation and training furnished to a patient whose ability to walk has been impaired by neurological, muscular or skeletal abnormality or other abnormality requires the skills of a qualified PT and constitute skilled PT and are considered reasonable and necessary if training can be expected to improve materially the patient's ability to walk.
4. **Range of Motion** - Range of motion exercises constitutes skilled PT only if they are part of an active treatment for a specific disease state, illness, or injury, that has resulted in a loss or restriction of mobility (as evidenced by PT notes showing the degree of motion lost and the degree to be restored).
5. **Maintenance Therapy** - Though Medicare and the word maintenance do not generally go together, it is important to note that this term "maintenance" is

listed as the fifth of seven listed coverable PT services in the Medicare *Manual*. Two examples explain the conditions that must be met for coverage and the documentation required that supports why the specialized skills (knowledge and judgment) of the PT are required to be safely carried out and the treatment aims of the physician achieved.

6. **Ultrasound, Shortwave, and Microwave Diathermy Treatments** - These treatments are listed in the Medicare *Manual* and are coverable PT services.

7. **Hot Packs, Infra-Red Treatments, Paraffin Baths and Whirlpool Baths** - Though the *Manual* states that heat treatments and baths of this type ordinarily do not require the skills of a qualified PT, it also states that the skills, knowledge and judgment of a qualified therapist might be required in the giving of such treatments or baths in a particular case, e.g., where the patient's condition is complicated by circulatory deficiency, areas of desensitization, open wounds, fractures, or other complications.

The seven above listed PT skills are described at length and with examples in Part Nine of this text, which is the physical therapy portion of the "coverage of services" section of the *HHA Manual* (HCFA Pub.-11). Readers are encouraged to review this material and to use the *Medicare Manual* as the source text for questions related to Medicare coverage. Explanations and examples accompany the Medicare language and clarify the specific coverage parameters.

Other interventions and services, based on the payer and the patient's individual condition may include postural drainage/chest percussion, home exercise regimens, strengthening and balance activities, edema management, bed mobility training, patient and caregiver education and instructions, prosthetic/orthotic training, electrical stimulation, teaching related to use of therapeutic equipment, safety precautions, wound and pain management, and others. Figures 1-9 and 1-10 are examples of PT care plans and PT revisit notes respectively. Readers are referred to Part Six, the specific care guides for examples of interventions and goals for additional PT care planning and documentation.

Speech-Language Pathology Services in Home Care

Patients present for SLP services with problems including impaired speech production, swallowing or voice disorders, impaired oral function or verbal expression and numerous other speech and swallowing problems related to their disease.

Speech-language pathology services are furnished only by a qualified speech-language pathologist (SLP) and "are those services necessary for the diagnosis and treatment of speech and language disorders that result in communication disabilities and for the diagnosis and treatment of swallowing disorders (dysphagia), regardless of the presence of a communication disability."

Figure 1-9

PHYSICAL THERAPY CARE PLAN

SOC DATE ___/___/___

DIAGNOSIS _____ ONSET ___/___/___
PROBLEM(S) _____

PATIENT/CLIENT DESIRED OUTCOMES	SHORT TERM OUTCOMES	Time Frame	LONG TERM OUTCOMES	Time Frame

PLAN OF CARE (Mark all applicable with an "X".)

Evaluation (B1)	Pulmonary Physical Therapy (B6)	Functional mobility training
Establish rehab. program	Ultrasound (B7)	Teach bed mobility skills
Establish home exercise program	Electrotherapy (B8)	Teach hip safety precautions
☐ Copy given to patient/client	Prosthetic training (B9)	Teach safe/effective use of adaptive/assist
☐ Copy attached to chart	Preprosthetic training	device (specify)
Patient/Client/Family education	Fabrication of orthotic device (B10)	Teach safe stair climbing skills
Therapeutic exercise (B2)	Muscle re-education (B11)	Other:
Transfer training (B3)	Management and evaluation of care plan (B12)	
Home program (B4) Establish / Upgrade	TENS	
Gait training (B5)	Cardiopulmonary PT	
Balance training/activities	CPM (specify)	

MODALITIES _____ REHAB POTENTIAL ☐ Good ☐ Fair ☐ Poor
FREQUENCY AND DURATION _____
EQUIPMENT RECOMMENDATIONS _____
SAFETY ISSUES/INSTRUCTION/EDUCATION _____

COMMENTS/ADDITIONAL INFORMATION _____

PATIENT/CLIENT/CAREGIVER RESPONSE TO PLAN OF CARE _____

DISCHARGE DISCUSSED WITH: ☐ Patient/Client/Family ☐ Care Manager ☐ Physician ☐ Other (specify) _____
CARE COORDINATION: ☐ Physician ☐ PT ☐ OT ☐ ST ☐ SS ☐ SN ☐ Other (specify) _____

APPROXIMATE NEXT VISIT DATE ___/___/___
PLAN FOR NEXT VISIT _____

PLAN DEVELOPED BY (signature/title/date) _____ ___/___/___

CARE PLAN REVIEW

DATE	REVIEWED/REVISED BY (signature/title)	COMMENTS

PART 1 — Clinical Record   PART 2 - Therapist   PART 3 - Care Coordination

PATIENT/CLIENT NAME – Last, First, Middle Initial   ID#

Form 3592/3P © 1994 Briggs Corporation, Des Moines, IA 50306
To order, phone 1-800-247-2343 PRINTED IN U.S.A.   **PHYSICAL THERAPY CARE PLAN**

Reprinted with permission from Briggs Health Care Products, Des Moines, Iowa, 1999.

Figure 1-10

PHYSICAL THERAPY REVISIT NOTE

DATE OF SERVICE _____ / _____ / _____
TIME IN _____ OUT _____

HOMEBOUND REASON: ☐ Needs assistance for all activities ☐ Residual weakness
☐ Requires assistance to ambulate ☐ Confusion, unable to go out of home alone
☐ Unable to safely leave home unassisted ☐ Severe SOB, SOB upon exertion
☐ Dependent upon adaptive device(s) ☐ Medical restrictions
☐ Other (specify) _____

TYPE OF VISIT:
☐ Revisit
☐ Revisit and Supervisory Visit
☐ Other (specify) _____
SOC DATE _____ / _____ / _____

TREATMENT DIAGNOSIS/PROBLEM _____

EXPECTED TREATMENT OUTCOME(S) _____

PHYSICAL THERAPY INTERVENTIONS/INSTRUCTIONS (Mark all applicable with an "X".)

Evaluation (B1)	Pulmonary Physical Therapy (B6)	Functional mobility training
Establish rehab. program	Ultrasound (B7)	Teach bed mobility skills
Establish home exercise program	Electrotherapy (B8)	Teach hip safety precautions
☐ Copy given to patient/client	Prosthetic training (B9)	Teach safe/effective use of adaptive/assist
☐ Copy attached to chart	Preprosthetic training	device (specify)
Patient/Client/Family education	Fabrication of orthotic device (B10)	Teach safe stair climbing skills
Therapeutic exercise (B2)	Muscle re-education (B11)	Other:
Transfer training (B3)	Management and evaluation of care plan (B12)	
Home program (B4) Establish / Upgrade	TENS	
Gait training (B5)	Cardiopulmonary PT	
Balance training/activities	CPM (specify)	

OBSERVATIONS, INSTRUCTIONS AND MEASURABLE OUTCOMES _____

EVALUATION AND PATIENT/CLIENT/CAREGIVER RESPONSE _____

CARE PLAN: ☐ Reviewed/Revised with patient/client involvement.
If revised, specify _____
☐ Outcome/Instruction achieved (describe) _____
☐ PRN order obtained
APPROXIMATE NEXT VISIT DATE: _____ / _____ / _____
PLAN FOR NEXT VISIT _____
DISCHARGE DISCUSSED WITH: ☐ Patient/Client/Family
☐ Care Manager ☐ Physician ☐ Other (specify) _____
BILLABLE SUPPLIES RECORDED? ☐ N/A ☐ Yes (specify) _____
CARE COORDINATION: ☐ Physician ☐ PT ☐ OT ☐ ST ☐ SS
☐ SN ☐ Other (specify) _____

SUPERVISORY VISIT (Complete if applicable)
☐ PT Assistant ☐ Aide / ☐ Present ☐ Not present
SUPERVISORY VISIT: ☐ Scheduled ☐ Unscheduled
OBSERVATION OF _____
TEACHING/TRAINING OF _____
PATIENT/CLIENT/FAMILY FEEDBACK ON SERVICES/CARE
(specify) _____
NEXT SCHEDULED SUPERVISORY VISIT _____ / _____ / _____
CARE PLAN UPDATED? ☐ No ☐ Yes (specify) _____
If PT assistant/aide **not present**, specify date he/she was
contacted regarding updated care plan: _____ / _____ / _____

SIGNATURES/DATES

Complete TIME OUT (above) prior to signing below.

X _____
Patient/Client/Caregiver (if applicable)   Date _____ / _____ / _____
Therapist (signature/title)   Date _____ / _____ / _____

PART 1 — Clinical Record   PART 2 — Therapist   PART 3 — Care Coordination

PATIENT/CLIENT NAME — Last, First, Middle Initial   ID#

Form 3578/3P   © 1994 Briggs Corporation, Des Moines, IA 50306
To order, phone 1-800-247-2343 PRINTED IN U.S.A.

PHYSICAL THERAPY REVISIT NOTE

Reprinted with permission from Briggs Health Care Products, Des Moines, Iowa, 1999.

[Medicare *HHA Manual* (HCFA Pub.-11) (205.2C)]

The following are the acceptable or coverable services for SLP according to Medicare:

1. **Assessment [of speech, language, voice, rhythm and swallowing disorders]** - The skills of a SLP are required for the assessment of a patient's rehabilitation needs (including the causal factors and severity of the speech and language disorders), and rehabilitation potential.

2. **Speech-voice production services** - The services of a SLP would be covered if they are needed as a result of an illness or injury and are directed towards specific speech/voice production.

3. **Communicative activities of daily living** - SLP would be covered where the service can only be provided by a SLP and where it is reasonably expected that the service will materially improve the patient's ability to independently carry out any one or combination of communicative activities of daily living in a manner that is measurably at a higher level of attainment than that prior to the initiation of the services.

4. **The establishment of a hierarchy of speech-voice-language communication tasks and cueing** - The services of a SLP to establish a hierarchy of speech-voice-language communication tasks and cueing that directs a patient toward speech-language communication goals in the plan of care would be covered SLP services.

5. **The training of the patient, family, or other caregivers to augment communication** - The services of a SLP to train the patient, family, or other caregivers to augment the speech-language communication, treatment or to establish an effective maintenance program would be covered SLP services.

6. **Aphasia** - The services of a SLP to assist patients with aphasia in rehabilitation of speech and language skills are covered when needed by a patient.

7. **Voice disorders** - The services of a SLP to assist patients with voice disorders to develop proper control of the vocal and respiratory systems for correct voice production are covered when needed by a patient.

Each of the seven above listed SLP skills is addressed in the *Medicare HHA Manual* (HCFA - Publication 11) and is reprinted in its entirety for review in Part Nine of this text. Readers are encouraged to review this material and use these pages as the source text for questions related to Medicare coverage.

Other interventions and services, based on the payer and the patient's individual condition, may include assessment of a speech, language, voice, rhythm and swallowing disorders, aphasia therapy programs, oral-motor exercises, patient/family education, dysphagia therapy, establishment of an effective home program of compensatory and safety strategies including problems such as cognitive deficits, communication interventions, swallowing programs, rehabilitation of speech and language skills and communication services, voice therapy for esophageal speech, progressive treatment for speech, language, voice, rhythm, and swallowing disorders, developing and teaching progressive home program, training in the use of augmentative communication devices, modification of food/fluid consistency, and others. Examples of a ST care plan and revisit note follow for review in Figures 1-11 and 1-12. Oftentimes the SLP or ST works in collaboration with the dietitian or medical nutrition therapist (MNT).

Dietitian Services in Home Care

Dietitians have a very important role in home care although their services are not one of the six coverable Medicare home care services. The coordination between the SLP and the dietitian is key to patients meeting their goals related to nutrition. The dietitian in home care works with a wide range of patients, including patient populations with diabetes mellitus, congestive heart failure, renal disease or failure. They are oftentimes consulted in wound and ostomy management, malnutrition, cancers, and enteral and parenteral feedings and nutritional support. The scope also extends to patients experiencing difficulty swallowing, weight loss, and eating disorders. All clinicians must consider the patient's need for the dietitian on admission and throughout care should the patient's nutritional status be compromised and need intervention to achieve desired goals. Most organizations have a list of clinical indicators that necessitate the need for these specialized services. Readers are referred to Figure 1-15 for a listing of Care Management/Consult/Referral Criteria that lists the Medical Nutrition Therapist (MNT) and indicators that may necessitate a referral.

Occupational Therapy Services In Home Care

Occupational therapists (OT) and certified occupational therapy assistants (COTAs), who practice under the supervision of an OT, provide OT services in home care. The plan of care is developed by the OT after conducting the patient assessment, and the COTA can assist in carrying out the plan. Some states require state certification or licensure of COTAs. The organization who employs the OT practitioner, whether OT or COTA, is responsible for verifying that all OTs and COTAs have current regulation credentials. Some states have licensure and practice acts that define the specific duties and scope of function for COTAs practicing in those states.

Occupational Therapy Coverage: Special Considerations

A requirement for a Medicare beneficiary to qualify for home health services is that a beneficiary must have a need for skilled nursing care on an intermittent basis, or physical therapy, or speech therapy, or a continuing need for OT. Any

Figure 1-11

SPEECH THERAPY
CARE PLAN

SOC DATE ___/___/___

DIAGNOSIS _____ ONSET ___/___/___
ANALYSIS OF EVALUATION/TEST SCORES _____

PATIENT/CLIENT DESIRED OUTCOMES	SHORT TERM OUTCOMES	Time Frame	LONG TERM OUTCOMES	Time Frame

PLAN OF CARE (Mark all applicable with an "X".)

Evaluation (C1)	Aural rehabilitation (C6)	Speech dysphagia instruction program
Establish rehab. program	Non-oral communication (C8)	Care of voice prosthesis including
Establish home maintenance program	Alaryngeal speech skills	removal, cleaning, site maintenance
☐ Copy given to patient/client	Language processing	Teach/Develop communication system
☐ Copy attached to chart	Food texture recommendations	Trach. instruction and care
Patient/Client/Family education	Safe swallowing evaluation	Other:
Voice disorders (C2)	Therapy to increase articulation,	
Speech articulation disorders (C3)	proficiency, verbal expression	
Dysphagia treatments (C4)	Lip, tongue, facial exercises to	
Language disorders (C5)	improve swallowing/vocal skills	

FREQUENCY AND DURATION _____ REHAB POTENTIAL ☐ Good ☐ Fair ☐ Poor
EQUIPMENT RECOMMENDATIONS _____
SAFETY ISSUES/INSTRUCTION/EDUCATION _____

COMMENTS/ADDITIONAL INFORMATION _____

PATIENT/CLIENT/CAREGIVER RESPONSE TO PLAN OF CARE _____

DISCHARGE DISCUSSED WITH: ☐ Patient/Client/Family
☐ Care Manager ☐ Physician ☐ Other (specify)_____
CARE COORDINATION: ☐ Physician ☐ PT ☐ OT ☐ ST ☐ SS
☐ SN ☐ Other (specify)_____

APPROXIMATE NEXT VISIT DATE ___/___/___
PLAN FOR NEXT VISIT _____

PLAN DEVELOPED BY (signature/title/date) _____ ___/___/___

CARE PLAN REVIEW

DATE	REVIEWED/REVISED BY (signature/title)	COMMENTS

PART 1 — Clinical Record   PART 2 - Therapist   PART 3 - Care Coordination

PATIENT/CLIENT NAME — Last, First, Middle Initial | ID#

Form 3596/3P   © 1994 Briggs Corporation, Des Moines, IA 50306
To order, phone 1-800-247-2343 PRINTED IN U.S.A.

SPEECH THERAPY CARE PLAN

Reprinted with permission from Briggs Health Care Products, Des Moines, Iowa, 1999.

Figure 1-12

SPEECH THERAPY REVISIT NOTE

DATE OF SERVICE ____/____/____

TIME IN _____ OUT_____

HOMEBOUND REASON: ☐ Needs assistance for all activities ☐ Residual weakness
☐ Requires assistance to ambulate   ☐ Confusion, unable to go out of home alone
☐ Unable to safely leave home unassisted ☐ Severe SOB, SOB upon exertion
☐ Dependent upon adaptive device(s)   ☐ Medical restrictions
☐ Other (specify) ____

TYPE OF VISIT:
☐ Revisit
☐ Revisit and Supervisory Visit
☐ Other (specify) ____

SOC DATE ____/____/____

TREATMENT DIAGNOSIS/PROBLEM ____

EXPECTED TREATMENT OUTCOME(S) ____

SPEECH THERAPY INTERVENTIONS/INSTRUCTIONS (Mark all applicable with an "X".)

Evaluation (C1)	Aural rehabilitation (C6)	Speech dysphagia instruction program
Establish rehab. program	Non-oral communication (C8)	Care of voice prosthesis including
Establish home maintenance program	Alaryngeal speech skills	removal, cleaning, site maintenance
☐ Copy given to patient/client	Language processing	Teach/Develop communication system
☐ Copy attached to chart	Food texture recommendations	Trach. instruction and care
Patient/Client/Family education	Safe swallowing evaluation	Other:
Voice disorders (C2)	Therapy to increase articulation,	
Speech articulation disorders (C3)	proficiency, verbal expression	
Dysphagia treatments (C4)	Lip, tongue, facial exercises to	
Language disorders (C5)	improve swallowing/vocal skills	

OBSERVATIONS, INSTRUCTIONS AND MEASURABLE OUTCOMES ____

EVALUATION AND PATIENT/CLIENT/CAREGIVER RESPONSE ____

CARE PLAN: ☐ Reviewed/Revised with patient/client involvement.
If revised, specify ____

☐ Outcome/Instruction achieved (describe) ____

☐ PRN order obtained
APPROXIMATE NEXT VISIT DATE: ____/____/____
PLAN FOR NEXT VISIT ____

DISCHARGE DISCUSSED WITH: ☐ Patient/Client/Family
☐ Care Manager ☐ Physician ☐ Other (specify) ____
BILLABLE SUPPLIES RECORDED? ☐ N/A ☐ Yes (specify) ____

CARE COORDINATION: ☐ Physician ☐ PT ☐ OT ☐ ST ☐ SS
☐ SN ☐ Other (specify) ____

SUPERVISORY VISIT (Complete if applicable)

☐ ST Assistant ☐ Aide / ☐ Present ☐ Not present
SUPERVISORY VISIT: ☐ Scheduled ☐ Unscheduled
OBSERVATION OF ____

TEACHING/TRAINING OF ____

PATIENT/CLIENT/FAMILY FEEDBACK ON SERVICES/CARE
(specify) ____

NEXT SCHEDULED SUPERVISORY VISIT ____/____/____
CARE PLAN UPDATED? ☐ No ☐ Yes (specify) ____

If ST assistant/aide **not present**, specify date he/she was
contacted regarding updated care plan: ____/____/____

SIGNATURES/DATES

Complete **TIME OUT** (above) prior to signing below.

X _____   ____/____/____
Patient/Client/Caregiver (if applicable)   Date

_____   ____/____/____
Therapist (signature/title)   Date

PART 1 — Clinical Record   PART 2 — Therapist   PART 3 — Care Coordination

PATIENT/CLIENT NAME — Last, First, Middle Initial | ID#

Form 3580/3P   © 1994 Briggs Corporation, Des Moines, IA 50306
To order, phone 1-800-247-2343 PRINTED IN U.S.A.

SPEECH THERAPY REVISIT NOTE

Reprinted with permission from Briggs Health Care Products, Des Moines, Iowa, 1999.

one of these qualifying services will establish the patient's eligibility for Medicare home health services. It is important to note that since it is a "continuing need" for OT, **OT is not a qualifying service to start (or initiate) care or services, but is a qualifying skilled service to continue care** when other skilled services have been discontinued. For an example, if a patient begins services with skilled intermittent nursing and OT, but later skilled nursing is no longer required but OT continues to provide services, OT would be the qualifying skilled service which would allow the agency to continue billing Medicare. So although the OT cannot initiate home care services from a Medicare perspective, the OT can continue to provide services after the other qualifying "stand-alone" services of either nursing, PT, or SLP have opened the case.

The following are the Medicare acceptable or coverable services provided by OTs:

1. **Assessment** - [The assessment and reassessment of a patient's rehabilitation and potential or to develop and/or implement an OT program] are covered when they are reasonable and necessary because of the patient's condition.

2. **Planning, Implementing, and Supervision of Therapeutic Programs** - The planning, implementing and supervision of therapeutic programs including, but not limited to: selecting and teaching task oriented therapeutic activities designed to restore function, tasks and activities designed to restore sensory-integrative function, therapeutic activity programs as a part of an overall "active treatment" program for a patient with a diagnosed psychiatric illness, teaching compensatory techniques to improve the level of independence in the activities of daily living, the designing, fabricating, and fitting of orthotic and self-help devices, and vocational and prevocational assessment and training that is directed toward the restoration of function in the activities of daily living lost due to illness or injury.

Other interventions and services, based on the payer and the patient's individual condition may include instruction in adaptive techniques and use of assistive devices for activities of daily living (ADL) training/retraining, homemaking, addressing safety and functioning related to significant safety concerns, therapeutic exercise for improving upper extremity function, instruction in use of assistive devices to increase independence in self-care such as bathing, dressing, grooming, energy conservation to increase functional activity level, self-care training, functional mobility training for ADL, home management training, work simplification, balance training, motor coordination training, perceptual motor training, joint protection, splinting/orthotics and fabrication, neuro-muscular re-education, life skills training, retraining and compensation for cognitive/perceptual impairment, patient/family education and others. Examples of an OT care plan and revisit note follow for review in Figures 1-13 and 1-14.

Figure 1-13

OCCUPATIONAL THERAPY CARE PLAN

SOC DATE ___/___/___

DIAGNOSIS _____ ONSET ___/___/___

PROBLEM(S) _____

PATIENT/CLIENT DESIRED OUTCOMES	SHORT TERM OUTCOMES	Time Frame	LONG TERM OUTCOMES	Time Frame

PLAN OF CARE (Mark all applicable with an "X".)

Evaluation (D1)	Neuro-developmental training (D7)	Therapeutic exercise to right/left hand
Establish rehab. program	Sensory treatment (D8)	to increase strength, coordination,
Establish home exercise program	Orthotics/Splinting (D9)	sensation and proprioception
☐ Copy given to patient/client	Adaptive equipment (fabrication	Other:
☐ Copy attached to chart	and training) (D10)	
Patient/Client/Family education	Teach alternative bathing skills	
Independent living/ADL training (D2)	(unable to use tub/shower safely)	
Muscle re-education (D3)	Retraining of cognitive, feeding	
Perceptual motor training (D5)	and perceptual skills	
Fine motor coordination (D6)	Body image training	

MODALITIES _____ REHAB POTENTIAL ☐ Good ☐ Fair ☐ Poor

FREQUENCY AND DURATION _____

EQUIPMENT RECOMMENDATIONS _____

SAFETY ISSUES/INSTRUCTION/EDUCATION _____

COMMENTS/ADDITIONAL INFORMATION _____

PATIENT/CLIENT/CAREGIVER RESPONSE TO PLAN OF CARE _____

DISCHARGE DISCUSSED WITH: ☐ Patient/Client/Family
    ☐ Care Manager   ☐ Physician   ☐ Other (specify)_____
CARE COORDINATION: ☐ Physician   ☐ PT   ☐ OT   ☐ ST   ☐ SS
    ☐ SN   ☐ Other (specify)_____

APPROXIMATE NEXT VISIT DATE ___/___/___
PLAN FOR NEXT VISIT _____

PLAN DEVELOPED BY (signature/title/date) _____ ___/___/___

CARE PLAN REVIEW

DATE	REVIEWED/REVISED BY (signature/title)	COMMENTS

PART 1 — Clinical Record   PART 2 - Therapist   PART 3 - Care Coordination

PATIENT/CLIENT NAME — Last, First, Middle Initial   ID#

Form 3594/3P © 1994 Briggs Corporation, Des Moines, IA 50306
To order, phone 1-800-247-2343 PRINTED IN U.S.A.

OCCUPATIONAL THERAPY CARE PLAN

Reprinted with permission from Briggs Health Care Products, Des Moines, Iowa, 1999.

Figure 1-14

OCCUPATIONAL THERAPY REVISIT NOTE

DATE OF SERVICE ____/____/____

TIME IN _____ OUT_____

HOMEBOUND REASON: ☐ Needs assistance for all activities ☐ Residual weakness
☐ Requires assistance to ambulate ☐ Confusion, unable to go out of home alone
☐ Unable to safely leave home unassisted ☐ Severe SOB, SOB upon exertion
☐ Dependent upon adaptive device(s) ☐ Medical restrictions
☐ Other (specify) _____

TYPE OF VISIT:
☐ Revisit
☐ Revisit and Supervisory Visit
☐ Other (specify)_____
SOC DATE ____/____/____

TREATMENT DIAGNOSIS/PROBLEM _____

EXPECTED TREATMENT OUTCOME(S) _____

OCCUPATIONAL THERAPY INTERVENTIONS/INSTRUCTIONS (Mark all applicable with an "X".)

Evaluation (D1)	Neuro-developmental training (D7)	Therapeutic exercise to right/left hand to increase strength, coordination, sensation and proprioception
Establish rehab. program	Sensory treatment (D8)	
Establish home exercise program	Orthotics/Splinting (D9)	Other:
☐ Copy given to patient/client	Adaptive equipment (fabrication and training) (D10)	
☐ Copy attached to chart		
Patient/Client/Family education	Teach alternative bathing skills (unable to use tub/shower safely)	
Independent living/ADL training (D2)		
Muscle re-education (D3)	Retraining of cognitive, feeding and perceptual skills	
Perceptual motor training (D5)		
Fine motor coordination (D6)	Body image training	

OBSERVATIONS, INSTRUCTIONS AND MEASURABLE OUTCOMES _____

EVALUATION AND PATIENT/CLIENT/CAREGIVER RESPONSE _____

CARE PLAN: ☐ Reviewed/Revised with patient/client involvement.	**SUPERVISORY VISIT (Complete if applicable)**
If revised, specify _____	☐ OT Assistant ☐ Aide / ☐ Present ☐ Not present SUPERVISORY VISIT: ☐ Scheduled ☐ Unscheduled
☐ Outcome/Instruction achieved (describe)_____	OBSERVATION OF_____
☐ PRN order obtained APPROXIMATE NEXT VISIT DATE: ____/____/____ PLAN FOR NEXT VISIT _____	TEACHING/TRAINING OF _____
	PATIENT/CLIENT/FAMILY FEEDBACK ON SERVICES/CARE (specify)_____
DISCHARGE DISCUSSED WITH: ☐ Patient/Client/Family ☐ Care Manager ☐ Physician ☐ Other (specify)_____ BILLABLE SUPPLIES RECORDED? ☐ N/A ☐ Yes (specify)____	NEXT SCHEDULED SUPERVISORY VISIT ____/____/____ CARE PLAN UPDATED? ☐ No ☐ Yes (specify) _____
CARE COORDINATION: ☐ Physician ☐ PT ☐ OT ☐ ST ☐ SS ☐ SN ☐ Other (specify) _____	If OT assistant/aide **not present**, specify date he/she was contacted regarding updated care plan: ____/____/____

SIGNATURES/DATES

Complete **TIME OUT** (above) prior to signing below.

X_____ ____/____/____   _____ ____/____/____
Patient/Client/Caregiver (if applicable)   Date   Therapist (signature/title)   Date

PART 1 — Clinical Record   PART 2 — Therapist   PART 3 — Care Coordination

PATIENT/CLIENT NAME — Last, First, Middle Initial	ID#

Form 3579/3P © 1994 Briggs Corporation, Des Moines, IA 50306
To order, phone 1-800-247-2343 PRINTED IN U.S.A.   **OCCUPATIONAL THERAPY REVISIT NOTE**

Reprinted with permission from Briggs Health Care Products, Des Moines, Iowa, 1999.

Readers are referred to the *HHA Manual* (HCFA Pub-11), Section 205.2 in Part Nine of this text. Coverage of services for patients and seven coverage examples for OT services are reprinted here in its entirety. Readers are encouraged to review this material and use the *HHA Manual* as the source text for questions related to Medicare home health coverage.

The Role of the Therapist as Case Manager

There are varied definitions for case management and differing roles for the case manager. Case management can succinctly be defined as a process for coordinating and managing across geography, the care continuum, and care sites to achieve pre-determined and agreed-upon patient outcomes. Usually in medical case management, such as for Medicare, this role is assumed by a nurse or a therapist and provided during the patient's length of stay in home care. Part of the reason nurses or therapists may be the case manager is for efficiency as these are the only clinicians who can open or initiate Medicare home care services. This is important to note as currently for Medicare home care, the medical social worker cannot "stand-alone". However, social workers may be case managers in some models, usually more psychosocial or social models.

Effective case management includes the prudent use of resources and coordination of all aspects of care related to developing and achieving outcomes for the specified patient-population or case load. Simply put, the case manager is accountable for meeting outcomes within an appropriate time frame while adhering to preestablished standards. Key responsibilities include: the effective use of resources; collaboration and coordination with other members of the health care team; establishing a partnership with the patient and caregivers/family members to accomplish those outcomes. One of the hallmarks of effective case management is an indepth evaluation. Throughout the course of care, the case manager acts as a patient advocate to facilitate meeting identified patient/family needs. The following lists sources of data that must be assessed and evaluated for the creation of an effective case management plan.

Sources of Data Needed for Holistic Case Management

- The patient's medical history
- The patient's prior level of care
- The patient's environment and home/safety risk factors
- The patient's and family's dynamics
- The patient's and family's abilities related to care
- The primary caregiver's capabilities, availability, and willingness to provide care

- The patient's medications (e.g., prescribed, OTC, other remedies, etc.)
- The patient's resources and ability to access resources
- The patient's need for other services (e.g., nursing, physical or occupational therapy, speech-language pathology services, home health aide services, social work services, nutritional assessment, hospice care, etc.)

"Therapy Only" Case Considerations

A challenge in home care has historically been the "therapy only" patients. The classic patient is an elderly man who has had a new cerebral vascular accident (CVA), is homebound, confined to a wheelchair from a prior stroke. The patient now needs a SLP assessment and intervention due to a change in speech and communication skills as reported by the patient and family who told the referring doctor that "he is using different words and the wrong words (only) since this last stroke." The role assumed by the therapist has sometimes been determined by the state licensure act for home care or in some states, the specific practice act. In other words, in some states all cases are opened by registered nurses or as specified by licensing or another regulatory body. In other states though, therapists have been opening and case managing home care "therapy only" cases for years. Another impediment to therapists assuming this role has been the availability of therapists in certain geographic parts of the country. Whatever the role of the therapist related to admissions at a particular organization, the emerging roles for both nurses and therapists will be as case managers. The most important component of effective case management revolves around identifying the patient's specific care needs. It is in this capacity that the admitting case manager therapist must know the roles of the other team members and when a referral to another team member may be appropriate and mandated from quality and risk management perspectives.

Patient Example: Identifying Other Patient Needs

An example is the patient that was referred to a home care organization from an insurance company case manager who authorized three physical therapy visits. The referral information noted the reason for referral as "new left-sided paresis." This patient was a 39-year-old man and after speaking with the physician to validate the therapy assessment and specific orders, it was learned that the patient was on steroids and other medications and had an aggressive brain tumor. The organization was located in a state where therapy only cases are allowed per law, but the nurse manager and the therapist were concerned that this patient may also have nursing needs such as a need for observation and assessment of the patient's neurological status, risk for seizures, and medication management. The patient had a seizure prior to leaving the hospital and nursing was then also authorized. *It is important that all team members know each others' roles and more importantly, when to collaborate and question if another service should be involved for safety or scope of practice reasons.* Figure 1-15 assists case managers in the early identification of appropriate indicators for referral to another discipline or specialty.

Medicare Skilled Nursing Services

Not surprisingly, nursing and home health aide visits account historically for the highest numbers of home visits. When we think of the medical Medicare model and the Medicare patient population it is easy to understand why this is true. We know that these patients are on numerous medications for numerous health problems and most have co-morbidities. Sometimes in home care you think every elder has a urinary catheter and shoeboxes full of prescription and over-the-counter (OTC) medications needing to be reviewed. In reality this is not the case, but the number of elders needing home care continues to grow. According to Medicare, "to be covered as skilled nursing services, the services must require the skills of a registered nurse or a licensed practical nurse under the supervision of a registered nurse, must be reasonable and necessary to the treatment of the beneficiary's illness or injury as discussed in Section 205.1A and B, and must be intermittent as discussed in Section 205.1C." (*HHA Manual* HCFA Pub.-11).

There are fifteen (15) skilled nursing services that are coverable under the Medicare home care program. It is important to note that Medicare states: "a person expected to need more or less full-time skilled nursing care over an extended period of time; i.e. a patient who requires institutionalization, would usually **not** qualify for home health benefits." (Section 205.1C3). Some of the most frequently used services include:

- Observation and assessment of patient's condition when only the specialized skills of a medical professional can determine a patient's status
- Management and evaluation of a patient care plan
- Teaching and training activities
- Administration of medications
- Tube feedings
- Nasopharyngeal and tracheostomy aspiration [suctioning]
- Catheters
- Wound care (may include three skills - observation and assessment of the wound site, signs and symptoms of infection, the hands-on wound care such as a dressing change, and teaching and training of the wound care to the beneficiary or family)

- Ostomy care
- Medical gasses
- Rehabilitative nursing
- Venipuncture (Not a stand-alone qualifying service pursuant to the Balanced Budget Act of 1997. May be provided and covered only if another skilled service [such as another nursing or therapy services] is being provided.)
- Student nurse visits
- Psychiatric evaluation and therapy

It goes without saying that all team members need to identify when they do not feel comfortable with a particular task or assessment, or think assessment by another specialty may be appropriate. The previous example about the man with the brain tumor is an example where the prudent therapist, after providing their PT evaluation and realizing the multiple medications and the patient's illness trajectory, spoke with the supervisor and the doctor about this patient's other health service needs and the doctor then initiated orders for a nursing assessment and plan.

Like the therapy section of the *Home Health Agency Manual* (HCFA Pub.-11), there are also general principles that govern reasonable and necessary skilled nursing care with numerous examples. Readers are encouraged to review the 15 covered nursing services in the Medicare *Home Health Agency Manual*. For an in-depth text on home care nursing, care planning and documentation, readers are referred to the *Handbook of Home Health Standards and Documentation Guidelines for Reimbursement* (Mosby, 1997).

Regardless of the clinician's specialty area, the following are the care processes that must occur to provide skillful and compassionate care to all patients. The following highlights the activities of the therapist or nurse case manager.

Managing the Patient's Care: The Care Process

- Performs the initial assessment
- Defines the plan of treatment (or care)
- Identifies the team members
- Clarifies an understanding of each person's role
- Understands and prepares for variations in the process
- Reassesses every visit and other times throughout the episode of care
- Changes the plan, based on patient findings and needs, and
- Communicates, coordinates and documents!

Figure 1-15   CASE MANAGEMENT / CONSULT / REFERRAL CRITERIA

REHAB & ANCILLARY

C A R E M G M T R E F E F F A L	Physical Therapist	Speech Therapist	Occupational Therapist

	❏ Rehab intensive diagnosis
	❏ Functional limitations:
	    ❏ Total hip/knee
	    ❏ Fracture
	    ❏ Laminectomy
	❏ No skilled nursing needs (teaching, assessment, treatments)
	❏ Medically stable
	❏ Independent in medication management
		❏ Dysphagia
		❏ Cognitive impairment
		❏ Communication impairment
		❏ Independent in functional activities
		❏ Ambulates safely
		❏ No skilled nursing needs (teaching, assessment, treatments)
		❏ Medically stable
		❏ Independent in medication management
			For reasons below when other skilled services not required
			
			❏ No skilled nursing needs (teaching, assessments, treatments)
			❏ Medically stable
			❏ Independent in medication management

	❏ Impaired balance
	❏ Impaired ambulation
	❏ Impaired ability to transfer
	❏ Impaired bed mobility
	❏ Weight bearing restriction
	❏ Poor endurance for functional activity
	❏ Decreased ROM/joint contracture
	❏ Decreased muscle strength
	❏ Home safety/modification
	❏ Prosthetic/orthotic training
	❏ Impaired stair climbing
	❏ Caregiver instruction/establish home program
	❏ Frequent falls
	❏ Pain with movement
	❏ Use of assistive devices
		❏ Impaired swallowing
		❏ Impaired expression
		❏ Impaired comprehension
		❏ Impaired cognition/memory
		❏ Impaired voice
		❏ Non-verbal communication
		❏ Oral/facial muscle weakness
		❏ Caregiver instruction/establish home program
		❏ Loss of phonation (S/P trach, laryngectomy)
			❏ Impaired dexterity/coordination
			❏ Decreased UE ROM/strength
			❏ Cognitive/perceptual impairment
			❏ Need for adaptive equipment/training
			❏ Energy conservation/work simplification
			❏ Impaired ability for self care:
			    ❏ Feeding
			    ❏ Bathing
			    ❏ Grooming
			    ❏ Dressing
			    ❏ Homemaking
			❏ Caregiver instruction/establish home program
			❏ Communication difficulty (writing/phone use)
			❏ Need for adaptive home environment
			❏ HCA seeing patient for assist w/ADLs

Figure 1-15   CASE MANAGEMENT / CONSULT / REFERRAL CRITERIA (cont'd)

REHAB & ANCILLARY

Medical Social Worker	Medical Nutrition Therapist	Home Care Aide

❏ Placement
❏ Community resources
❏ Psychosocial assessment (general)
❏ Family member out of control
❏ Caregiver stressed/inappropriate; patient at risk
❏ Suspected neglect/abuse
❏ Assist with advance directives
❏ Financial assessment
❏ Request for Application for Assistance by Reimbursement
❏ Frequent hospitalization
❏ End stage illness
❏ Contracting with patients/families
	❏ Diagnosis of:
	  ❏ Diabetes Mellitus
	  ❏ Congestive Heart Failure
	  ❏ Renal Failure
	❏ Malnutrition
	❏ Difficulty swallowing
	❏ Ostomy
	❏ Wound (stage II-IV)
	❏ Enteral feedings
	❏ Parenteral nutrition
	❏ Recent unplanned weight loss (>= 5% usual body weight)
	❏ Any identified knowledge deficit related to diet/ nutrition requirements
	❏ Eating disorders
	❏ Cancer patients receiving treatment (chemo, radiation)
		❏ Not independent in self care
		❏ Recently discharged from hospital/nursing home
		❏ Self care is unsafe due to physical/mental status
		❏ Unkempt patient
		❏ Neglected patient
		❏ Stressed caregiver
		❏ Requires assistance with light housekeeping, meal preparation, eating, exercises, normally self-administered medications

Figure 1-15   CASE MANAGEMENT / CONSULT / REFERRAL CRITERIA (cont'd)

NURSING

	Behavioral Health	Rehabilitation	Cardiac

C A R E M G M T	❏ Primary Psychiatric Diagnosis (DSM IV)	❏ Rehab-intensive diagnosis with skilled nursing needs
		❏ Primary rehabilitation diagnosis or procedure:
		  ❏ CVA
		  ❏ Joint Replacement
		  ❏ Fracture
		  ❏ Laminectomy
		  ❏ Spinal cord injury
		  ❏ Traumatic brain injury
		  ❏ Brain or spinal cord surgery
		  ❏ Limb amputation
		  ❏ Multiple Sclerosis
		  ❏ Parkinson's Disease
		  ❏ Amyotrophic Lateral Sclerosis
		❏ Patient requires close coordination of nursing and multiple therapy services in order to meet maximum rehabilitation potential
			❏ Primary cardiac diagnosis:
			  ❏ Angina
			  ❏ Atrial fibrillation
			  ❏ Cardiomyopathy
			  ❏ Congestive Heart Failure
			  ❏ Post-Myocardial Infarction
			  ❏ Pre-/post-cardiac bypass or valve replacement surgery
			❏ Implantable defibrillator
			❏ New pacemaker inserted
			❏ Complex cardiac therapies:
			  ❏ Cardiac event monitoring
			  ❏ EKG monitoring
			  ❏ IV inotropic

C O N S U L T	❏ Experiencing emotional distress
	❏ "Difficult" patients/families
	❏ Experiencing symptoms of mental disorder:
	  ❏ Pervasive, lingering sad mood
	  ❏ Mood swings
	  ❏ Lack of energy
	  ❏ Isolation
	  ❏ Loss of appetite
	  ❏ Insomnia
	  ❏ Delusions
	  ❏ Panic
	  ❏ Hallucinations (auditory, visual, other)
	  ❏ Excessive/inappropriate guilt
	  ❏ Mania
	  ❏ Unrealistic/excessive anxiety or worry
	❏ Demonstrated self-destructive behavior
	❏ Dysfunctional grieving
	❏ Substance abuse
	❏ Non-compliant behavior (when unable to determine reason for non-compliance)
		❏ Secondary rehab diagnosis impacting primary diagnosis
		❏ Knowledge deficit regarding disease process and management
		❏ Patient with primary rehabilitation diagnosis who develops skilled nursing needs after admission to therapy service
			❏ Multiple cardiac medication changes
			❏ Secondary cardiac diagnosis impacting primary diagnosis
			❏ Knowledge deficit re: cardiac status/treatments

Figure 1-15   CASE MANAGEMENT / CONSULT / REFERRAL CRITERIA (cont'd)

NURSING

Diabetes Education	Enterostomal Therapy	Infusion Therapy	Pulmonary
❑ New to insulin ❑ Newly-diagnosed Diabetes Mellitus ❑ New to blood glucose monitoring ❑ Uncontrolled diabetes ❑ Diabetics with an infectious process and known blood sugar alterations ❑ Diagnosis of hypoglycemia ❑ Changed from oral agents to insulin	❑ Learning ostomy irrigation procedure ❑ New ostomies and continent diversions ❑ Experiencing problems with ostomy or appliance ❑ Complex/problematic wounds requiring frequent changes in wound management supplies/ technique	❑ Any patient admitted with an IV ❑ IV antibiotics ❑ IV hydration ❑ IV pain control ❑ IV chemotherapeutics ❑ IV inotropics ❑ IV diuretics ❑ Line flushes ❑ TPN ❑ Intraspinal narcotics ❑ Central line port care	❑ Primary Pulmonary Diagnosis 　❑ Asthma 　❑ Asthmatic Bronchitis 　❑ Black Lung Disease 　❑ Bronchitis 　❑ COPD 　❑ Cor Pulmonale 　❑ Cystic Fibrosis 　❑ Emphysema 　❑ Interstitial Pulmonary Fibrosis 　❑ Kyphoscoliosis 　❑ Obesity Hypoventilation Syndrome 　❑ Obstructive Sleep Apnea 　❑ Sarcoidosis 　❑ Silicosis ❑ Requires complex respiratory treatment modalities 　❑ BiPAP 　❑ CPAP 　❑ Trach care/management 　❑ Transtracheal oxygen therapy ❑ Tracheostomy ❑ New laryngectomy
❑ Unstable blood sugars identified after admission to service ❑ Primary diagnosis related to diabetes complication ❑ Poor wound healing with diabetes diagnosis ❑ Old meter/need for new equipment ❑ Poor self-management/hygiene (e.g., foot care) ❑ Patient with multiple questions about diabetes management ❑ Poor technique with blood glucose monitoring or injections ❑ Knowledge deficit or change in caregiver that impacts diabetes management	❑ Wound assessment and evaluation of treatment ❑ At risk for skin breakdown/altered skin integrity ❑ Evaluation and recommendations for support surfaces (e.g., bed, wheelchair) ❑ Skin rash(es) present ❑ Concerns related to incontinence (urinary/fecal) or urinary catheter ❑ New onset of incontinence ❑ Ostomy assessment and evaluation of current appliance and need for change in type of appliance ❑ Demonstrates deficit in self-management (i.e., questionable wound care technique, appliance changes etc.) ❑ Knowledge deficit or change in caregiver that impacts ostomy or wound management ❑ Nephrostomy tubes	❑ Difficult blood draw ❑ Monthly port flush ❑ Placement of access device ❑ Patient education ❑ Assess appropriateness of patient for home infusion	❑ Changes in pulmonary medication regime ❑ Secondary pulmonary diagnosis impacting primary diagnosis ❑ Knowledge deficit regarding pulmonary status/ treatments ❑ Need specialized respiratory testing and assessment ❑ Evaluate response to respiratory treatment modality ❑ Patient teaching relative to pulmonary condition and/or respiratory treatment modality

Reprinted with permission from Meridia Home Care Services, Mayfield Village, Ohio, 1999.

11 Patient-Directed Roles of the Effective Case Manager

1. Assumes responsibility for the patient's care from intake (though sometimes may meet new patients in the hospital or other care sites before inpatient discharge) through discharge.

2. Performs the initial assessment, completes related documentation such as the OASIS and initiates ordered care and care coordination activities (e.g,. OASIS, confirmation and/or clarification of doctor orders, HCFA Form 485, physician telephone orders, etc.)

3. Completes the plan of care after thoughtful analysis of the assessment and other data collected and individualizes the standardized care plan, protocol, or path as per organizational policy.

4. Communicates effectively about the progress of the plan on an ongoing basis with the patient and caregiver, physician(s), nurses, aides, social workers, therapists, and other involved team members in the patient's/family's care.

5. Assumes accountability for projected agreed-upon outcomes for patients, including use of resources, time on service, and others as specified by organizational data management standards.

6. Identifies variances in standardized care or protocols and care processes to identify areas for improved performance related to patient care and the organization.

7. Advocates for needed patient services or resources, based on clearly communicating quantifiable, objective information.

8. Documents communications and clinical findings in the patient record per organizational requirements and standards that support quality, coverage, and reimbursement.

9. Acts as a positive role model or preceptor for therapy, nursing and other team members new to home or hospice home care.

10. Coordinates care with others involved in patient care (e.g., insurance company nurse, volunteer, home medical equipment or prosthetic or orthotic technician, and others).

11. Collaborates with all patients, family and team members, and otherwise provides services and activities needed to achieve patient and program goals.

The Case Manager's Roles as Supervisor and Educator

Administrative roles of the case manager are the supervisory and educational components. The home health aide team members look to the case manager for scheduling and providing supervisory visits and care direction, as well as ongoing education about the patient's needs and the care they provide. The following discussion addresses the home health aide's role and important contribution to patients and the care team in the Medicare home care program.

Home Health Aide Services: Making the Difference for Patients

If you have been practicing in home care for any length of time, you know that patients always say they will miss their aide the most upon discharge. Another way the aide's intrinsic value is expressed by patients and families is on the organization's patient satisfaction tools or surveys. More times than I can count the written narrative section reads something like this: "I loved my nurse, Sally. She helped me take a shower, helped wash my hair after my stroke when I couldn't use my right arm. She was also a great cook and prepared my special diabetes breakfasts three mornings a week. I still miss her." Sounds like a great comment for feedback to the nurse for her thoughtful care; only Sally is not a nurse, she is an aide.

The home health aide provides services to support the patient's treatment plan through assistance with personal care (e.g., assist with bathing), basic physiological monitoring (e.g., taking vital signs), and some services "incidental" to the personal care tasks (e.g., light cleaning, preparation of a meal, taking out the trash, shopping). The reason for the visits by the home health aide must be to provide hands-on personal care to the patient or services that are needed to maintain the patient's health or to facilitate treatment of the patient's illness or injury (e.g., the incidental services).

In cases where patients receive therapy and aide services, it is imperative that the patient's functional progress toward therapy goals be identified and communication with the aide be effective and on an ongoing basis. In such cases, the timely review and revision or updating of the aide care plan will enable the aide to provide a dynamic, but appropriate level of assistance to the patient, thus facilitating the achievement of maximum or optimal independent functioning. An example occurs when the OT is training the patient in tub transfers with bathing. The aide should then follow the OT's program, as taught to the patient, to support and empower the patient to be safe and independent and follow the plan of care. The aide's feedback to the therapist on patient follow-through also assists the therapist to determine appropriate direction and progression of the patient's goals.

It is particularly important that the therapist team members have an indepth knowledge of the home health aide's multifaceted roles, because as case manager the services of an aide could be helpful for patient safety, hygiene, and overall helping the patient achieve the agreed-upon goals. It goes without saying that therapists should review their particular state's regulation and practice acts to determine supervisory requirements, as they relate to the therapist's specific activities and timelines related to the supervision of home health aides.

Medicare and Home Health Aide Services

For home health aide services to be covered, the beneficiary must meet the qualifying criteria as specified in Section 204 of the *HHA Manual* (HCFA Pub-11), the services which are provided by the home health aide must be part-time or intermittent as discussed in Section 206.7 of the *HHA Manual* (HCFA Pub-11); the services must meet the definition of home health aide services, and the services must be reasonable and necessary to the treatment of the beneficiary's illness or injury. *The reason for the visits by the home health aide must be to provide hands-on personal care of the beneficiary or services which are needed to maintain the beneficiary's health or to facilitate treatment of the beneficiary's illness or injury.*

The physician orders should indicate the frequency of the home health aide services required by the beneficiary. These services may include but are not limited to:

- Personal care means bathing, dressing, grooming, caring for hair, nail and oral hygiene which are needed to facilitate treatment or to prevent deterioration of the beneficiary's health, changing the bed linens of an incontinent beneficiary, shaving, deodorant application, skin care with [non-medicated] lotions and/or powder, foot care, and ear care.
- Feeding, assistance with elimination (including enemas unless the skills of a licensed nurse are required due to the patient's condition, routine catheter care and routine colostomy care), assistance with ambulation, changing position in bed, assistance with transfers.
- Simple dressing changes which do not require the skills of a licensed nurse.
- Assistance with medications which are ordinarily self-administered and which do not require the skills of a licensed nurse to be provided safely and effectively. **(Author Note: This means that aides do not generally give or administer medications. They may, depending on state licensure and practice acts, remind or tell the patient what time it is or assist with child-proof medication lids when patients are unable to twist them open and request this assistance.)**

- Assistance with activities which are directly supportive of skilled therapy services but do not require the skills of a therapist to be safely and effectively performed such as routine maintenance exercises, assistance with ADL home programs as instructed by the therapist, and repetitive speech routines to support speech therapy.

When a home health aide visits a patient to provide a health related service as discussed above, the home health aide may also perform some incidental services which do not meet the definition of a home health aide service (e.g., light cleaning, preparation of a meal, taking out the trash, shopping). However, the purpose of a home health aide visit may not be to provide these incidental services since they are not health related services, but rather are necessary household tasks that must be performed by anyone to maintain a home. (Section 206.2, *HHA Manual* HCFA Pub-11).

For an indepth discussion on home health aide services and care planning readers are referred to the handbook *Home Health Aide: Guidelines for Care* (Marrelli, 1996) and its companion text for aide managers *Home Health Aide: Guidelines for Care Instructor Manual* (Marrelli, 1997).

Home Health Aide: Supervisory Visits: The Law

The Medicare law requires that if the patient receives skilled nursing care, the RN must perform the supervisory visit. If the patient is not receiving skilled nursing care, but is receiving another skilled service (e.g., PT, OT, or SLP) supervision may be provided by the appropriate therapist. The RN or therapist must make an on-site visit to the patient's home no less frequently than every two weeks.

Other Supervisory Activities

Nurse case managers may also supervise licensed vocational or practical nurses, similar to the therapist supervising the PTA or COTA team members. See the following "Supervisory Visit Note" Figure 1-16 for a documentation example to assist in maintaining compliance related to supervision. Many of these requirements, including the frequency of the supervision, how often on-site supervision must occur and other specific standards are directed by state practice acts or state law language.

Figure 1-16

SUPERVISORY VISIT NOTE

DATE OF VISIT ____/____/____

TIME IN _____ OUT _____

Phoenix Health Care Corporation/Americare of Oklahoma 1998

HOME HEALTH AIDE SUPERVISORY VISIT
Complete When HHA Supervisory Visit is
NOT Made in Conjunction With Another Skilled Visit

VISIT: ☐ Scheduled ☐ Unscheduled
AIDE: ☐ Present ☐ Not Present
TYPE: ☐ Routine ☐ Aide Assist Vs

If Present Skills Observed: ☐ Vital Signs ☐ Personal Care ☐ Elimination ☐ Activity Assist ☐ Nutrition ☐ Household
☐ Medication Reminder ☐ Infection Control ☐ Other _____

If Present Safety Observation:
Back support belt worn? ☐ Yes ☐ No If "no" explain: _____
Proper body mechanics demonstrated? ☐ Yes ☐ No If "no" explain: _____

Care Plan Present? ☐ Yes ☐ No   Care Plan Reviewed? ☐ Yes ☐ No   Care Plan Revised? ☐ Yes ☐ No
Care Rendered According to Plan? ☐ Yes ☐ No If "no" explain: _____

Add'l Teaching/Training Provided? ☐ Yes ☐ No
Describe:

Approx. date next SV ____/____/____
Plan: ☐ Continue HHA visits
☐ Decrease HHA to _____

Patient/client/caregiver satisfied with care? ☐ Yes ☐ No Comments: _____
☐ D/C HHA on _____

LICENSED NURSE SUPERVISORY VISIT
Complete for LPN Supervisory Visit

VISIT: ☐ Scheduled ☐ Unscheduled
LPN: ☐ Present ☐ Not Present
TYPE: ☐ Routine ☐ Other

If Present Skills Observed: ☐ Vital Signs ☐ Wound Care ☐ Diabetic Care ☐ Venipuncture ☐ Teaching ☐ Ostomy Care
☐ Medication Mgmt. ☐ Infection Control ☐ Respiratory Care ☐ IM Injection ☐ IV Care ☐ General Assessment
☐ Psychiatric Support ☐ Bowel/Bladder Care ☐ Other _____

If Present Safety Observed: Proper body mechanics demonstrated? ☐ Yes ☐ No If "no" explain:

Care Plan Present? ☐ Yes ☐ No   Care Plan Reviewed? ☐ Yes ☐ No   Care Plan Revised? ☐ Yes ☐ No
Care Rendered According to Plan? ☐ Yes ☐ No If "no" explain: _____

Add'l Teaching/Training Provided? ☐ Yes ☐ No
Describe:

Approx. date next SV ____/____/____
Plan: ☐ Continue SN visits
☐ Decrease SNV to _____

Patient/client/caregiver satisfied with care? ☐ Yes ☐ No Comments: _____
☐ D/C SNV on _____

OT – ST – PT – MSS ASSISTANT SUPERVISORY VISIT
Complete When OT, ST, PT, MSS Supervisory Visit is
NOT Made in Conjunction With Another Skilled Visit

If Present Describe Skills Observed: _____

VISIT: ☐ Scheduled ☐ Unscheduled
SV FOR: ☐ PTA ☐ OTA ☐ STA ☐ MSS
ASSISTANT ☐ Present ☐ Not Present
TYPE: ☐ Routine ☐ Other (describe)

If Present Safety Observed: Proper body mechanics demonstrated? ☐ Yes ☐ No If "no" explain:

Care Plan Present? ☐ Yes ☐ No   Care Plan Reviewed? ☐ Yes ☐ No   Care Plan Revised? ☐ Yes ☐ No
Care Rendered According to Plan? ☐ Yes ☐ No If "no" explain: _____

Add'l Teaching/Training Provided? ☐ Yes ☐ No
Describe:

Approx. date next SV ____/____/____
Plan: ☐ Continue with POT
☐ Other (describe) _____

Patient/client/caregiver satisfied with care? ☐ Yes ☐ No Comments: _____

HOMEMAKER – COMPANION - SITTER - SUPERVISORY VISIT
Complete for Homemaker, Companion, Sitter Other Non-Personal Care
Supervisory Visit

If Present Describe Service Observed: _____

VISIT: ☐ Scheduled ☐ Unscheduled
SV FOR: ☐ Homemaker ☐ Companion
☐ Sitter ☐ Other _____
STAFF ☐ Present ☐ Not Present
TYPE: ☐ Routine ☐ Other

If Present Safety Observed: Proper body mechanics demonstrated? ☐ Yes ☐ No If "no" explain:

Plan Of Service Present? ☐ Yes ☐ No   Plan Reviewed? ☐ Yes ☐ No   Plan Revised? ☐ Yes ☐ No
Care Rendered According to Service Plan? ☐ Yes ☐ No If "no" explain: _____

Add'l Teaching/Training Provided? ☐ Yes ☐ No Describe:

Patient/client/caregiver satisfied with service? ☐ Yes ☐ No Comments:

Approx. date next SV ____/____/____
Plan: ☐ Continue with Service Plan
☐ Other (describe) _____

SIGNATURE/TITLE/DATE OF INDIVIDUAL COMPLETING SUPERVISORY VISIT

_____
Nurse/Therapist/Social Worker Signature/ Title ☐ RN ☐ PT ☐ OT ☐ ST ☐ MSS   *Date*

PART 1 – Clinical Record   PART 2 – Care Manager

Patient/Client Name – Last, First   *Medical Record Number AND Unit Number*

Reprinted with permission from Phoenix Health Care Corporation/Americare of Oklahoma, 1998.

Team Communications and Care Coordination: Keys to Success

The litmus test of care coordination can be best described in the following scenario. If something would happen to one of your peer colleagues (e.g, if you are a SLP, a SLP, if an OT an OT, an RN an RN, etc.) and they had to visit your patients this morning (and with no verbal report!) would your clinical documentation tell the story of your patient? Does it list the information about the caregivers and other team members who also visit, have an accurate and up-to-date medication list, say exactly what the current plan of care is and numerous other details that comprise effective documentation and clearly communicate the needs of the patient? In cases where patients receive aide services, the patient's functional progress directed toward therapy must be identified and effectively communicated to the aide(s) on an ongoing basis. What is the mechanism at your organization to facilitate this process? It is easy to see that the provision of quality home care is hinged upon care coordination activities and the associated documentation that reflects these efforts.

The documentation must be able to tell any reviewer, peer, or state or accreditation surveyor the exact details of the care for each particular patient. This is much easier said than done. If you have ever been in the scenario where a colleague needed emergency surgery or had to leave town unexpectedly and it was hard to determine the patient's specific ordered visit frequency, the exact repetitions in the home rehab program delegated to the aide (and who the specific aide to be supervised that day was), you have been in that uncomfortable position. Chart in your patient's clinical records with the thought that other team members do not have the base of knowledge that you have from actually being there and providing care to patients. Write all the information that provides for the best continuity and care coordination across and among the team.

Examples of Effective Care Coordination

- Calling the case manager and updating him/her on the patient's progress and your findings
- Attending interdisciplinary team meetings
- Calling the physician and updating him/her on your findings/concerns
- Validating that the patient understands the discharge instructions by being able to list the taught actions for self-care
- Planning a joint visit with another team member (eg., nurse, aide, other therapist or assistant)
- Calling in report on the aide or nurse's voice mail after the therapy visit to update the team members on the patient's progress and documenting this call

- Communications with patients, family members, and caregivers
- Documenting all of the above types of communications, as well as other phone calls, meetings, and communications related to your patient's care
- Others, as numerous as the creativity of the team to facilitate this important component of quality home care

Summary

Patient care planning and related processes are the nuts and bolts of the provision of home care services. The knowledge base of the first three domains all come together into a practical plan for patient care that will most effectively assist in achievement of desired patient outcomes.

One way to assist in facilitating outcomes is the model of case management and the case manager role. Case management will be the emerging role in the changing vision of home care practice for the future.

PART TWO
Specialty Therapy Practices

Pediatrics and Therapy:
Making A Difference in Young Lives

Specialized care of infants and children continues to be an area of growth in home care. Neonatal intensive care (NICU) preemies, children after trauma with head injuries or extensive rehabilitation needs, developmentally challenged children and those with life-limiting cancers are some of the children cared for in this rewarding home care therapy specialty.

One of the best parts of a pediatric-focused practice and organization is the emphasis on the parents, siblings and other primary caregivers in the provision of family-system based care. This chapter presents an overview of the specialization and unique competencies needed by therapists and nurses caring for young patients with various rehabilitation needs.

Children Seen in Home Care Therapy Practice

The infants and children cared for by therapists in home care have a wide range of diagnoses and problems and may include those with cerebral palsy, torticollis, failure-to-thrive, communication problems, and developmental delays. As important as direct treatment is the information provided to the parents or caregivers about resources available. Information about equipment and other aids to support mobility and optimal function as well as management of contractures and deformities, and other supportive services may also need to be provided.

ICD-9 Codes For Pediatric Therapy

The following is a list of some of the most common therapy-related problems seen by home care therapists. This list is not all-inclusive, but is intended as a helpful reference site for clinicians as they seek common codes to correctly identify and code specific patient problems. Readers are referred to coding experts or their regional home health intermediary for specific coding questions or concerns related to accurate coding documentation.

Anoxia	799.0
Arthritis, juvenile rheumatoid	714.30

Asthma	439.90
Astrocytoma	191.9
Bone marrow transplant	41.00
Bronchiolitis	466.19
Cerebral palsy	343.9
Cerebral vascular accident	436
Chronic myelogenous leukemia	205.10
Chronic obstructive pulmonary disease	496
Chronic respiratory disease	770.7
Cleft lip	749.10
Cleft palate	749.00
Congenital heart disease	428.1
Cystic Fibrosis	277.00
Developmental disorder	315.9
Down's syndrome	758.0
Encephalitis	323.9
Ewing's sarcoma	170.9
Failure to thrive	783.4
Guillain-Barre Syndrome	357.0
Heart failure	428.9
Immaturity, extreme	765.00
Juvenile rheumatoid arthritis	714.30
Leukemia	
Acute lymphoblastic leukemia	204.00
Acute myelogenous leukemia	205.00
Chronic myelogenous leukemia	205.10
Medulloblastoma	191.6
Mental retardation	319
Meningitis	322.9
Muscular dystrophy	359.1
Neuroblastoma	194.0
Normal development, lack of	783.4
Osteosarcoma	170.9
Preterm infant	765.10
Respiratory problems, post birth	770.8
Retinoblastoma	190.5
Rhabdomyosarcoma	171.9
Rheumatoid arthritis, juvenile	714.30
Scoliosis, infantile	737.31

Seizure disorder	780.3
Sickle cell anemia	282.60
Sickle cell crisis	282.62
Sickle cell trait	282.5
Spina bifida	741.90
Spinal cord injury	952.9
Torticollis, congenital	754.1
Torticollis, due to birth injury	767.8
Torticollis, traumatic current	847.0
Trachea/bronchus	519.1
Tracheal stenosis	519.1
Tracheomalacia	519.1
Tracheostomy, attention to	V55.0
Wilms' tumor	189.0
Ventilator, dependence on	V46.1

Infection Control and Safety in Children: The Drool Factor

Kids are oral and they gum, drool and suck on anything, as do their sick or well siblings. For these reasons, infection control is more important than ever when caring for sick children and their families. Toys, plastic kitchen containers, or whatever else is used therapeutically with children receiving treatment must be cleaned on an ongoing basis. Organizations have varying policies for this important infection control activity. The following, Figures 2-1 and 2-2 are for review. They are an infection control policy with a corresponding log that tracks toys used by therapists and the dates of cleaning and disinfection.

Children are Different: 12 Tips for Success

The following are some of the areas in which rehabilitation team members must be aware and proficient when caring for pediatric patients and their families.

1. The work of children is play. For this reason, toys are often used in intervention directed toward achievement of milestones or identified rehabilitation goals. *The Magic Years by Fraiberg* is a very readable and helpful book for all team members who work with children. This book and other resources related to pediatric therapy are listed at the end of the book, in Part Ten in the "Directory of Resources" under the header of "Pediatrics."

Figure 2-1

HOME HEALTH AND HOSPICE
WHIDDEN MEMORIAL HOSPITAL
POLICY MANUAL

POLICY: Equipment Cleaning Policy

SCOPE: All equipment belonging to the agency be properly cleansed between patients.

OBJECTIVE: To ensure any equipment, especially toys, are cleaned between uses.

PROCEDURE:

1. Equipment owned by the agency and used for patient care, teaching or assessment must be returned to the agency and cleaned between patients.

2. The cleaner wears gloves while washing/cleaning the equipment/toys. Handwashing is done per agency policy.

3. Integrity of equipment is checked and inspected for proper working order and cleanliness before being distributed to patients by clinicians.

4. Equipment can be left on the table in the women's rest room in the agency, toys can be left in the blue plastic bin.

5. The equipment is cleaned by the cooperative student assigned to in-patient Rehab Services. The Rehab secretary may be utilized as backup, if needed.

6. The equipment is cleaned with a solution per organization policy and rinsed with water.

7. The equipment cleaning is noted as completed with the date and initials of the cleaner in the notebook hanging from the door.

8. Each cleaned item is tagged and returned to the rehab closet.

Reprinted with permission from Whidden Memorial Hospital, Hallmark Health Home Care, Everett, Massachusetts, 1995.

Figure 2-2   HOME HEALTH & HOSPICE CARE
WHIDDEN MEMORIAL HOSPITAL

EQUIPMENT CLEANING LOG PEDIATRIC PROGRAM

DATE	THERAPIST'S INITIALS	EQUIPMENT

Reprinted with permission from Whidden Memorial Hospital, Hallmark Health Home Care, Everett, Massachusetts, 1995.

2. The parents may be working through or processing their own grief and the presence of a nurse or therapist heightens the fact that they have a child with specialized needs. Clinicians will be more successful if they can work therapeutically with the parent or other primary caregiver. The parent may need to have the therapist be a caring listener and someone they trust to facilitate their child meeting certain milestones. The therapist can also be the health professional who can make medical jargon that the parent may have heard at the last doctor appointment "make sense" from their parental perspective. All of these roles are very important.

3. The goals don't change as frequently as for adult patients. In fact, progress itself toward goals occurs at a much slower pace. Pediatric goals usually need to be measured or reassessed approximately every two months. The progress may be slow, but may be measured or quantified with a percentage of success, such as "child transfers from sitting to standing from chair with one arm support 50% of trials" or gains noted in function such as "child stands for 30 seconds versus 15 seconds at last assessment." The goals themselves may be very small and the effectiveness may be apparent only (especially initially) to the mother or other direct caregivers. "Baby steps" are realistic when defining goals and interventions in effective pediatric therapy practice.

4. The parent, oftentimes the mother, may be the case manager. This is a significant change from the historical role of the clinician "expert" as the case manager. The mother, father, or other caregiver knows the most about their particular child's moods, changes, communications and other small facets that only they can identify. This ongoing assessment and reporting of identified changes to the therapists or nurses is key to the best home or hospice care for the entire family system.

Parent teaching is also an important component of quality pediatric therapy. The learning needs assessment, baseline knowledge, and parental readiness to learn and absorb information must all be addressed. At the same time, the parent may not be on the same "timeline" as the payer and therapist, and must be motivated to learn new skills or behaviors as identified by the treatment plan.

Parents who have been in the case management role may also be overwhelmed or "burned out" with the ongoing communication, scheduling and associated care coordination responsibilities while also trying to care for and nurture their special child. There may also be other children in the household who need these same parenting skills and time commitment. The therapist and nurse can play key roles in identifying this stressful state and perhaps providing respite from this sometimes overwhelming role by assuming or assisting with the case manager role.

5. The team approach is essential to the child's care. The therapist and the parent may co-case manage, again based on the situation, the parents, and their capabilities. This interdisciplinary team will bring together all team members in common efforts directed toward achievement of developmental milestones or other agreed-upon and clearly defined goals.

6. Age-appropriate considerations, interventions and even toys are key to success for both therapists and families. It goes without saying that whether caring for infants, toddlers, school-aged children, or adolescents, the tasks and milestones of childhood must be second-nature and measured as a standard part of holistic quality therapy practice. This includes a knowledge of the developmental milestones, such as those measured through tools such as the Denver Developmental Screening Test (DDST) and others. The following Figure 2-3 entitled "Developmental Competencies Reference Sheet" identifies these reference points through chronological age.

Besides the child being cared for with age-appropriate considerations, we must also review the parental situation. For example, it is not unusual for a developmentally delayed infant in our care to have parents who are teenagers themselves. These teenage parents are also working from their own framework and the interventions, care plan, and educational initiatives must consider this information as the teenage parents confront the situation and work toward successfully meeting the special needs of their child. The therapists and their communications can be key to facilitating the achievement of patient goals. The interactions noted between the child and parents or caregiver are also an important part of the pediatric assessment. Figure 2-4 "Items to be Considered When Assessing Pediatric Patients" lists these components.

7. The organization should have specific forms or documentation tools that are used just for the specialized pediatric patient population. For example, the information collected about an infant would be different from that of the school-age child and that of the teenager. Some forms address the very different stages and the corresponding developmental tasks and milestone achievements and are very useful in measuring progress and identifying the achievement of agreed-upon and realistic outcomes. Examples of pediatric therapy visit reports for PT, SLP, OT, and Figures 2-5, 2-6, and 2-7 respectively follow for review.

Figure 2-3   Developmental Competencies Reference Sheet

1 to 2 MONTHS
Able to be comforted
Tracks face and past midline
Social smiling
Brief periods of eye contact
Responds to voice or sounds
Head-righting reaction
Hands mostly fisted or partially open (hand grasp)
Head lag (pull to sit)
Movements symmetrical
Placing reaction
Nasal cry
Sucking/swallowing
Rooting reflex
Bite reflex
Toe grasp
Pick head up to clear face in prone

3 TO 4 MONTHS
Coos, gurgles, and squeals
Vocal babbling
Sits supported
Slight effort at head control
Head in midline
Flexor control in neck (pull to sit)
Chest up with forearm support in prone
Bears weight on legs
Hands predominately open
Arms come to midline
Regards hands and feet
Responds to parent's smile and talk
Listens to voices
Looks for sound source
Simultaneous vocalizing with parent
Vocal play
Beginning to form constant sounds
Repeats actions
Rhythmic sucking with lip closure
Stops sucking to listen
Looks and sucks at the same time
Smiles spontaneously
Expressive alternatives with face
Swipes at objects
Attempt to touch objects offered
Tracks objects 90 or more
Watches place where moving object disappears
Eyes start to converge
May have asymmetrical tonic neck reflex (ATNR)
May have toe grasp

5 TO 6 MONTHS
Integrated
Moro reflex
ATNR
Symmetrical tonic neck reflex (STNR)
Grasp reflex
Rooting reflex
No head lag in pull to sit
Sits momentarily leaning on hands
Rolls prone to supine
Rolls supine to prone
Head and chest raise to 90 with forearm support in prone
Uses ulnar palmer prehension
May use radial palmer prehension (thumb and two fingers)

Uses bilateral hand movements
Plays with feet and toes
Smiles at image in mirror
Reaches to familiar people
Exhibits differentiated crying/vocalizes emotion
Repeats action in play
Uses hands and mouth for sensory exploration of objects
Sucks and swallows pureed foods from spoon
Coordinates sucking, swallowing, and breathing

7 TO 8 MONTHS
Parachute reaction
Prone and supine equilibrium reactions
Lateral head righting (emerging equilibrium reaction)
Sits unsupported for up to 60 seconds
Protective extension to the sides
Integration of neck righting (body rotates as a whole) and emerging body on body rotation (segmental rotation)
Legs in extension in pull to sit
Easily pulls to stand
May pull self to stand
Stands with support
Will pivot in prone
May crawl (backward and then forward)
Transfers object from hand to hand
Reaches for objects with open hand
Uses inferior pincer grasp with raisin
Complete thumb opposition with block
Retains two of three objects offered
Thumb out of palm in prone weight-bearing
Takes textured food from a spoon
Gums and swallows
Holds bottle to drink
Drinks from cup (sip) with help
Begins finger feeding
Plays with toy 2 to 3 minutes
Finds hidden object
Looks for family members/pets when name is called
Responds to own name
Waves bye-bye
Babbles with inflections similar to adult speech
Forms bisyllabic repetitions (ma-ma, da-da)
Shows anxiety over separation from mother/father/caregiver
Laughs at pattycake and peekaboo games
Pats and touches mirror image
Sleeps through the night

9 TO 11 MONTHS
Assumes quadruped position from prone, supine, or sitting
Creeps
Sits alone and steady 10 minutes
All sitting equilibrium reactions
Protective extension to the rear
Pivots in sitting to pick up objects
Pulls to standing using furniture
May cruise by holding on to furniture

Lowers self to floor by fall
Pokes with isolated index finger
Uses neat pincer grasp with raisin
Takes object out of container
Bangs two cubes (objects) together
Removes pegs from a board
Responds to simple verbal request
Waves or claps when only verbal (not visual) cue is given
Pulls string to secure ring and succeeds
Imperfectly imitates sounds and movements never performed before
Understand and reacts to "no"
Enjoys looking at pictures in books
Participates in pattycake and peekaboo games
Repeats vocalizations and activities when laughed at
Offers but does not release
Explores environment
Holds, bites, and chews cookie
Holds spoon
Drinks from regular cup held for him

12 TO 14 MONTHS
Sits independently for extended period of time
Attains sitting position independently
Walks by self or with one hand held
Creeps up stairs (based on home environment)
Gets down from standing
Squats and stoops in play
Sideways walking
Builds two- or three-cube tower
Places one or two pegs in pegboard
Scribbles spontaneously (no demonstration) with crayon
Points with index finger
Imitates words inexactly
Uses two or three words meaningfully
Uses gestures and points to communicate
Names one or two familiar objects
Follows two-word commands
Helps dress self (extending arm or leg)
Removes hat and socks
Indicates discomfort over soiled diaper verbally or with gestures
Repeatedly finds toy when hidden under one of several covers
Puts eight 1-inch cubes in a coffee cup
Inverts container to find tiny object
Uses simple problem-solving skills
Shows affection
Displays tantrums
Eats three meals a day
Attempts to use spoon to feed self
Picks up and drinks from a cup (some spilling)
Initiates ball playing or social games
Offers and releases toy to adult

15 to 19 MONTHS
Runs stiffly
Walks up stairs held by one hand (no rail)
Creeps backward down stairs

Figure 2-3 (cont'd)

Standing, seats self in small chair
Climbs into adult size chair, turns, and sits
All equilibrium reactions in standing
Walks backward and sideward
Balances on one foot with assist
Throws ball overhand/attempts to kick ball
Pushes and pulls large toys around floor
Moves on ride on toys without pedals

20 to 23 MONTHS
Walks downstairs with one hand held
Walks upstairs stair to stair holding railing
Squats in play resumes standing position
Does not fall over picking up toy
Walks independently on 8-inch board
Walks a few steps with one foot on 2-inch balance beam
Throws ball overhand landing within at least 3 feet of target (large box)
Runs fairly well
Jumps in place both feet
Stands from supine by rolling to side

24 to 29 MONTHS
Significant decrease in base of support when walking on level surfaces
Catches large ball
Rides tricycle
Imitates simple bilateral movements of limbs head and trunk
Walks upstairs alone, stair to stair
Walks downstairs holding rail, stair to stair
Goes up and down slide

Jumps a distance of 8 inches
Jumps from bottom step
Runs, stops without holding or falling, avoids obstacles
Walks on line in general direction
Walks between parallel lines 8 inches apart
Stands on 2-inch balance beam with both feet
Attempts step on beam
Jumps backward
Walks on tip toes a few steps
Able to stand on one foot briefly

30 to 36 MONTHS
Walks backward at least 10 feet
Jumps sideward
Walks upstairs alone alternating feet
Walks downstairs alone, stair to stair
Walks downstairs alternating feet (34 m)
Jumps over string 2- to 8-inches high
Hops on one foot
Stands on one foot up to 5 seconds
Walks on tip toes 10 feet
Stands from supine using a sit up
Jumps a distance of at least 14 inches
Keeps feet on line for 10 feet
Uses pedals on tricycle alternately
Climbs jungle gyms and ladders
Catches 8-inch ball
Avoids obstacles in path
Able to run on toes
Makes sharp turns around corners when running

PRESCHOOLERS (AGE 3 TO 5 YEARS)
Self help
Eating and drinking
Toileting
Grooming
Dressing/undressing
Oral and nasal hygiene
Self identification

Motor development
Sensory perception
Fine motor
Gross motor
Child in wheelchair
Mobility aids needed

Communication
Auditory perception
Language comprehension
Language expressive
Alternative communication needs

Social Skills
Adaptive behaviors
Responsible behaviors
Interpersonal relationships
Personal welfare
Social manners

Learning/Cognitive
Attention span
Basic reading
Math
Writing skills
Reasoning skills

Figure 2-4   Items to Be Considered When Assessing Pediatric Patients

HISTORY
Behavior (Social/Emotional)
Mental status
Crying
Eye contact
Smile

Appearance/Structural Deformities/Muscle Length
Flaring of ribs
Head size/shape
Bone deformities
Coloring

Postural Control/Alignment
Symmetry/asymmetry
Sitting posture
Head control in all positions/planes

Muscle Tone
At rest
With effort
Associated reactions
Clonus
Tremors

Evoked Responses
Righting reactions
Equilibrium (tilting) responses
Protective (parachute) reactions

PRIMITIVE REFLEXES
Motor Skills
In assessing motor development look for movement patterns, synergy, dissociation, uncoordination, symmetry versus asymmetry, and establish an age level at which the patient is functioning.

Gross motor
Fine motor
Oral motor

Response to Sensory Input
Visual (tracking)
Auditory
Handling

ANY OTHER NOTEWORTHY ITEMS
Parents/care givers interaction with child
Appropriateness of toys
Medical response to therapy or positions
Mobility devices used

Figures 2-3 and 2-4. *Reprinted with permission from Carr, M. ed.,* **Community Home Health Report***, 33:4, 1998.*

Figure 2-5

HOME HEALTH AND HOSPICE of WHIDDEN MEMORIAL HOSPITAL
PHYSICAL THERAPY VISIT REPORT — PEDIATRIC

NAME: _____   ID # _____   DATE: _____

Record Activities Performed, Assist Needed, and Measurements:
Check mark indicates activity performed by therapist.

___ EVALUATION

___ THERAPEUTIC ROM EX:
___ P   ___ Stretching   ___ AA   ___ A

___ THERAPEUTIC STRENGTHENING EX:
___ AA   ___ A   ___ Resistive
___ Pre   ___ Muscle Re-Education

___ ENDURANCE TRAINING

___ DEVELOPMENT-GROSS MOTOR: ___ Developmental Sequence
___ Inhib-Relax   ___ Facilitation   ___ Coordination

___ CHEST PT

___ POSTURAL TRAINING

___ BALANCE ACTIVITIES:
___ Sit   ___ Stand   ___ Ambulation

___ TRANSFER TRAINING:
___ Supine to Sit   ___ Sit to Stand   ___ Sit to Supine
___ Side-Side   ___ Side-Sit   ___ Prone-Supine
___ Side-Supine

___ MOBILITY TRAINING:
___ Bed   ___ Floor   ___ W/C   ___ Other

___ GAIT TRAINING: ___ Device   ___ Assist
___ Level   ___ Uneven   ___ Stairs

___ MODALITY:
___ U.S.   ___ Ice   ___ E-Stim

___ EQUIPMENT:
___ Consult   ___ Train   ___ Adapt
___ Positioning   ___ Orthotic   ___ Prosthetic
___ Mobility   ___ Bath   ___ Other

___ SAFETY

___ PATIENT/CAREGIVER EDUCATION:
___ Return Demonstration

___ HHA INSTRUCTION/SUPERVISION:
___ Return Demonstration

___ CARE PLAN REVIEW

___ FREQUENCY OF VISITS: Duration _____
HAEIP _____

___ OTHER:

SIGNATURE: _____   DATE: _____

NARRATIVE:
Clinical Finding ___
Change Orders ___

See Addendum ___

Care Plan:
Reviewed ___ Revised ___
Prob.#s addressed _____

Reprinted with permission from Whidden Memorial Hospital, Hallmark Health Home Care, Everett, Massachusetts, 1995.

Figure 2-6

HOME HEALTH AND HOSPICE of WHIDDEN MEMORIAL HOSPITAL
SPEECH/LANGUAGE THERAPY VISIT REPORT — PEDIATRIC

NAME: _____ ID # _____ DATE: _____

Record Activities Performed, Assist Needed, and Measurements:
Check mark indicates activity performed by therapist.

___ EVALUATION

___ PRE-LANGUAGE/COGNITION:
  ___ Respond to Sound   ___ Tracking Level
  ___ Object Permanence   ___ Cause & Effect
  ___ Participate in Play   ___ Symbolic
    ___ Representational   ___ Cooperative
  ___ Object Use
  ___ Other:

___ RECEPTIVE LANGUAGE:
  ___ Single Word   ___ Sentence Level
  ___ Follow Directions   ___ Simple   ___ Complex
  ___ Body Part Identification
  ___ Respond to Questions   ___ Yes/No   ___ WH
  ___ Concept Development   ___ Other:

___ EXPRESSIVE LANGUAGE:
  ___ Babbling   ___ Reciprocal Vocal Play
  ___ Vocabulary Development
  ___ Production: ___ Words ___ Phrases
    ___ Sentences
  ___ Syntax   ___ Sign Language
  ___ Other:

___ ORAL MOTOR:
  ___ Stimulation   ___ Mobility
  ___ Dysphagia
  ___ Other:

___ ARTICULATION:
  ___ Sound Production:
    ___ Syllable   ___ Word   ___ Sentence
  ___ Rate:
  ___ Other:

___ FLUENCY:

___ PATIENT/FAMILY EDUCATION:

___ FREQUENCY OF VISITS:

___ OTHER: Duration _____
    HAEIP _____

SIGNATURE: _____ DATE: _____

NARRATIVE:
Clinical Finding ___
Change Orders ___

See Addendum ___

Care Plan:
Reviewed ___ Revised ___
Prob.#s addressed _____

Reprinted with permission from Whidden Memorial Hospital, Hallmark Health Home Care, Everett, Massachusetts, 1995.

Figure 2-7

HOME HEALTH AND HOSPICE of WHIDDEN MEMORIAL HOSPITAL
OCCUPATIONAL THERAPY VISIT REPORT — PEDIATRIC

NAME: _____ ID # _____ DATE: _____

Record Activities Performed, Assist Needed, and Measurements:
Check mark indicates activity performed by therapist.

___ EVALUATION
___ COGNITIVE ACTIVITIES:
   ___ Object Permanence   ___ Attending to Task
   ___ Cause and Effect   ___ Following Commands
   ___ Imitation   ___ Other

___ PERCEPTUAL ACTIVITIES:
   ___ Eye Control Fixation   ___ Depth Perception
   ___ Visual Pursuits   ___ Form Perception
   ___ Body Scheme   ___ Part/Whole Concepts
   ___ Bilateral Integration   ___ Spacial Relations
   ___ Figure Ground   ___ Color Concepts
   ___ Other

___ DEVELOPMENTAL - GROSS MOTOR:
   ___ Inhib-Relax   ___ Facilitation   ___ Coordination

___ POSTURAL TRAINING

___ BALANCE ACTIVITIES:
   ___ Sit   ___ Stand   ___

___ THER. ROM EX:
   ___ P   ___ Stretching   ___ AA   ___ A

___ THER. STRENGTHENING EX:
   ___ AA   ___ A   ___ Resistive   ___ PRE
   ___ Muscle Re-education

___ SELF-HELP ACTIVITIES:
   ___ Feeding   ___ Dressing/Undressing   ___ Other

___ SENSORIMOTOR:
   ___ Tactile   ___ Vestibular   ___ Proprioceptive
   ___ Kinesthesis

___ EQUIPMENT:
   ___ Consult   ___ Train   ___ Adapt
   ___ Positioning   ___ Orthotic   ___ Prosthetic
   ___ Mobility   ___ Bath   ___ Other

___ PATIENT/CAREGIVER EDUCATION:
   ___ Return Demonstration

___ HHA INSTRUCTION/SUPERVISION:
   ___ Return Demonstration

___ CARE PLAN REVIEW:

___ FREQUENCY OF VISITS: Duration _____
                        HAEIP _____

___ OTHER:

SIGNATURE: _____ DATE: _____

NARRATIVE:
Clinical Finding ___
Change Orders ___

See Addendum ___

Care Plan:
Reviewed ___ Revised ___
Prob.#s addressed _____

Reprinted with permission from Whidden Memorial Hospital, Hallmark Health Home Care, Everett, Massachusetts, 1995.

8. A specialized orientation and competency assessment identifying tasks and interventions directed to caring for children with special needs is a hallmark of quality. The competencies may include family systems theory, varying tools to monitor developmental progress (such as the DDST), care coordination with parent case managers and other team members, infection control with toys used in therapy intervention and many others.

9. Boundary and co-dependency issues may emerge in pediatric practice as we strive to care for children with complex needs in sometimes compromised settings and circumstances. It may be very frustrating to realize that sometimes we can only impact to the extent that is appropriate for a given patient problem. It is very easy to get very attached to these special children and see our role as more comprehensive and important than it can be from a longer-term perspective. This can be particularly difficult given problematic family systems and challenging interactions and (mis)communications that may occur among family members. Also difficult are the unusual home settings that do not facilitate what we consider the best or optimal care and dismal economic situations that are outside the professional purview of our roles. In these situations, or in situations of possible neglect or abuse, it is important that we involve the physician, the social worker and appropriate authorities in the community to effectively follow-up and address problems that adversely impact the plan of care and ensure the child's safety.

10. In the care cycle, the child is evaluated by the therapist, a specialized care plan is developed, detailed baseline findings are documented and the plan is reevaluated, based on the child's process and the organization's policies related to the provision of specialized high quality pediatric care. The care cycle itself may be long in some of these children as it may take months before appreciable change can be measured or objectively quantified since the last assessment or evaluation. It is also important to note that even though a child may benefit from ongoing service the payer or payment source may not want to pay for this continued care. The clinicians and organizations may need to identify other ways to facilitate goal achievement with the home program. Considerations include working collaboratively with other team members to continue the treatment program, and referrals to outside agencies or other community resources.

11. An empathic understanding of the longterm impact of having an ill child has an effect on the entire family system. The mother may sorely need a break from her responsibilities and this information may not be communicated in a clear manner. A classic example is when the sibling of the sick

child has a cold and the mother has to take that child to the pediatrician and forgets to call the therapists to reschedule visits. The compassionate skill of "patience" is perhaps why we call our patients that!

12. Safety in the home environment is an important component of the assessment and is reviewed during ongoing visits. Most organizations have their own safety assessment tool, but common concerns to be included are that the area be free from common hazards (e.g., poisons, paint chips, chemicals, stairs, electrical outlets, ferocious pets, availability of utilities, fire safety, child safety seats, where to ride in the car) and numerous others.

Summary

Caring for children with special care needs and their families is emerging as an important specialized component of home care and hospice practice. It goes without saying that children do better at home and development is promoted in the familiarity and comfort of the child's home environment. The therapist as care coordinator and case manager can assist patients and families in achieving growth and development or other therapeutic goals. The family-centered care provided and plan developed can make all the difference to these special children in attaining optimal function and development. Effective collaboration with other team members and family members, age appropriate communication with the child and an overall enjoyment of children are all ingredients to being successful in home care pediatric therapy practice.

Specialty Therapy Practices

Home Hospice Care and the Therapist:
Efforts Directed Toward Comfort and Safety

We only have to pick up the newspaper or watch television to see issues related to the general dissatisfaction with end-of-life care in our "medicalized" model of death in the U.S. Compassionate, skillful, holistic care for dying patients and their family members needs to be a goal of all health care providers. Home care and hospice organizations provide much of this care in the privacy of the patient's and family's home.

Hospice Care: An Introduction

Hospice is a holistic philosophy of care that transcends care sites. This means that hospice services can be provided at home, in the hospital, in a nursing home, or in another setting of the patient and family's choosing. The basic tenets of hospice include focusing on the quality of life, patients and families are the unit of care (instead of only the patient in traditional medical models), symptom and pain relief are the specialties of hospice with the intent of making every day the best it can be for patients and their loved ones (how we should all live every day), and hospice seeks not to extend life nor hasten or postpone death. Hospice then affirms life and sees dying as a natural, normal process. With these fundamentals in mind, patients and families choose hospice as a life-affirming array of services that traditionally are not found in other care models.

Services that hospice provides and patients and families receive include: medically-directed care, nursing, medical social services, dietary counseling services, therapy, aide, homemaker services as well as spiritual and psychosocial support and bereavement services for the patient's loved ones and other survivors.

The services are truly interdisciplinary and the patient's physician is a key member of the team. Care plan development, coordination and implementation is achieved through ongoing communication among the interdisciplinary team or group (IDT or IDG). In addition, referrals to hospice can be initiated by anyone (not just physicians). Medicare and other hospice insurance programs also cover medications, medical equipment and supplies related to the life-limiting illness, any related hospitalizations, respite if needed and other organized benefits of a holistic comprehensive package of services created to assist patients through this final phase of physical life while supporting family members. One of the most special aspects of hospice support are the cadre of specially-trained volunteers, who are often referred to as "the heart of hospice." These caregivers provide multifaceted and important duties and these roles are as varied as the patients and families served by the hospice. They may provide personal care, transportation to doctor office visits, be an accessible and nonjudgmental sounding board for patients and families, and provide numerous other activities and tasks that are valued for the more compassionate aspects of the best caring.

Still other services and fundamentals provided by hospice include education for the patient and especially the caregivers on what to expect and how to cope during this stressful time, 24-hour accessibility to hospice team members for visits or phone intervention and support, access to inpatient services should the patient's symptoms be distressing or difficult to manage at home, and other services, such as music, art, pet, or massage therapy, again depending on the hospice and its own philosophy and the specific services offered.

One of the more creative aspects of the Medicare hospice benefit (for an insurance benefit) is that the patients do not have to be "homebound," a major qualifying criteria for Medicare home health agency patients as discussed in Part One. Hospices may have specialty areas, such as pediatrics, end-stage cardiac supportive care or others, but whatever the model and the hospice, patients and their family members are encouraged to make all decisions (e.g., such as continuing to work, travel to a certain location before death, or other wishes) and have input into the plan and the actual care.

Why (or Why Not) Hospice

Many of us have cared for patients who were dying and were in the Medicare home health agency program and not receiving hospice care. It is important to note that not all patients choose or "elect" the Medicare hospice benefit, as it is required that patients elect to "give up" their regular Medicare benefit and the Medicare-certified hospice becomes the true case manager. This means that the hospice oversees the entire plan of care, including care sites, and coordinates any needed care across and among care settings and providers. Also the patient may wish to continue aggressive and (hopefully) still available curative treatment options.

The following patient example and Figure 2-8 seeks to explain some of the similarities and differences from the patient/family and clinician's perspectives. It is important that patients should have the final say in the choice of which program they are provided care through; be it the home health agency or the Medicare certified hospice.

Mr. Walker - A Patient Example

Mr. Walker is a 67-year-old man with an advanced prostate cancer. As you assess his rehabilitation needs and speak with Mr. Walker and his wife, you learn that this cancer is thought to be a reoccurrence as he reports he had surgery for cancer of the prostate six years ago. His wife reports that the doctor thought at some point they may want "hospice support" but they are not sure what that really means or if they want it. "Maybe we should continue with these treatments; the doctor says sometimes they kick in." Mr. Walker moves very slowly, is frail, and needs a cane and the support of his wife to walk. Mr. Walker also clearly states that he is on a new pain medication regimen. Mr. Walker could be either a home care patient or hospice patient sometime in his course of care and illness. What are the differences and similarities? The intersection of the "common" areas of intervention and care are shown in the intersection of the two circles below.

Figure 2-8   Dually-Certified Organizations Providing End-Of-Life Care

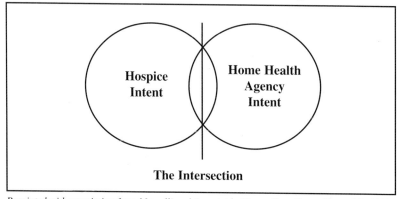

*Reprinted with permission from Marrelli and Associates, **Home Care Nurse News,** 6:3, 1999.*

According to data from the 1996 National Home and Hospice Care survey published by the by the National Center for Health Statistics, and displayed below in Figure 2-9, it is shown that 48.9% of organizations providing services to patients are dually-certified as both hospice and home care agencies. Because this data is from the 1996 National Home and Hospice Care survey we may be able to reasonably estimate that this number has increased since 1996. From an organizational and patient/family perspective, the dually-certified programs may be able to offer a seamless continuum of care, without patients and families "switching" or losing the known care provider. This model then shows a model of the intersection of patients being cared for by those organizations who are dually-certified, and who can provide either (or both at different times in the patient's care continuum) home health or hospice services to patients with life-limiting illnesses.

**Figure 2-9   Percent of Agencies Providing Hospice Care
by Type of Certification: United States, 1996**

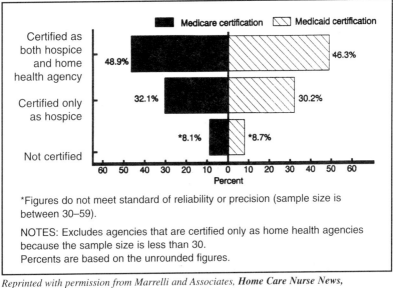

*Figures do not meet standard of reliability or precision (sample size is between 30–59).

NOTES: Excludes agencies that are certified only as home health agencies because the sample size is less than 30.
Percents are based on the unrounded figures.

Reprinted with permission from Marrelli and Associates, **Home Care Nurse News,**
Volume 5, No. 11, 1998.

Differences: A Review of the Intents of the Programs and Definitions

It is important for Medicare cost reporting and other compliance reasons that a differentiation be made throughout the admission process, and that patient and family choice and the intent of these two Medicare programs be reviewed by all involved in making this decision. The Medicare *State Operations Manual* (SOM) Section 2080 states that "hospice care is an approach to caring for terminally ill individuals that stresses palliative care (relief of pain and uncomfortable symptoms), as opposed to curative care. In addition to meeting the patient's medical needs, hospice care addresses the physical, psychosocial, and spiritual needs of the patient, as well as the psychosocial needs of the patient's family/caregiver. The emphasis of the hospice program is on keeping the hospice patient at home with family and friends as long as possible." *The Home Health Agency(HHA) Manual* (HCFA Pub.-11) in Section 200 states: "A home health agency (HHA) is a public agency or private organization that ... is primarily engaged in providing skilled nursing services and other therapeutic services, such as physical therapy (PT), speech-language pathology (SLP) services, or occupational therapy (OT), medical social services (MSS), and home health aide (HHA) services. Figure 2-10, "A Comparison of the Medicare Home Health Benefit and Hospice Benefit" follows for review.

There are varying models for the therapy team members in the provision of hospice care. Specialized hospice team members are provided with a hospice orientation prior to providing care to patients and families. In addition, like home care, therapists are competency assessed and attend ongoing education seminars to provide the best hospice care services.

Other differences between home care and hospice include that hospice care goes across care sites and is a holistic philosophy of care where the patient and family comprise the unit of care, whereas the HHA benefit is generally more beneficiary-directed. Other unique hospice differences include bereavement and the volunteer support that is considered the unique and special "heart" of hospice that supports patients and their loved ones through a usually difficult time in their lives. Keep in mind that both programs have benefits for the patient and family.

Similarities in the Intersection of the Two Spheres

- Compassionate end-of-life care
- Skillful comprehensive assessments (e.g., physical, spiritual [e.g., JCAHO accredited], caregiver ability, capability, etc.)
- Interdisciplinary focus - hospice - the interdisciplinary (IDG) team members home health agency (HHA) - nurse, SW, OT, PT, SLP, aide

Figure 2-10

A Comparison of the Medicare Home Health Benefit and Hospice Benefit

Service	Medicare Home Health Benefit*	Medicare Hospice Benefit**
Nurse	Covered for skilled care, if part time or intermittent	Covered for skilled and supportive care
Physician	Not covered under home care, but 80% of approved charge covered under Part B	Attending physician 80% covered under Part B; consulting physician 100% covered under Hospice Benefit; hospice medical director consultations covered 100%
Social Work and Counseling Services	Covered for patient	Covered for patient and family (persons who play a significant role in the patient's life, including individuals who may or may not be legally related to the patient)
Pastoral Counseling and Chaplain Services	Not covered	Covered
Home Care Aide	Covered, if part time or intermittent	Covered, as specified in Hospice Plan of Care
Volunteers for Patient and Caregivers	Not included	Included
Physical Therapy Occupational Therapy Speech Language Pathology	Covered, with some limitations on Occupational Therapy	Covered, as specified in Hospice Plan of Care
Dietitian	Not covered for individual patients	Covered, as specified in Hospice Plan of Care
Respiratory Therapy	Not covered for individual patients	Covered, as specified in Hospice Plan of Care
Inpatient Care	Not covered	Covered, as specified in Hospice Plan of Care
Respite Care	Not covered	Covered, as specified in Hospice Plan of Care
Continuous Care	May be covered where the need is finite and predictable	Covered, as specified in Hospice Plan of Care, during a period of medical crisis
Services to Nursing Facility Residents	Not covered	Covered if patient is hospice-eligible and facility and hospice have a written agreement

Figure 2-10 (cont'd)

Service	Medicare Home Health Benefit*	Medicare Hospice Benefit**
24-hour On-call Services	Not required, but frequently included	Covered
Bereavement Counseling	Not included	Included
Medications Related to Primary Illness	Not covered	Covered
Durable Medical Equipment (DME)	80% approved amount covered under Part B	100% covered, as specified in Hospice Plan of Care
Medical Supplies	Covered	100% covered, as specified in Hospice Plan of Care
Service Periods and Certification Requirements	Unlimited services if qualifying and coverage criteria are met. Recertification every 60-62 days	The Medicare hospice benefit is divided into benefit periods: • an initial 90-day period; • a subsequent 90-day period; and • subsequent 60-day periods of indefinite duration. The beneficiary must be recertified as terminally ill at the beginning of each benefit period.
Homebound status	Required	Not required

* There are additional services that can be provided in the home but that are not included in the home health benefit. Medicare will pay for reasonable and necessary home health visits if the following requirements are met:
1. Patient needs skilled care.
2. Patient is homebound.
3. Care is authorized by physician.
4. Home health agency is Medicare certified.

** Medicare will pay for hospice care if the following requirements are met:
1. Terminal illness with a prognosis of 6 months or less, certified by a physician.
2. Patient elects hospice benefit.
3. Hospice program is Medicare certified.

Hospice Association of America • 228 Seventh Street, SE • Washington, DC 20003-4306 • 202/546-4759

Reproduced by permission of the Hospice Association of America, Washington, D.C., 1999. Not for further reproduction.

- Roles of the nurse in both programs may include that of:
  educator, assessor of patient/family health status, coordinator of care, case
  manager, planner of care, evaluator of care, supervisor of nursing staff
  (e.g., LPN/LVN, HHA team members) and advocate for patient and family
- Roles of the therapist may include rehabilitation interventions, safety related
  to function and mobility, family/caregiver training and education, assistance
  with pain reduction modalities and others, based on the patient and family's
  unique needs and the individualized plan of care

For Both Programs the Quality and Customer Service Imperatives Are That:

1) The organizations and team members are in compliance with Medicare
   and other laws and rules (e.g., state practice acts, OSHA, CDC guidelines,
   that patient rights and wishes are respected, etc.)
2) There be a comprehensive orientation provided for all team members,
   based on their responsibilities and a program of ongoing education.
3) There be a framework for the provision of home-based care services
   (e.g., includes community knowledge, staffing guidelines, safety/
   environment of care considerations, etc.)
4) There be a broad-base of clinical expertise, especially those directed
   toward pain (the "fifth vital sign") and symptom assessment and practice
   skills (e.g., pain management, congestive heart failure, etc.) Readers are
   referred to the "Pain Management" care guide in Part Six.
5) Both programs within the organization strive for the standardization of
   care and care processes across the organization.
6) Care planning and care coordination be provided and documented on an
   ongoing basis and include the patient, family and the entire team involved
   in the patient's care.
7) Patient and family wishes are respected and patient rights and the
   addressing of ethical challenges be heard and handled in a sensitive
   and timely manner.
8) Clinical documentation is accurate, detailed, and meets the standards of
   documentation generally and creates a written picture of the patient and
   family, the environment, and where the care is directed for care planning
   and discharge.
9) Efforts are ongoing and directed toward improving the quality, such
   as performance improvement of the organization, including clinical
   operations, customer service, patient education, timely return of
   physician orders, and other components of what the best hospice home
   care looks like.

10) Patients are admitted to either the HHA or hospice program with a clear understanding of the benefits and services of the program chosen and the role of the patient and family/caregiver related to care planning and involvement in care.

Palliative Care

At the same time, there has been much discussion about palliative care. Palliative care can be defined as a service of care for patients with progressive and incurable illness which provides treatment of physical, emotional and spiritual pain and symptomology. Palliative care is provided under the auspices of hospice. The goal of palliative care is to achieve comfort, improve the patient's quality of life while providing support to the patient's family or care-givers. Comfort care and effective case management are oftentimes key components of a palliative program of care. The World Health Organization defines palliative care as "active total care of patients whose disease is not responsive to curative treatment. The goal of palliative care is to achieve the best quality of life for terminally ill patients." Whichever the model or term used, the clinicians role in providing competent and skillful care is the same.

Therapy Coverage and Care Planning Considerations: A Case Study

I remember being a new home care hospice nurse and having a patient who had a pathologic hip fracture from her lung cancer metastasis. The family had called me after the patient, a kind, elderly woman complained of pain after getting back to bed earlier that morning. Upon review of my findings on the visit and in talking to the patient and her daughter, it was clear that she may have fractured her hip. I still keep in touch with the skillful, compassionate therapist who worked with myself, the aide and the physician to allow this patient to stay home - which is what she requested every visit. Effective pain management, teaching the aide, the nursing team members and the family how to safely move and care for this patient were all provided by the PT. The patient and family teaching, the observation and assessment and communications with the physician and the IDG, and numerous other activities were coordinated with the therapist to assist this patient and family in meeting their unique needs, while always respecting and honoring the patient's wishes.

Whether the patient is in the home care or hospice program, the therapist must have an understanding of the coverage and documentation requirements, including the forms used by the organization and guidelines for their correct and accurate completion. The following information and checklist, Box 2-1 can provide assistance in the documentation of effective care that supports coverage and compliance.

Box 2-1

A Checklist for Hospice Documentation

✔ Does your documentation paint a picture from the onset of care through continuation of hospice services?

✔ Does your documentation distinguish clearly between the chronic and terminal phases of a disease, especially if it is long and chronic in nature?

✔ Are any patient periods of exacerbation, stabilization, and further deterioration specified?

✔ Does documentation show how treatments and medication play a palliative role in the plan of care?

✔ Does documentation in all notes complete the picture of the terminally ill patient? Remember that what is "normal" and "stable" to a hospice nurse or other team member may still indicate a clearly terminal patient if the details are provided in the documentation.

✔ Are generalizations such as "no change" or "as tolerated" avoided? (The payers pay for covered care and the nurse's documentation plays an important role.)

✔ Are the physician's certification, assessments, and recertification(s) of terminal illness complete and included?

✔ Are all discipline visit notes and/or telephone calls signed, dated, legible, and descriptive of the course of care related to the patient, family, and caregivers?

✔ Has the physician provided written material covering the patient's course of illness and care to date?

✔ Are all the laboratory and other test results included?

✔ Is the hospice election form signed and dated by the hospice provider and the patient/family or other responsible party?

✔ Is the effective date for the care clearly marked?

✔ Is there a discharge summary, history, and physical from the hospital?

✔ Is the plan of care established, updated, and being followed?

✔ Has a copy of the election form been left with the patient/family or other responsible party?

✔ If and when different levels of care are used, is there documentation of the date, time, and reason for the change in the level of care and services?

✔ Have the patient's assessments been performed, painting a clear picture of the patient's status, including these core aspects of hospice care: functional, spiritual, nutritional, clinical, emotional, psychological, and physical assessments and plans?

✔ Are handwritten notes or other entries legible to team members or others who may require the information?

✔ Are data elements or areas needing completion addressed in an understandable manner? For example, is there a legend or a list of acceptable abbreviations in instances where abbreviations occur?

✔ Does the care plan reflect the problems identified during the comprehensive assessment?

✔ Overall, does the hospice record and the documentation pass the test of effective care planning and coordination? Could another colleague, in your absence, review the record and be able to effectively continue with the hospice plan of care?

*Reprinted with permission from Marrelli and Associates, **Home Care Nurse News**, Volume 5, No. 2, 1998.*

Documentation Problems to Avoid

Problems with therapy documentation occur when the documentation does not support the patient's terminal illness. Other problems with therapy documentation include:

- The documentation looks like hospice care for non-terminal patients,
- Missing or illegible documentation
- Check boxes without any narrative to explain the patient's problems and needs
- Therapy interventions appears to be not "medically reasonable and necessary" because the documentation did not explain the patient's problems, current status and where the care was directed for safety or stability
- No valid physician certification or recertification as required by law
- Assessment/admission documentation did not explain or document the patient's prior level of function
- A lack of or no documented objective functional measures
- Documentation does not support the patient's terminal illness

Summary

Hospice care is a special way of caring for patients and their families when the decision has been made to end curative treatment endeavors. In hospice, we say the shift has changed focus from "cure" to "care." Medicare and many other insurers have identified a bundle or comprehensive group of services to address the unique needs of this patient population and their families during this difficult time. Therapists providing care interventions directed toward comfort, safety and stability have an important contribution to make that assists these patients and their families to oftentimes remain at home either longer or more comfortably. Gait strengthening or training, teaching family members safe mobility tips and how to use a transfer board safely are just some of the services that the PT may be providing in the community. The OT provides important services directed toward improving or maintaining functionality while identifying methods to improve quality of life related to ADLs. The SLP's important contributions to the hospice patient population include improving swallowing safety and recommendations for caregivers and alternative communication methods at a time when patients and family members must communicate for effective closure with family and friends.

For indepth information about hospice and care planning, readers are referred to the *Hospice and Palliative Care Handbook: Quality, Compliance, and Reimbursement* (Mosby, 1999) and *Mosby's Home Care and Hospice Drug Handbook* (Mosby, 1999) for indepth discussions related to hospice care documentation, care planning and clinical practice issues. All of these services and interventions together assist hospice patients and patients in palliative care programs to achieve their best level toward the end-of-life.

PART THREE
The Rehabilitation Team: The Big Picture
Practice Standards, Guidelines, and Considerations for PT, SLP, and OT from the National Professional Associations

PHYSICAL THERAPY SERVICES

Information in this section is based on information from documents published and available through the American Physical Therapy Association.

Providers

Physical therapy services are provided by a physical therapist (PT) or physical therapist assistant (PTA) under the direction and supervision of a physical therapist.

From 1960 to the present, physical therapists are graduates of a professional physical therapist education program accredited by the Commission on Accreditation in Physical Therapy Education (CAPTE). Graduates from 1926 to 1959 completed physical therapy curricula approved by appropriate accreditation bodies. Physical therapists must be licensed in the state or states in which they practice.

Physical therapists may achieve clinical specialist certification through the American Board of Physical Therapy Specialties (ABPTS). Certification areas for clinical specialization include Cardiopulmonary, Clinical Electrophysiology, Geriatrics, Neurology, Orthopaedics, Pediatrics, and Sports Physical Therapy.

Physical therapist assistants are graduates of a physical therapist assistant associate degree program accredited by an agency recognized by the Commission on Accreditation in Physical Therapy Education (CAPTE). State law, third-payer coverage requirements, personnel availability and individual home health agency policy will determine the extent to which assistants are used in delivering home care services in a given demographic area.

The *Home Health Agency Manual (HIM-11)* outlines care delivered by the physical therapist assistant, under the delegation and supervision of a physical therapist, as a covered service under the Medicare home health benefit. When determined appropriate by the physical therapist, the physical therapist assistant may be assigned to perform selected therapeutic interventions, communication and documentation activities. The supervising physical therapist should be actively involved in ongoing assessment of the physical therapist assistant's level of competency, to ensure that professional activities are appropriately delegated, and based on the individual assistant's performance capacity.

Scope of Practice

Physical therapy is the care and services provided by or under the direction and supervision of a physical therapist. As shown in Figure 3-1, the physical therapist integrates five elements into patient care: examination, evaluation, diagnosis, prognosis, and intervention in an effort to maximize outcomes.

Figure 3-1   The Elements of Patient Care

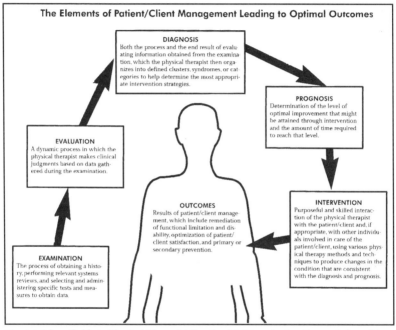

*Reprinted from **Guide to Physical Therapist Practice** (1997), p. 1 - 4, with permission of the American Physical Therapy Association.*

Examination

The examination is the process of obtaining a patient health history, performing relevant systems reviews, and selecting and administering specific tests and measures. The types of tests and measures selected by the physical therapist are based on information gathered from the health history and systems review. See Box 3-1 for specific measures and tests. Other factors affecting tests and measures selection include the complexity of the condition and the purpose of the referral or visit.

Box 3-1
Specific Tests and Measures Performed by Physical Therapists

Aerobic Capacity and Endurance
Aerobic capacity and endurance are measures of the ability to perform work or participate in activity over time using the body's oxygen uptake and delivery and energy release mechanisms. During activity, the physical therapist uses tests ranging from simple determinations of blood pressure, heart rate, and respiratory rate to complex calculations of oxygen consumption and carbon dioxide production to determine the appropriateness of the response to increased oxygen demand. Monitoring responses at rest and during and after activity may indicate the degree and severity of impairment, identify cardiopulmonary deficits that result in functional limitation, and indicate the need to use or recommend other tests and measures and specific interventions.

Anthropometric Characteristics
Anthropometric characteristics describe human body measurements such as height, weight, girth, and body fat composition. The physical therapist uses these tests and measures to test for muscle atrophy, gauge the extent of edema, and establish a baseline to allow patients/clients to be compared to national norms on such variables as weight and body fat composition. Results of these tests and measures may indicate the need to use or recommend other tests and measures.

Arousal, Attention, and Cognition
Arousal is the stimulation to action or to physiologic readiness for activity. *Attention* is selective awareness of a part or aspect of the environment or selective responsiveness to one class of stimuli. *Cognition* is the act or process of knowing, including both awareness and judgment. The physical therapist uses specific tests and measures to assess responsiveness; orientation to time, person, place, and situation; and ability to follow directions. These tests and measures guide the physical therapist in the selection of interventions by indicating whether the patient/client has the cognitive ability to participate in the plan of care.

Assistive and Adaptive Devices
Assistive and adaptive devices include a variety of implements or equipment used to aid patients/clients in performing tasks or movements. *Assistive devices* include crutches, canes, walkers, wheelchairs, power devices, long-handled reachers, and static and dynamic splints. *Adaptive devices* include raised toilet seats, seating systems, and environmental controls. The physical therapist uses specific tests and measures to determine whether a patient/client might benefit from such a device or, when such a device already is in use, to determine how well the patient/client performs with it.

Community and Work (Job/School/Play) Integration or Reintegration (Including Instrumental Activities of Daily Living)

Community and work (job/school/play) integration or reintegration is the process of assuming roles in the community or at work. The physical therapist uses the following tests and measures to (1) make an informed judgment as to whether a patient/client is currently prepared to assume community or work roles, including all instrumental activities of daily living (IADL), or (2) determine when and how such integration or reintegration might occur. The physical therapist also uses these tests and measures to determine whether an individual is a candidate for a work hardening or work conditioning program. The physical therapist considers patient/client safety, perceptions, and expectations while performing the test and measures.

Cranial Nerve Integrity

Cranial nerve integrity involves somatic, visceral, and afferent and efferent components. The physical therapist uses cranial nerve integrity tests and measures to localize a dysfunction in the brain stem and to identify cranial nerves that merit an in-depth examination. The physical therapist uses a number of these tests to assess sensory and motor functions, such as taste, smell, and facial expression.

Environmental, Home, and Work (Job/School/Play) Barriers

Environmental, home, and work (job/school/play) barriers are the physical impediments that keep patients/clients from functioning optimally in their surroundings. The physical therapist uses the barriers tests and measures to identify any of a variety of possible impediments, including safety hazards (e.g., throw rugs, slippery surfaces), access problems (e.g., narrow doors, thresholds, high steps, absence of power doors or elevators), and home or office design barriers (e.g., excessive distances to negotiate, multistory environment, sinks, bathrooms, counters, placement of controls or switches). The physical therapist uses these tests and measures, often in conjunction with portions of other tests and measures, to suggest modifications to the environment (e.g., grab bars in the shower, ramps, raised toilet seats, increased lighting) that will allow the patient/client to improve functioning in the home, workplace, and other settings.

Ergonomics and Body Mechanics

Ergonomics refers to the relationships among the worker, the work that is done, the tasks and activities inherent in that work, and the environment in which the work is performed. Ergonomics uses scientific and engineering principles to improve the safety, efficiency, and quality of movement involved in work. *Body mechanics* refers to the interrelationships of the muscles and joints as they maintain or adjust posture in response to environmental forces.

The physical therapist uses the ergonomics and body mechanics tests and measures to examine the work environment on behalf of patients/clients and to determine the potential for trauma or repetitive stress injuries from inappropriate workplace design. These tests and measures may be conducted after a work injury or as a preventive measure, particularly when a patient/client is returning to the work environment after an extended absence.

Gait, Locomotion, and Balance

Gait is the manner in which a person walks, characterized by rhythm, cadence, step, stride, and speed. *Locomotion* is the ability to move from one place to another. Balance is the ability to maintain the body in equilibrium with gravity both statically (e.g., while stationary) and dynamically (e.g., while walking). The physical therapist uses gait, locomotion, and balance tests and measures to investigate disturbances in gait, locomotion, and balance because they frequently lead to decreased mobility, a decline in functional independence, and an increased risk of falls. Gait, locomotion, and balance problems often involve difficulty in integrating sensory, motor, and neural processes. The physical therapist also uses these tests and measures to determine whether the patient/client is a candidate for assistive, adaptive, orthotic, protective, supportive, or prosthetic devices or equipment.

Integumentary Integrity

Integumentary integrity is the health of the skin, including its ability to serve as a barrier to environmental threats (e.g., bacteria, parasites). The physical therapist uses integumentary integrity tests and measures to assess the effects of a wide variety of problems that result in skin and subcutaneous changes, including pressure and vascular, venous, arterial, diabetic, and necropathic ulcers; burns and other traumas; and a number of diseases (e.g., soft tissue disorders). These tests and measures also are used to obtain more information about circulation through inspection of the skin or the nail beds.

Joint Integrity and Mobility

Joint integrity is the conformance of a joint to expected anatomic and biomechanical norms. *Joint mobility* involves the capacity of a joint to be moved passively in certain ways that take into account the structure and shape of the joint surface in addition to characteristics of the tissue surrounding the joint. The assessment of joint mobility involves the performance of accessory joint movements by the physical therapist because these movements are not under the voluntary control of the patient. The physical therapist uses the joint integrity and mobility tests and measures to determine whether there is excessive or limited motion of the joint. Excessive joint motion necessitates a program of protection, whereas limited joint motion calls for interventions to increase mobility and enhance functional capability.

Motor Function (Motor Control and Motor Learning)

Motor function is the ability to learn or demonstrate the skillful and efficient assumption, maintenance, modification, and control of voluntary postures and movement patterns. The physical therapist uses motor function tests and measures in the diagnosis of underlying impairments and their contributions to functional limitation and disability. Deficits in motor function reflect the type, location, and extent of the impairment, which may be the result of pathology or other disorders. Weakness, paralysis, dysfunctional movement patterns, abnormal timing, poor coordination, clumsiness, involuntary movements, or dysfunctional postures may be manifestations of impaired motor function.

Muscle Performance (Including Strength, Power, and Endurance)

Muscle performance is the capacity of a muscle to do work (force x distance). Muscle strength is the (measurable) force exerted by a muscle or a group of muscles to overcome a resistance in one maximal effort. Muscle power is work produced per unit of time or the product of strength and speed. Muscle endurance is the ability to contract the muscle repeatedly over a period of time. The performance of an individual muscle depends on its characteristics of length, tension, and velocity. Integrated muscle performance over time is mediated by neurologic stimulation, fuel storage, and fuel delivery in addition to balance, timing, and sequencing of contraction. The physical therapist uses muscle performance tests and measures to determine the ability to produce movements that are prerequisite to functional activity.

Neuromotor Development and Sensory Integration

Neuromotor development is the acquisition and evolution of movement skills throughout the life span. Sensory integration is the ability to integrate information from the environment to produce movement. The physical therapist uses neuromotor development and sensory integration tests and measures to assess motor capabilities in infants, children, and adults. The tests and measures may be used to assess mobility, achievement of motor milestones and healthy responses, postural control, and voluntary and involuntary movement. The physical therapist also uses these tests and measures to test balance, righting and equilibrium reactions, eye-hand coordination, and other motor capabilities.

Orthotic, Protective, and Supportive Devices

Orthotic, protective, and supportive devices are used to support weak or ineffective joints or muscles and may serve to enhance performance. *Orthotic devices* include splints, braces, shoe inserts, and casts. *Protective devices* include braces, protective taping, cushions, and helmets. *Supportive devices* include supportive taping, compression garments, corsets, slings, neck collars, serial casts, elastic wraps, and oxygen. The physical therapist uses specific tests and measures to determine the need for orthotic, protective, and supportive devices in patients/clients not currently using them and to evaluate the appropriateness and fit of those devices already in use. The physical therapist correlates patient/client problems with available devices to make a choice that best serves the individual. For example, the physical therapist may have to choose between an orthosis that provides maximum control of motion and one that allows considerable movement.

Pain

Pain is a disturbed sensation that causes suffering or distress. The physical therapist uses pain tests and measures to determine the intensity, quality, and temporal and physical characteristics of any pain that is important to the patient. The physical therapist may determine a cause or a mechanism for the pain through these tests and measures. The tests and measures also may be used to determine whether referral to another health care professional is appropriate.

Posture

Posture is the alignment and positioning of the body in relation to gravity, center of mass, and base of support. The physical therapist uses posture tests and measures to assess structural abnormalities in addition to the ability to right the body against gravity. "Good posture" is a state of musculoskeletal balance that protects the supporting structures of the body against injury or progressive deformity. Findings from these tests and measures may lead the physical therapist to perform additional tests and measures (e.g., joint integrity and mobility, respiration, ventilation [gas exchange], and circulation).

Prosthetic Requirements

A *prosthesis* is an artificial device used to replace a missing part of the body. Physical therapists use specific tests and measures for patients/clients who might benefit from a prosthesis or for patients wearing a prosthesis. The physical therapist selects a prosthesis that will allow optimal freedom of movement and functional capability with minimal discomfort and inconvenience.

Range of Motion (Including Muscle Length)

Range of motion (ROM) is the space, distance, or angle through which movement occurs at a joint or a series of joints. *Muscle length* is measured at various joint angles through the range. Muscle length, in conjunction with joint integrity and soft tissue extensibility, determines flexibility. The physical therapist uses ROM tests and measures to determine the arthrokinematics and biomechanics of a joint, including flexibility and movement characteristics. Adequate ROM is valuable for injury prevention because it allows the tissues to adjust to imposed stresses. Loss of ROM is associated in most cases with loss of function.

Reflex Integrity

A *reflex* is a stereotypic, involuntary reaction to any of a variety of sensory stimuli. The physical therapist uses reflex integrity tests and measures to determine the excitability of the nervous system and the integrity of the neuromuscular system.

Self-Care and Home Management (Including Activities of Daily Living and Instrumental Activities of Daily Living)

Self-care includes activities of daily living (ADL), such as bed mobility, transfers, gait, locomotion, developmental activity, dressing, grooming, bathing, eating, and toileting. *Home management* includes more complex instrumental activities of daily living (IADL), such as maintaining a home, shopping, cooking, performing heavy household chores, managing money, driving a car or using public transportation, structured play (for infants and children), and negotiating school environments. The physical therapist uses tests and measures to determine the level of performance of the tasks necessary for independent living. The results of these tests and measures may lead the physical therapist to determine that the patient/client needs assistive and adaptive, orthotic, protective, supportive, or prosthetic devices or equipment; body mechanics training; organized functional training programs; or therapeutic exercise programs. The physical therapist considers patient/ client safety, perceptions, and expectations while performing the tests and measures.

Sensory Integrity (Including Proprioception and Kinesthesia)

Sensory integrity includes peripheral sensory processing (e.g., sensitivity to touch) and cortical sensory processing (e.g., two-point and sharp/dull discrimination). *Proprioception* includes position sense and the awareness of the joints at rest. *Kinesthesia* is the awareness of movement. The physical therapist uses sensory integrity tests and measures to determine the integrity of the sensory, perceptual, or somatosensory processes. Sensory, perceptual, or somatosensory abnormalities are frequent indicators of pathology.

Ventilation, Respiration (Gas Exchange), and Circulation

Ventilation is the movement of a volume of gas into and out of the lungs. *Respiration* refers primarily to the exchange of oxygen and carbon dioxide across a membrane into and out of the lungs and at the cellular level. *Circulation* is the passage of blood through the heart, blood vessels, organs, and tissues; it also describes the oxygen delivery system. The physical therapist uses ventilation, respiration, and circulation tests and measures to determine whether the patient has an adequate ventilatory pump and oxygen uptake and delivery system to perform activities of daily living (ADL), ambulation, and aerobic exercise.

*Reprinted from: **Guide to Physical Therapist Practice**, APTA (1997), Chapter 2, pages 2-2 through 2-24, with permission of the American Physical Therapy Association.*

Evaluation

The evaluation is the dynamic process in which the physical therapist makes clinical judgments based on data gathered during the examination. The evaluation process reflects patient specific findings and needs, taking into account the extent and duration of functional loss and the level and likelihood of benefit from therapeutic interventions.

Diagnosis

The diagnosis, or label describing a presentation of signs and symptoms, is reached after organizing the examination findings and evaluation results into clusters, syndromes, or categories for interpretation. The physical therapist utilizes the diagnosis as a guide in developing a treatment plan to alleviate symptoms and/or remediate deficits.

Prognosis

The prognosis is the predicted level of functional improvement and the associated time frames necessary to achieve anticipated goals and desired outcomes.

Interventions

Interventions are the purposeful and skilled interaction of the physical therapist with the patient or caregiver, using various physical therapy procedures and techniques to produce changes in the patient's condition. Physical therapy interventions can be grouped into three categories: 1) coordination, communication, and documentation; 2) patient-related instruction; and 3) direct interventions.

Coordination, communication and documentation functions ensure that appropriate care is delivered in a coordinated and comprehensive manner, and documented to meet care planning, care coordination, outcome, regulatory, and reimbursement demands.

Patient and/or caregiver-related instruction is the process of presenting information and developing skills to promote achievement of desired functional and health outcomes. Emphasis is placed on empowering the patient and/or caregiver(s) to gain competence in as much of the therapeutic activities as they can reasonably, safely, and effectively perform.

Direct Interventions

Based on the patient's functional limitations, the physical therapist selects, and applies or modifies one or more direct interventions to achieve the desired outcomes. Figure 3-2 outlines categories of direct interventions physical therapists utilize, with the first three (therapeutic exercise, functional training in self-care and home management, and functional training in community and work integration/reintegration) representing the core elements of most physical therapy plans of care. Box 3-2 provides detailed descriptions of physical therapy interventions.

Figure 3-2   Physical Therapy Interventions

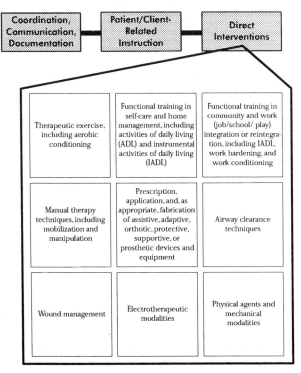

*Reprinted from **Guide to Physical Therapist Practice**, (1997) p. 3 - 1, with permission of the American Physical Therapy Association.*

Box 3-2   Descriptions of Physical Therapy Interventions

Coordination, Communication, and Documentation
Coordination, communication, and documentation are processes that ensure (1) appropriate, coordinated, comprehensive, and cost-effective services between admission and discharge and (2) cost-effective and efficient integration or reintegration into home, community, or work (job/school/play) environments. These processes involve collaborating and coordinating with agencies; coordinating and monitoring the delivery of available resources; coordinating data on transition; coordinating the patient/client management provided by the physical therapist; ensuring and facilitating access to health care services and resources and to appropriate community resources; facilitating the development of the discharge plan; facilitating timely delivery of available services; identifying current resources; providing information regarding the availability of advocacy services; obtaining informed consent; protecting patient/client rights through procedural safeguards and services; providing information, consultation, and technical assistance; and providing oversight for outcomes data collection and analysis.

Patient/Client-Related Instruction
Patient/client-related instruction is the process of imparting information and developing skills to promote independence and to allow care to continue after discharge. Instruction should focus not only on the patient but on the family, significant others, and caregivers regarding the current condition, plan of care, and transition to roles at home, at work, or in the community, with the goal of ensuring (1) short-term and long-term adherence to the interventions and (2) primary and secondary prevention of future disability. The development of an instruction program should be consistent with the goals of the plan of care and may include information about the cause of the impairment, functional limitation, or disability; the prognosis; and the purposes and benefits and risks of the intervention. All instruction should take into consideration the influences of patient/client age, culture, gender roles, race, sex, sexual orientation, and socioeconomic status.

Therapeutic Exercise (Including Aerobic Conditioning)
Therapeutic exercise includes a broad group of activities intended to improve strength, range of motion (ROM) (including muscle length), endurance, breathing, balance, coordination, posture, motor function (motor control and motor learning), motor development, or confidence when any of a variety of problems constrains the ability to perform a functional activity. The physical therapist targets problems with performance of a movement or task and specifically directs therapeutic exercise to alleviate impairment, functional

limitation, or disability. Therapeutic exercise includes activities to improve physical function and health status (or reduce or prevent disability) resulting from impairments by identifying specific performance goals that will allow patients/clients to achieve a higher functional level in the home, school, workplace, or community. Also included: activities that allow well clients to improve or maintain their health or performance status (for work, recreational, or sports purposes) and prevent or minimize future potential health problems. Therapeutic exercise also is a part of fitness and wellness programs designed to promote overall well-being or, in general, to prevent complications related to inactivity or overuse. This intervention may be used during pregnancy and the postpartum period to improve function and reduce stress. It also may be used (with proper guidance) in patients with hematologic and oncologic disorders to combat fatigue and systemic breakdowns. Therapeutic exercise may prevent further complications and decrease utilization of health care resources before, during, and after surgery or hospitalization. Therapeutic exercise is performed actively, passively, or against resistance. When the patient/client cannot participate actively due to weakness or other problems, passive exercise may be necessary. Resistance may be provided manually, by gravity, or through use of a weighted apparatus or of mechanical or electromechanical devices. Aquatic physical therapy uses the physical and hydrodynamic properties of water to facilitate performance.

Functional Training in Self-Care and Home Management (Including Activities of Daily Living and Instrumental Activities of Daily Living)
Functional training in self-care and home management includes a broad group of performance activities designed to (1) enhance neuromusculoskeletal, cardiovascular, and pulmonary capacities and (2) integrate or return the patient/client to self-care or home management as quickly and efficiently as possible. Functional training is used to improve the physical function and health status of patients/clients with physical disability, impaired sensorimotor function, pain, injury, or disease. Functional training also is used for well clients. It frequently is based on activities associated with growth and development. The physical therapist targets problems with performing a movement or task and specifically directs the functional training to alleviate impairment, functional limitation, and disability. The physical therapist may select from a number of options, including training in the following: activities of daily living (ADL); instrumental activities of daily living (IADL); body mechanics; therapeutic exercise; and use of therapeutic assistive, adaptive, orthotic, protective, supportive, or prosthetic devices or equipment. Organized functional training programs such as back schools also may be selected.

Functional Training in Community and Work (Job/School/Play) Integration or Reintegration (Including Instrumental Activities of Daily Living, Work Hardening, and Work Conditioning)

Functional training in community and work (job/school/play) integration or reintegration includes a broad group of activities designed to integrate or to return the patient/client to community, work (job/school/play), or leisure activities as quickly and efficiently as possible. It involves improving physiologic capacities to facilitate the fulfillment of community and work-related roles. Functional training is used to improve the physical function and health status of patients/clients with physical disability, impaired sensorimotor function, pain, injury, or disease; it also is used for well individuals. It frequently is based on activities associated with growth and development. The physical therapist targets the problems in performance of movements, community activities, work tasks, or leisure activities and specifically directs the functional training to enable return to the community, work, or leisure environment. A variety of approaches may be taken, depending on patient/client needs; for example, the physical therapist may provide training in instrumental activities of daily living (IADL) to a patient/client who needs to live more independently, and body mechanics and posture awareness training to a patient/client who is deficient in those areas.

Work hardening and work conditioning are specialized functional training programs designed to reduce the impairment, functional limitation, or disability associated with work-related injuries.

Manual Therapy Techniques (Including Mobilization and Manipulation)

Manual therapy techniques consist of a broad group of passive interventions in which physical therapists use their hands to administer skilled movements designed to modulate pain; increase joint range of motion (ROM); reduce or eliminate soft tissue swelling, inflammation, or restriction; induce relaxation; improve contractile and noncontractile tissue extensibility; and improve pulmonary function. These interventions involve a variety of techniques, such as the application of graded forces. Physical therapists use manual therapy techniques to improve physical function and health status (or reduce or prevent disability) resulting from impairments by identifying specific performance goals that allow patients/clients to achieve a higher functional level in self-care, home management, community and work (job/school/play) integration or reintegration, or leisure tasks and activities.

Prescription, Application, and, as Appropriate, Fabrication of Devices and Equipment (Assistive, Adaptive, Orthotic, Protective, Supportive, and Prosthetic)

Prescription, application, and, as appropriate, fabrication of assistive, adaptive, orthotic, protective, supportive, and prosthetic devices and equipment include the use of a broad group of therapeutic appliances, implements, devices, and equipment to enhance performance of tasks or movements, support weak or ineffective joints or muscles, protect body parts from injury, and adapt the environment to facilitate activities of daily living (ADL) and instrumental activities of daily living (IADL). These devices and equipment often are used in conjunction with therapeutic exercise, functional training, work conditioning and work hardening, and other interventions and should be selected in the context of patient/client needs and social and cultural environments. The physical therapist targets the problems in performance of movements or tasks and selects (or fabricates) the most appropriate device or equipment, then fits it and trains the patient/client in its use and application. The goal is for the patient/client to function at a higher level and to decrease functional limitation.

Airway Clearance Techniques

Airway clearance techniques include a broad group of activities used to manage or prevent consequences of acute and chronic lung diseases and impairment, including those associated with surgery. Airway clearance techniques may be used with therapeutic exercise, manual therapy techniques, or mechanical modalities to improve pulmonary function. The physical therapist performs airway clearance techniques to improve physical function and health status (or reduce or prevent disability) resulting from impairments, functional limitations, and disabilities by identifying specific performance goals that allow the patient/client to achieve a higher functional level in home management, community and work (job/school/play) integration or reintegration, and leisure movements, tasks, and activities.

Wound Management

Wound management includes procedures used to achieve a clean wound bed, promote a moist wound environment, facilitate autolytic debridement, absorb excessive exudate from a wound complex, and enhance perfusion and oxygen and nutrient delivery to tissues in addition to management of the resulting scar. As a component of wound management, *debridement* is a therapeutic procedure involving removal of nonviable tissue from a wound bed, most often by the use of instruments, autolysis, therapeutic modalities, or enzymes. The desired effects of wound management may be achieved in a variety of ways. The physical therapist may use physical agents, electrotherapeutic and mechanical modalities, dressings, topical agents, debridement, and oxygen therapy as part of a plan of care to alter the function of tissues and organ systems required for repair. Wound management interventions are used directly by the physical therapist, based on patient/client needs and the direct physiological effects that are required.

Electrotherapeutic Modalities

Electrotherapeutic modalities, which include a broad group of agents involving electricity, are used by physical therapists to augment other active or functionally oriented procedures in the plan of care. Specifically, these modalities are used to help patients/clients modulate or decrease pain; reduce or eliminate soft tissue swelling, inflammation, or restriction; maintain strength after injury or surgery; decrease unwanted muscular activity; assist muscle contraction in gait or other functional training; or increase the rate of healing of open wounds and soft tissue.

Physical Agents and Mechanical Modalities

Physical agents and mechanical modalities are used by physical therapists in conjunction with or in preparation for other interventions, such as therapeutic exercise and functional training. Physical agents which involve thermal, acoustic, or radiant energy are used by physical therapists in increasing connective tissue extensibility; modulating pain; reducing or eliminating soft tissue swelling, inflammation, or restriction caused by musculoskeletal injury or circulatory dysfunction; increasing the healing rate of open wounds and soft tissue; remodeling scar tissue; or treating skin conditions. Mechanical modalities include a broad group of procedures used by physical therapists in modulating pain; stabilizing an area that requires temporary support; increasing range of motion (ROM); or applying distraction, approximation, or compression.

*Reprinted from: **Guide to Physical Therapist Practice**, APTA (1997), Chapter 3, pages 3-2 through 3-14, with permission of the American Physical Therapy Association. (Note: Interventions are listed in the order of preferred usage according to the American Physical Therapy Association).*

Outcomes

The outcomes that physical therapy interventions intend to impact are remediation of functional limitation and disability, maximization of patient/client satisfaction, and achievement of primary or secondary prevention.

Indications

A referral for physical therapy may be indicated for patients experiencing impairment, functional limitations, disabilities, or changes in physical functional and health status resulting from injury, disease, or other causes. Box 3-3 lists some of the problems addressed by physical therapists.

Box 3-3   Sample List of Potential Diagnoses for Physical Therapy Referrals

- Amputation
- Amyotrophic Lateral Sclerosis (ALS)
- Asthma
- Coronary artery bypass graft (CABG)
- Cancer (CA)
- Cerebral vascular accident (CVA)
- Closed head injury (CHI) or Head trauma
- Collagen disorders
- Congestive Heart Failure (CHF)
- Chronic Obstructive Pulmonary Disease (COPD)
- Fractures
- Frequent falls
- Hypertension (HTN)
- Joint replacement
- Mastectomy
- Multiple Sclerosis (MS)
- Myocardial Infarction (MI)
- Neuropathies
- Osteoarthritis (OA)
- Osteoporosis
- Rheumatoid arthritis (RA)
- Pain
- Paraplegia
- Parkinson's Disease
- Post-surgical care
- Quadriplegia
- Wound care

ADDITIONAL RESOURCES FOR PHYSICAL THERAPY

Excerpts reprinted from *Guidelines for the Provision of Physical Therapy in the Home*, (1996) APTA, Alexandria, VA., pages 1-6, 12-18, with permission of the American Physical Therapy Association.

Guidelines for the Provision of Physical Therapy in the Home

These guidelines are intended to provide a basic foundation for the provision of physical therapy to clients in their place of residence. Consistent with the American Physical Therapy Association's (APTA) terminology, the guidelines represent *Board-approved, nonbinding statements of advice* pertaining to the specifics of home health. The Community Home Health Section of APTA, in conjunction with the Section's Quality Assurance and Practice committees, initiated the process of developing the guidelines in 1982. Input regarding the guidelines was obtained from APTA staff members and Community Home Health Section members, committee chairs and Executive Board.

The guidelines do represent statements of conditions that reflect *minimum performance criteria* for the administration of physical therapy in the home. These criteria can be used to assess the process of physical therapy within the agency. The guidelines established are subject to changes and modifications given the dynamics of the profession and are not intended to supersede established home-health-related rules and regulations.

Role of the Physical Therapist in the Home

Guideline: The physical therapist will provide client care:

1. In accordance with APTA's *Standards of Practice*;

2. In accordance with APTA's *Guide for Professional Conduct*;

3. In accordance with APTA's Code of Ethics;

4. In accordance with applicable municipal, state, and federal laws; and

5. In coordination with the client's other care providers.

Criteria: 1. Provide the evaluation/assessment visit upon referral.

2. Provide services that require the skills of a physical therapist consistent with the established plan of care.

3. Act as a consultant to other care providers as appropriate.

4. Participate in:

    4.1 Client care conferences,

    4.2 Inservices,

    4.3 Chart audit activities,

    4.4 Quality improvement activities, and

    4.5 Peer review activities.

5. Provide instruction to the client/caregiver:

    5.1 Verbal and

    5.2 Written

6. Provide documentation to the agency for inclusion in the client's clinical record (refer to criterion 10 below).

    6.1 Submission of documentation should be in a timely manner in compliance with applicable state and federal home-health-related rules and regulations, agency requirements, and/or third-party payer requirements.

7. Perform physical therapist assistant supervisory visits:

    7.1 In accordance with applicable municipal, state, and federal rules and regulations.

    7.2 To:

        7.2.1 Evaluate the client's progress,

        7.2.2 Update the plan of care as applicable,

        7.2.3 Assess the client's progress toward the established outcomes,

        7.2.4 Document the client's response to treatment, and

        7.2.5 Provide skilled treatment when coordinated with the physical therapist assistant.

    7.3 In accordance with APTA's policy on *Direction, Delegation, and Supervision in Physical Therapy Services*, revised HOD 06-95-08-09.

    7.4 Upon the request of the physical therapist assistant, for reexamination of the client, in instances of:

       7.4.1 A noted change in the client's response to treatment,

       7.4.2 A noted change in the client's medical status, or

       7.4.3 A planned discharge of the client from physical therapy.

8. Assess competence of support personnel to perform assigned/delegated activities.

9. Be accessible by telecommunications to the physical therapist assistant at all times while the physical therapist assistant is treating the client.

10. Maintain confidentiality of information relating to the physical therapist-client relationship in accordance with:

    10.1 The agency's confidentiality policies and procedures and

    10.2 APTA's *Guide for Professional Conduct.*

11. Support physical therapy education through the acceptance of interns and through participation in established intern education programs as appropriate.

12. Demonstrate knowledge of available community resources/services.

    12.1 Make recommendations for follow-up care in coordination with the agency that admitted the client, and

    12.2 Utilize other agency care providers to assist with referrals to community resources.

Role of the Physical Therapist Assistant in the Home

Guideline: The physical therapist assistant will provide client care:

1. In accordance with APTA's *Standards of Practice*;

2. In accordance with APTA's *Guide for Conduct of the Affiliate Member*;

3. In accordance with APTA's *Standards of Ethical Conduct for the Physical Therapist Assistant*;

4. In accordance with APTA's policy on *Direction, Delegation, and Supervision in Physical Therapy Services*, revised HOD 06-95-08-09;

5. In accordance with APTA's policy on *Physical Therapy Services: Access, Admission, and Patient's Rights*, HOD 06-93-16-22;

6. In accordance with applicable municipal, state, and federal rules and regulations;

7. In coordination with the supervision physical therapist; and

8. In coordination with the client's other care providers.

Criteria:

1. Perform skilled procedures and related tasks that have been selected and delegated by the supervising physical therapist.

2. Provide instruction to the client/caregiver:

    2.1 Verbal and

    2.2 Written

3. Provide documentation to the agency for inclusion in the client's clinical record.

    3.1 Submission of documentation should be in a timely manner in compliance with applicable municipal, state, and federal home-health-related rules and regulations, agency requirements, and/or third-party payer requirements.

4. Monitor and communicate to the supervising physical therapist any changes in the client's condition.

5. Monitor and document the client's response to therapeutic physical therapy intervention.

    5.1 Communicate to the supervising physical therapist the client's:

        5.1.1 Progress/lack of progress and

        5.1.2 Response to physical therapy intervention.

6. Participate in, as appropriate:

    6.1 Individual and multidisciplinary care conferences,

6.2   Inservices/continuing education,

6.3   Chart audit activities,

6.4   Quality improvement activities, and

6.5   Peer review.

7.   Maintain confidentiality of information relating to the physical therapist assistant-client relationship in accordance with:

7.1   The agency's confidentiality policies and procedures and

7.2   APTA's *Standards of Ethical Conduct for the Physical Therapist Assistant.*

8.   Demonstrate knowledge of available community resources/services.

Examination/Evaluation Visit

Guideline: The physical therapist will provide examination/evaluation information consistent with the:

1.   Nature of referral to home health services and

2.   Needs of the client for coordinated care.

Criteria: 1.   The examination/evaluation should include, but not be limited to:

1.1   Aerobic capacity or endurance:

1.1.1   Blood pressure,

1.1.2   Respiratory rate, and

1.1.3   Pulse.

1.2   Anthropometric characteristics:

1.2.1   Edema,

1.2.2   Height,

1.2.3   Weight, and

1.2.4   Girth.

1.3   Arousal, mentation, and cognition:

1.3.1   Ability to learn and

1.3.2   Communication skills.

1.4   Assistive, adaptive, supportive, and protective devices:

    1.4.1   Short-term/long-term requirements for durable medical equipment (DME) and assistive devices, and

    1.4.2   Need for and proper use of assistive devices for ambulation and activities of daily living (ADLs).

1.5   Balance:

    1.5.1   All applicable surfaces and

    1.5.2   Different environmental conditions.

1.6   Community and work reintegration.

1.7   Cranial nerve integrity:

    1.7.1   Auditory function and

    1.7.2   Visual function.

1.8   Environmental, home, and workplace barriers:

    1.8.1   Prior and present functional status:

        1.8.1.1   In household,

        1.8.1.2   In community, and

        1.8.1.3   In workplace, if applicable;

    1.8.2   Homebound status, if applicable; and

    1.8.3   Home safety and physical environment:

        1.8.3.1   Emergency plan of care and

        1.8.3.2   Architectural barriers.

1.9   Ergonomics or body mechanics.

1.10 Gait:

    1.10.1   All applicable surfaces,

    1.10.2   Stairs, and

    1.10.3   Weight-bearing status.

1.11 Integumentary integrity.

1.12   Joint integrity and mobility.

1.13   Motor function:

    1.13.1   Posture,

    1.13.2   Coordination, and

    1.13.3   Administration of physical performance scales.

1.14   Muscle performance:

    1.14.1   Strength/force production and

    1.14.2   Motor control/movement quality.

1.15   Neuromotor development and sensory integration.

1.16   Orthotic requirements.

1.17   Pain:

    1.17.1   Use of appropriate pain measurement scale.

1.18   Posture:

    1.18.1   All applicable positions.

1.19   Prosthetic requirements.

1.20   Range of motion/muscle length.

1.21   Reflex integrity.

1.22   Self-care and home management:

    1.22.1   Bed mobility,

    1.22.2   Transfer status to all applicable surfaces,

    1.22.3   Gait analysis,

    1.22.4   Wheelchair mobility,

    1.22.5   Self-care activities, and

    1.22.6   Need for referrals to additional care providers and community resources.

1.23   Sensory integration examination.

1.24   Ventilation, respiration, and circulation.

1.25   Review of client's medical history:

    1.25.1 Current complaints with date of onset,

    1.25.2 Medication utilization, and

    1.25.3 Pertinent past history/complaints.

  1.26 Social and emotional environment:

    1.26.1 Identify client's support system,

    1.26.2 Assess ability of client's support system to care for client, and

    1.26.3 Identify client's financial resources.

2. The examination/evaluation is to be documented within APTA's Guidelines for Physical Therapy Documentation, third-party payer, and/or agency requirements, including but not limited to:

 2.1 The identified client problems that indicate the need for skilled physical therapy intervention;

 2.2 Measurable client outcomes that are linked to the identified problems (prognosis);

 2.3 The frequency and duration of physical therapy intervention, for that specific period, which is required to achieve the stated outcomes;

 2.4 Therapeutic interventions to be provided to the client throughout the course of treatment; and

 2.5 The skilled physical therapy interventions provided to the client during the initial visit.

3. The examination/evaluation visit must:

 3.1 Be dated;

 3.2 Be signed with the physical therapist's full name;

 3.3 Indicate the appropriate professional designation (e.g., PT);

 3.4 Indicate the therapist's license number, if applicable; and

 3.5 If applicable, indicate:

    3.5.1 Time the visit started,

    3.5.2 Time the visit was completed, and

    3.5.3 Total time spent with the client.

<u>Physical Therapy Plan of Care</u>

Guideline: Physical therapy services shall be:

1. Provided by or under the supervision of a licensed physical therapist in accordance with APTA's policy on *Direction, Delegation, and Supervision in Physical Therapy Services,* revised HOD 06-95-08-09);

2. Performed in accordance with the established plan of care documented following the examination/evaluation visit; and

3. Documented in accordance with APTA's *Guidelines for Physical Therapy Documentation,* regulatory requirements, and consistent with the agency's policies and procedures related to documentation.

Criteria: 1. The physical therapist's treatment interventions will be of such a complex nature that the skills of a physical therapist or physical therapist assistant are required.

2. The physical therapist will evaluate, document, and implement program changes, at each visit, as indicated by the performance of the client/caregiver.

    2.1 The physical therapist assistant will:

        2.1.1 Perform physical therapy procedures and related tasks that have been selected and delegated by the supervising physical therapist, and

        2.1.2 Document the response to training and progress at each visit, as indicated by the physical therapist.

3. The physical therapist will review the written plan of care with the client/caregiver and the physician and update the plan as required by:

    3.1 Federal home health rules and regulations;

    3.2 State home health regulations;

    3.3 Third-party payers, as applicable; and

    3.4 The agency's policies and procedures.

4. The physical therapist shall communicate and document conferences with other care providers treating the client regarding the client's problems, progress, and outcomes:

   4.1 Following the examination/evaluation,

   4.2 Prior to the client's discharge from physical therapy,

   4.3 No less than monthly during the course of the plan of care,

   4.4 In accordance with the agency's conference schedule, and

   4.5 As required by the reimbursing agent.

5. All communication demonstrating coordination of care between members of the client's multidisciplinary team will be documented.

   5.1 All documentation entries are to be included as a permanent part of the client's medical record.

6. Treatment visits made by a physical therapist or physical therapist assistant will include, but are not limited to:

   6.1 Vital sign monitoring, as indicated.

   6.2 Therapeutic interventions as delineated in the plan of care.

   6.3 Instructions to the client/caregiver.

   6.4 Assessment of the client's/caregiver's comprehension of the instructions.

   6.5 Assessment of the client's response to the therapeutic interventions.

   6.6 Documentation of the client's:

      6.6.1 Problems,

      6.6.2 Progress,

      6.6.3 Concerns, and

      6.6.4 Response to the plan of care.

   6.7 Discharge plans as delineated by the physical therapist.

7. The client's plan of care shall be updated, as required by regulatory bodies, by the physical therapist when the content of the plan has changed.

   7.1   This is to occur at least every 30 days or as the client's condition warrants an update.

8. The physical therapist and physical therapist assistant shall be knowledgeable of available community resources/services.

   8.1   The physical therapist may make recommendations for follow-up care in coordination with the agency that admitted the client.

   8.2   The physical therapist may utilize other agency care providers to assist with referrals to community resources.

9. The physical therapist or physical therapist assistant may instruct the home health aide in procedures as taught to the client/caregiver.

   9.1   The physical therapist or physical therapist assistant will report to the individual who has direct responsibility for home health aide supervision regarding the instructions provided to the home health aide.

American Physical Therapy Association References:
(APTA, 1111 North Fairfax Street, Alexandria, VA 22314-1488, 1-703-684-2782).

Guide to Physical Therapist Practice, 1997, [Publication No. P-139].

Guidelines for the Provision of Physical Therapy in the Home, Section on Community Home Health/American Physical Therapy Association, 1996 [Publication No. p-131].

SPEECH-LANGUAGE PATHOLOGY SERVICES

Information in this section is based on information from documents published and available through the American Speech-Language-Hearing Association.

Providers

Speech-language pathology services are provided by speech-language pathologists educated at the master's or doctoral degree level, and holding the Certificate of Clinical Competence (CCC) from the American Speech-Language-Hearing Association (ASHA), and, where applicable, state licensure. As primary care providers of communication treatment and other services, speech-language pathologists are autonomous professionals, and as such, do not require physician's orders or prescriptions to deliver care, unless required by a specific third-party payer.

Scope of Practice

The practice of speech-language pathology includes referral identification, assessment, consultation and counseling, and treatment of individuals with speech and language disorders resulting in communication disabilities, and/or swallowing disorders (dysphagia). Communicative function includes underlying processes including cognitive skills, memory, attention, perception, and auditory processing. Functional communication includes the ability to convey or receive a message effectively and independently, regardless of the mode.

Referral

The SLP receives referrals for patients who are suspected of having communication and/or swallowing disorders and screens for appropriateness of referral. The initial identification of patients appropriate for SLP services may be made by hospital discharge planners, physicians, family members, intake nurses, or other professional or support members of the home care team.

Assessment

The assessment process focuses on determining the level of functional communicative ability or oral motor function. Speech-Language pathologists use norm and criterion-referenced evaluations to determine the existence of a speech, language, and/or oral pharyngeal disorders. Box 3-4 lists some of these specific assessments. Data collected during the assessment process is used to determine the patient's diagnosis, predict the rehabilitation potential, and establish a treatment plan.

Box 3-4   Specific Assessments Which May be Performed by the Speech-Language Pathologist

Articulation/Phonology Assessment	Procedures to assess speech articulation/phonology, delineating strengths, deficits, contributing factors, and implications for functional communication.
Augmentative and Alternative Communication (ACC) Assessment	Procedures to determine the appropriateness of aids, techniques, symbols and/or strategies to augment or replace speech and enhance communication of patients/clients with expressive and/or receptive communication disorders.
Cognitive-Communication Assessment	Procedures to assess cognitive-communication impairments, delineating strengths, deficits, contributing factors, and implications for functional communication.
Comprehensive Speech-Language Pathology Assessment	Procedures for detailed analysis of speech, language, cognitive communication, or swallowing function.
Fluency Assessment	Procedures to assess aspects of speech fluency, delineating strengths, deficits, contributing and concomitant factors, and implications for functional communication.
Language Assessment for Adults	Procedures to assess the language systems of adults, delineating strengths, deficits, contributing factors and social, academic and vocational needs for using language functionally to listen, speak, read and write; and related cognitive-communication processes.

Orofacial Myofunctional Assessment	Procedures to assess orofacial myofunctional patterns for speech and related functions, delineating strengths, deficits, contributing factors, and implications.
Prosthetic/Adaptive Device Assessment	Procedures to identify and determine the appropriateness of prosthetic/ adaptive device(s) used to enhance communication.
Resonance and Nasal Airflow Assessment	Procedures to assess oral, nasal, and velopharyngeal function for speech production, delineating strengths, deficits, contributing factors, and implications for functional communication.
Swallowing Function Assessment	Procedures to assess the oral pharyngeal and related upper digestive structures and functions to determine swallowing function, and oropharyngeal/respiratory coordination.
Voice Assessment	Procedures to assess vocal structure and function, identifying strengths, deficits, contributing factors, and implications for functional communication.

*Modified from: **Preferred Practice Patterns for the Profession of Speech-Language Pathology**, ASHA, (1997), used with permission from the American Speech-Language-Hearing Association.*

Consultation and Counseling

The speech-language pathologist serves as a resource to agencies and health care providers on communication disorders, educating on issues related to appropriate referrals for speech, language, swallowing, and cognition needs.

Treatment

The SLP develops a treatment plan and initiates the provision of treatment for the purpose of increasing the patient's ability to achieve functional communicative independence, to improve oral motor functioning (e.g., swallowing), and to achieve understanding, compliance, and competency of the patient and caregivers in daily participation in therapeutic activities. Box 3-5 lists some of the interventions performed by the SLP.

Box 3-5   Speech-Language Pathology Interventions

Augmentative and Alternative Communication (ACC) System and/or Device Treatment/Orientation	Procedures to assist individuals to understand and use their personalized augmentative and alternative communication systems.
Fluency Treatment	Procedures for addressing fluency disorders and concomitant features of fluency disorders.
Orofacial Myofunctional Treatment	Procedure to facilitate the patient's ability to use appropriate orofacial myofunctional patterns.
Prosthetic/Adaptive Device Treatment/Orientation	Procedures to assist individuals to understand and use their customized prosthetic/adaptive device.
Swallowing Function Treatment	Procedures to facilitate the patient's ability to masticate and swallow more safely and more efficiently.
Treatment of Central Auditory Processing Disorders (CAPD) in Adults	Procedures to improve the communication abilities of an individual with a central auditory processing disorder.
Voice Treatment	Procedures for addressing disorders of voice production, including possible organic, neurologic, behavioral, and psychosocial etiologies, and alaryngeal speech disorders.

*Modified from: **Preferred Practice Patterns for the Profession of Speech-Language Pathology**, ASHA, (1997), Used with permission of the American Speech-Language-Hearing Association.*

Indications

A referral for speech-language pathology services would be indicated for patients with identified speech and language disorders that result in communication disabilities, or for the diagnosis and treatment of swallowing disorders (dysphagia). Home care providers should recognize situations involving existing home care patients where SLP referrals would be appropriate. Box 3-6 lists some of the potential diagnoses necessitating a SLP referral. These situations include patients who demonstrate a change in functional speech, swallowing or motivation, clearing of confusion or the remission of some other medical condition that previously contraindicated SLP services.[1]

Box 3-6   Sample List of Potential Diagnoses for Speech-Language Pathology Referrals

- Alzheimer's disease
- Amyotrophic Lateral Sclerosis (ALS)
- Brain tumor
- Cancer (CA)
- Cerebral vascular accident (CVA)
- Closed head injury (CHI) or Head trauma
- Gastrostomy
- Laryngectomy
- Meningitis
- Multiple Sclerosis (MS)
- Parkinson's Disease
- Tracheostomy

Copyright Marrelli and Associates, 1999.

ADDITIONAL RESOURCES FOR SPEECH-LANGUAGE PATHOLOGY

Excerpts reprinted from *Delivery of Speech-Language Pathology and Audiology Services in Home Care - Position Statement,* (1988) ASHA, Vol. 30, pp 77-79. with permission of the American Speech-Language-Hearing Association.

Delivery of Speech-Language Pathology and Audiology Services in Home Care

Delivery of speech-language pathology and audiology services in home care encompasses components which are unique to this setting as well as components that are generic to the delivery of speech-language pathology and audiology services regardless of work setting. The following list describes selected generic and specialized components considered important to the home setting.

[1]HIM-11 205.2 C.1

Generic Components

- Referrals - The speech-language pathologist and audiologist receive referrals on patients who are suspected of having a speech-language-hearing disorder or who are in need of speech-language pathology and/or audiology services. In addition, they also recommend appropriate interagency and intraagency referrals.

- Assessment - Norm and criterion-referenced evaluations are used by speech-language pathologists and audiologists to determine if a speech-language-hearing disorder exists. Data are collected and used to determine the patient's diagnosis and rehabilitation potential. In addition, the data are used to develop the patient's treatment plan, expected frequency and duration of treatment, discharge goals, and other recommendations when indicated.

- Treatment - The speech-language pathologist and audiologist intervene based upon their established treatment plans. These treatment plans are reassessed and revised as indicated until discharge goals are achieved or the patient has reached maximum potential for benefit from treatment.

- Family Involvement - When appropriate, the speech-language pathologist and audiologist involve the people present in the home so as to maximize treatment effectiveness.

- Recordkeeping - The speech-language pathologist and audiologist provide appropriate documentation which clearly and succinctly reports services.

- Utilization of Supportive Personnel - The speech-language pathologist and audiologist may utilize supportive personnel (for example, home care aides, speech-language pathology aides) to provide services under their supervision.

- Supervision - Speech-language pathologists and audiologists are involved in supervision which primarily involves that tasks and skills of "clinical supervision" may involve supervising peers, clinical fellows, and/or students completing professional education requirements. Tasks involved in supervision, competencies for effective clinical supervision and preparation for clinical supervisors are found in ASHA's position statement, "Clinical Supervision in Speech-Language Pathology and Audiology" (ASHA, 1985). On-site supervision is provided to students whenever delivering clinical services.

- Cultural/Linguistic Factors - Cultural/linguistic factors may necessitate modification of materials, the format of the evaluation and diagnostic and treatment approaches as well as the use of a bilingual evaluator and/or translator.

- Interdisciplinary Management - The speech-language pathologist and audiologist work with other appropriate professionals to 1) coordinate services, goals, and plans, and 2) ensure appropriate services are provided and continuity of care is maintained.

- Quality Assurance - The speech-language pathologist and audiologist evaluate and monitor on an ongoing basis the quality and appropriateness of speech-language-hearing services provided. When problems are identified through peer review, action plans are developed by the speech-language pathologist and audiologist to resolve these problems. Follow-up evaluations are then conducted in order to demonstrate problem resolution.

Specialized Components of Home Care

- Travel - The speech-language pathologist and audiologist may travel extensively when providing services in the home. Documentation of time and distance is maintained.

- Safety/Infection Control - The speech-language pathologist and audiologist may experience unique environmental and/or health concerns when going into the home. Special precautions related to patient care and personal safety need to be made.

- Reimbursement - Third-party payers have varied and specific regulations that allow billing reimbursement for speech-language pathology and audiology services. Speech-language pathologists and audiologists need to familiarize themselves with these requirements.

Role of the Speech-Language Pathologist and Audiologist

Services in the home are generally provided by a team of professionals. The home care team may include the speech-language pathologist, audiologist, home care aide, homemaker, family member or caregiver, nurse, nutritionist, occupational therapist, physical therapist, physician, psychologist, respiratory therapist, social worker, and special education teacher. The home care team is coordinated by a patient care manager. While the registered nurse frequently coordinates the services of the home care team, the speech-language pathologist and audiologist also are qualified to serve as patient care managers.

The professional role of the speech-language pathologist includes, but is not limited to:
1. conducting speech, language, and/or oral pharyngeal evaluations;
2. developing and recommending appropriate individual treatment/ education programs;

3. providing treatment;
4. referring to other health professionals;
5. instructing and counseling family members, nurses, and other members of the home care team;
6. providing referral and follow-up with other community resources;
7. recommending prosthetic and augmentative communication devices;
8. conducting hearing screenings;
9. providing aural rehabilitation in consultation with an audiologist;
10. participating in admission /discharge planning;
11. providing appropriate documentation;
12. supervising peers, clinical fellows, supportive personnel, and students in training;
13. providing inservice training to agency staff;
14. providing public education;
15. conducting research;
16. developing and participating in prevention activities;
17. directing and administering home care services; and
18. maintaining quality control.

Personnel Preparation

The Certificates of Clinical Competence (CCC) in Speech-Language Pathology and Audiology indicate that speech-language pathologists and audiologists have basic knowledge and clinical training related to the provision of services to various patient populations. In order to assure the most efficient and effective delivery of speech-language-audiology services in home care, it is important for speech-language pathologists and audiologists to acquire additional special knowledge and practicum experiences in a number of areas unique to home care. This knowledge and experience may be obtained from a variety of sources including graduate education programs, clinical fellowship year, professional practice, and continuing education. Areas of professional knowledge with which speech-language pathologists and audiologists need to be familiar, but to which they are not restricted, include the following:

1. treatment of neurologically impaired children and adults in the home;
2. provision of services to persons with communication problems and oral pharyngeal disorders resulting from trauma, severe illness, and/or surgery;
3. provision of services to infants and children including knowledge of pre-speech and language development;
4. family intervention techniques;

5. observation of patients within the home environment;
6. drugs/medications/illnesses and disabilities and their effects on communication;
7. infection control;
8. roles and responsibilities of other health care professionals;
9. participation on an interdisciplinary team;
10. medical terminology;
11. documentation required in home care; and
12. reimbursement and legislative issues impacting service delivery in home care.

Summary

Due to changing demographics, consumer preference, and priorities of the United States health care and educational systems, home care services are an increasingly vital area. Consequently, the number of communicatively impaired persons who need home based speech-language pathology and audiology services is increasing. This paper addresses the range of speech-language pathology and audiology services that may be provided in the home regardless of the payer source. It is the position of the American Speech-Language-Hearing Association that home based speech-language pathology and audiology services should be conducted by certified (and licensed where applicable) speech-language pathologists and audiologists and individuals who meet the educational requirement for certification and are receiving the supervised experience required for certification. It is essential that speech-language pathologists and audiologists working in home care (1) be familiar with all of the components of service delivery, (2) assume the various roles and responsibilities, and (3) develop the knowledge and skills outlined in this position statement.

Excerpts beginning on the next page are reprinted from *Guidelines for the Delivery of Speech-Language Pathology and Audiology Services in Home Care*, (1990), ASHA, 33(Suppl. 5), 29-34. With permission of the American Speech-Language-Hearing Association.

Guidelines for the Delivery of Speech-Language Pathology and Audiology Services in Home Care

Basic components of speech-language pathology and audiology services in the home care setting include identification and referral, assessment, treatment, case management, and consultation/education for the full range of communication and related disorders.

A. Identification and Referral

The initial identification of clients, who need referral for speech-language pathology or audiology services is made by hospital discharge planners, intake nurses, physicians, and other home care providers. Certain medial diagnoses often will trigger a referral. In-service training provided by the speech-language pathologists and audiologists is critical to ensure appropriate and complete referrals.

B. Assessment

The purpose of assessment is to ascertain the level of functional communicative ability; to gather information needed to design or revise treatment programs; and to provide a baseline against which to document progress, regression, or plateau.

An assessment should include the following information:
- Pertinent medical, educational, vocational, and psychosocial history;
- Diagnoses of communication and related disorders with date of onset and/or exacerbation (latest episode or recurrence of relevant illness, regression or progression);
- Prior speech-language pathology and audiology services and outcome of those services if available;
- Formal and/or informal measures. These may include standardized tests, direct observation of client behaviors; nonstandardized tests, and interviews/consultations with family, friends, or other professionals. Measures should address all aspects of functional communication. Based on the client's medical diagnosis and pertinent clinical information, appropriate diagnostic measures can be selected;
- Interpretation of test scores and assessment data;
- Environmental factors including opportunities for communication, and level of stimulation;

- Functional limitations regarding communication and related processes;
- Rehabilitation/habilitation potential; and
- Recommendations for intervention including selection and training for augmentative communication/assistive listening devices or hearing aids, or for the need to establish a maintenance program. The audiologist faces particular challenges when providing assessment of a home care client. It often will be necessary to conduct audiologic assessment in a less than ideal environment.

The audiologist should take into account the noise levels of the test environment, the need for calibration and maintenance of equipment that is transported, the client's contributing health factors, and the client's communication needs.

An assessment of potential benefit from hearing aids and assistive listening devices should address the client's degree of independence, fine motor coordination, availability of help from family members and other caregivers, and the communication needs of the home environment.

C. Treatment

Treatment within the home care environment is based on acceptable methods of practice established by the professions of speech-language pathology and audiology. The focus must be to help the client become more communicatively functional within his/her environment. Interventions should be based on the client's medical history and diagnosis, the course of prior treatment, the findings of a current assessment, the needs and priorities of the client and his/her family/caregiver within the natural context of the home environment.

The purpose of treatment is to increase the client's ability to achieve functional communicative independence, to improve oral motor functioning (e.g., swallowing ability), and to ensure family/caregiver understanding, interaction and participation.

Family members/caregivers should have an understanding of the assessment, prognosis, and treatment provided to the client. The establishment of a treatment plan should be a cooperative activity through which each person's responsibilities and expectations are delineated. The treatment goals should be derived from the clinician's, client's, and family members'/caregiver's input. Counseling should provide strategies to increase the client's communication success in the home.

Treatment plans, home programs, and maintenance programs should be developed, documented in the clinical record, implemented and periodically reassessed and revised. Treatment should continue until goals have been achieved or until the client has reached maximum benefit from treatment.

Treatment provided by audiologists includes the recommendation and fitting of hearing aids, assistive listening devices, and other aural rehabilitation services. Evaluation and fitting procedures must be modified as appropriate for the home environment and the abilities of the client. Other family members and caregivers should be involved to ensure the successful use of hearing aids and assistive devices.

D. Case Management

Case management involves the coordination of the full range of service delivery to a particular client and is a primary feature of service delivery in home care. Therefore, as part of an interdisciplinary team, the speech-language pathologist and audiologist should collaborate with other health care providers involved in the client's care. Interdisciplinary communication, cooperation and coordination are considered essential to quality services. In some cases, the speech-language pathologist and audiologist may assume the responsibility of case manager. As case manager, the speech-language pathologist and audiologist would provide care that meets the needs of the client; coordinate the care provided by all professionals, so that all are working toward the same goals and reinforcing each other's goals; ensure that the client and family/caregiver are involved in and agree to the established goals, care plan, and discharge plan; and ensure that care provided meets any eligibility criteria.

As a general rule, the speech-language pathologist and audiologist should keep other health care providers informed about the treatment, goals, and progress in order to facilitate the overall care provided and be aware of all other health care services being provided and the goals of those services. This coordination of care should be done on an ongoing basis and at specified time intervals with coordination of care documented in the chart.

The speech-language pathologist and audiologist are responsible for communicating any change in the client's health status to the appropriate medical care provider, and refer to other health care providers as appropriate.

E. Consultation and Education

1) Consultation. The speech-language pathologist and audiologist serve as resources and consultants to community agencies and other health care providers on communication disorders and related issues. Information provided may pertain to appropriate referrals, admission/discharge, and the nature of speech, language, hearing swallowing, cognition, and related disorders. Consultation may involve administrative issues such as revising agency forms, conducting surveys, developing policies and procedures and participating in the claims appeal process.

2) Education. The speech-language pathologist and audiologist can provide in-services and workshops on communication and related disorders to other health care providers. These activities can help home care providers understand how to improve communication with their clients and how to make appropriate referrals.

American Speech-Language-Hearing Association References:

(ASHA, 10801 Rockville Pike, Rockville, MD 20852-3279, 1-301-897-5700).

Scope of Practice in Speech-Language Pathology (1996), <u>ASHA</u>, Vol. 38, (Suppl. 16), 16-20.

Guidelines for the Delivery of Speech-Language Pathology and Audiology Services in Home Care, (1990), <u>ASHA</u>, Vol. 33 (Suppl. 5), pp 29-34.

Position Statement. Delivery of Speech-Language Pathology and Audiology Services in Home Care, (1998), <u>ASHA</u>, Vol. 30, pp 77-79.

Preferred Practice Patterns for the Profession of Speech-Language Pathology, (1997).

ASHA Desk Reference, (1985).

OCCUPATIONAL THERAPY SERVICES

Information in this section is based on information from documents published and available through the American Occupational Therapy Association.

Providers

Occupational therapy services are provided by a registered occupational therapist (OTR) or a certified occupational therapy assistant (COTA) under the direction and supervision of an occupational therapist.

Occupational therapists are graduates of an occupation therapy curriculum accredited by the Accreditation Council for Occupational Therapy Education (ACOTE).

Occupational therapists may achieve board certification in the clinical areas of neurorehabilitation or pediatrics through the American Occupational Therapy Association.

Occupational therapy assistants are graduates of a two-year associate degree or one of a limited number of certificate programs. State law, third-payer coverage requirements, personnel availability and individual home health agency policy will determine the extent to which assistants are used in delivering home care services in a given demographic area. The *HIM-11* outlines care delivered by the occupational therapy assistant, under the delegation and supervision of an occupational therapist, as a covered service under the Medicare home health benefit, after eligibility for home health services has been established by virtue of a prior need for one of the primary/initial qualifying services (nursing, physical therapy, or speech-language pathology). When determined appropriate by the occupational therapist, the occupational therapy assistant may be assigned to perform selected therapeutic interventions, communication and documentation activities. The supervising occupational therapist should be actively involved in ongoing assessment of the occupational therapy assistant's level of competency, to ensure that professional activities are appropriately delegated, and based on the individual assistant's performance capacity.

Scope of Practice

Occupational therapy is the use of purposeful activity or interventions designed to achieve functional outcomes which promote health, prevent injury or disability, and which develop, improve, sustain or restore the highest possible level of independence of any individual who has an injury, illness, cognitive impairment, psychosocial dysfunction, mental illness, developmental or learning disability, physical disability, or other disorder or condition.[2]

---

[2] The American Occupation Therapy Association (1994, July) Definition of occupational therapy practice for state regulation. The American Occupational Therapy Association, Inc. policy manual

Occupational therapy services include patient screening, referral acceptance, evaluation, intervention planning, intervention implementation, transition and discontinuation of services.

Patient Screening

The occupational therapist, or occupational therapy assistant under the supervision of the occupational therapist, may participate in selection and administration of specific screening activities, obtaining and reviewing client-specific data to determine the need for further evaluation and intervention.

Referral Acceptance

A registered occupational therapist accepts and responds to referrals in accordance with AOTA's Statement of Occupational Therapy Referral[3], and in compliance with laws or regulations. When the needs of the client can best be served by the expertise of other professionals or services, the occupational therapists refers clients to appropriate resources.

Evaluation

The occupational therapist evaluates the client's level of function related to performance areas, performance components, and performance contexts. (See Boxes 3-7, 3-8 and 3-9).

Box 3-7 Uniform Terminology and Definitions for Occupational Therapy Patient Performance Evaluation

Performance areas	• Broad categories of human activity that are typically part of daily life. They are activities of daily living, work and productive activities, and play or leisure activities.
Performance components	• Elements of performance required for successful engagement in performance areas, including sensorimotor, cognitive, psychosocial, and psychological aspects

[3]American Occupational Therapy Association (1994), Statement of Occupational Referral. *American Journal of Occupational Therapy*, 48, 1034.

Performance contexts	• Situations or factors that influence an individual's engagement in desired and/or required performance areas. Performance contexts consist of temporal aspects (chronological, developmental, life cycle, disability status) and environmental aspects (physical, social, political, cultural)

Modified from American Occupational Therapy Association, Uniform terminology for Occupational Therapy-Third edition. *American Journal of Occupational Therapy*, 49, 1994, 1047-1054. Used with permission of the American Occupational Therapy Association.

Box 3-8   Specific Occupational Therapy Assessment Areas

• Cognitive assessment	Including general alertness and orientation to surroundings, attention span, memory, judgment, and the ability to follow directions
• Environmental contexts and safety assessment	Including the patient's ability to function safely in his or her own environment, presence of safety hazards or fall risks, and the need for environmental modifications or adaptive equipment
• Living situation assessment	Including availability of caregiver(s), and access to community services/supports
• Medical history	Including significant medical and psychiatric history
• Participation in major life roles and interests assessment	Includes role classifications such as homemaker, retiree, volunteer, or grandparent
• Physical limitations assessment	Range of motion, strength, limitations in endurance, and activity tolerance
• Recent psychosocial stressors assessment	Identification of stressors that are contributing to the patients functional decline
• Sensory and perceptual deficits assessment	Including deficits in vision, hearing, proprioception, and tactile areas

Modified from: *Guidelines for Occupational Therapy Practice in Home Health*, AOTA, 1995, pp. 47-8. Used with permission of the American Occupational Therapy Association.

The occupational therapist selects, performs, analyzes, interprets, and summarizes assessment data to determine the current functional status and drive the care plan development activities. The occupational therapist follows defined protocols when standardized assessments are used, and completes evaluation documentation within the time frames, formats and standards required by the practice settings, government agencies, payers, and external accreditation bodies.

Intervention Plan

Based on the findings of the evaluation and the desires and expectations of the patient and appropriate others, the occupational therapist develops the intervention plan. The care plan includes patient-centered, measurable goals, which are behavioral, functional and contextually relevant to the individual patient.

Intervention

The occupational therapist implements the care plan through use of specified purposeful activities or therapeutic methods. Purposeful activities refer to goal-directed behaviors or tasks that result in active participation in self-maintenance, work, leisure, and play. An activity is purposeful if the individual is an active, voluntary participant and if the activity is directed toward a goal that the individual considers meaningful. "The therapeutic purposes for which purposeful activity is used include mastery of a new skill, restoration of a deficient ability, compensation for functional disability, health maintenance, or prevention of dysfunction."[4]

The occupational therapist utilizes the practice of "grading" activities, or progressively changing the process, tools, or environment associated with a given activity to gradually increase or decrease the performance demands. Grading can be achieved by modifying an activity's temporal conditions (e.g. the duration or sequence), or environmental conditions (e.g., the position or location of the patient, or the use of supportive or assistive devices). Occupational therapists also utilize the strategy of adaptation to enable a patient to achieve a therapeutic goal or functional outcome. Adaptation is a process that changes an aspect of the activity or environment to facilitate successful patient performance in a particular functional task. Adaptation strategies may include the use of assistive devices and techniques to improve the level of patient performance.[5] Boxes 3-11, 3-12, and 3-13 provide examples of home adaptations which occupational therapists may utilize or suggest to improve patient function and safety.

[4]American Occupational Therapy Association, Position Paper. Purposeful Activity. *The American Journal of Occupational Therapy*, 47, 1993, 1081-1082.
[5]AOTA, Position Paper. Purposeful Activity.

Box 3-9   Occupational Therapy Interventions

Activities of daily living (ADLs) interventions	Techniques to improve deficits, or affects of deficits, in ADLs, including toileting, bathing, dressing, and eating
Cognitive status interventions	Techniques to improve deficits, or affects of deficits, in attention span, memory problem solving, sequencing and categorization
Environmental adaptation	Techniques to improve deficits, or the affects of deficits in functional mobility and/or safety through architectural barriers through home modification or durable medical equipment (DME) requirements
Functional communication interventions	Techniques to facilitate telephone use or emergency response mechanisms, also handwriting skills
Motor Coordination / Functional mobility ventions	Techniques to improve deficits, or affects of deficits, in gross and fine motor inter-coordination, dexterity, lateral and bilateral integration, range of motions measurements, muscle tone, postural control and alignment, transfer ability, and object manipulation
Instrumental activities of daily living (IADLs) interventions	Techniques to improve deficits, or affects of deficits, in IADLs, including housework, meal preparation, cooking, laundry, money management and community access
Medication administration	Techniques to improve patient's function in medication administration when cognitive or motoric deficits are identified
Perceptual processing interventions	Techniques to improve deficits, or affects of deficits, in body scheme, right-left discrimination, depth perception, spatial relations, eye/hand coordination, and figure ground awareness

Sensory status interventions	Techniques to improve deficits, or affects of deficits, in sensory awareness and processing abilities
Splinting interventions	Techniques to improve function, decrease pain and/or prevent deformity through recommendation, fabrication/fitting, monitoring and instruction in splint use

Modified from: *Guidelines for Occupational Therapy Practice in Home Health*, AOTA, (1995), Chapter 5, pages 31-35. Used with permission of the American Occupational Therapy Association.

Transition Services

With involvement of the patient, caregivers, family, team and community resources, the occupational therapist develops a formal transition plan to meet the patient's individual discharge planning needs.

Discontinuation of Services

The OT discharges the patient from services upon achievement of the predetermined therapy goals, achievement of the patient's maximum benefit from OT services, or request by the patient to discontinue OT services. Discontinuation activities follow an identified discharge plan that identifies and addresses appropriate follow-up activities and resources. The OT identifies and documents changes in the patient's status between the initial evaluation and discharge, or the treatment outcomes.

Indications

Referral for occupational therapy services is appropriate for those individuals with motor, sensory, cognitive, perceptual, emotional, or social deficits associated with illness or injury. See Boxes 3-10, 3-11, 3-12 and 3-13 for specific indications for occupational therapy interventions.

Box 3-10   Sample List of Potential Diagnoses
for Occupational Therapy Referrals

- Alzheimer's Disease
- Amputation
- Amyotrophic Lateral Sclerosis (ALS)
- Asthma
- Coronary Artery Bypass Graft (CABG)
- Cancer (CA)
- Cerebral vascular accident (CVA)
- Closed head injury (CHI) and Head trauma
- Collagen disorders
- Congestive Heart Failure (CHF)
- Chronic Obstructive Pulmonary Disease (COPD)
- Depression and Psychiatric disorders
- Development delay
- Fractures
- Hand and upper extremity (UE) injuries
- Joint replacement
- Mastectomy
- Multiple Sclerosis (MS)
- Myocardial Infarction (MI)
- Osteoarthritis (OA)
- Paraplegia
- Parkinson's Disease
- Psychological disorder (e.g. depression, schizophrenia)
- Quadriplegia
- Rheumatoid arthritis (RA)
- Spinal cord injury (SCI)
- Visual disorder

Box 3-11 Bathtub Barriers and Adaptations

Problem	Possible Solutions
Slippery bathtub floor	• Use rubber suction-grip tub mats
Bathtub sliding glass doors prevent easy entry to tub	• Remove doors from track. Substitute plastic curtain, hung with hooks and a spring tension bar.
Poor standing balance	• Use bathtub bench or transfer tub bench.
Unable to clean perianal area	• Use bathtub bench (often square shaped) with keyhole opening, combined with use of long-handled sponge.
Limited funds for bathtub bench or bathtub seat	• Use sturdy chair (e.g., molded plastic chair or metal kitchen chair with rubber crutch tips on feet; possibly covered with plastic trash bag, although watch safety due to slipperiness of plastic bag.)
Bathtub bench too low	• Utilize adjustable height bathtub bench legs.
Unstable sitting balance	• Bathtub bench with a back. *Note: Bathtub bench backs may be contraindicated for large individuals due to their tendency to push a person forward.
Unable to enter bathtub standing up	• Use bathtub bench with transfer board or transfer bench. Place one side in the tub and the other end placed outside tub; comes in padded or flat bench models.
Desire to sit in water, rather than on bathtub bench	• Order bathtub hydraulic lift chair, with swivel seat, to aid transfers. Inflatable bathtub chairs are less costly, but be careful of patient's stability if recommending use.
Desire to control water flow	• Recommend long-handled, hand-held shower hose with lightweight shower head. *Note: Control of water ideally

	located in showerhead handle for individual to control, rather than on the wall, due to fluctuating water pressure. Also helps individual remain seated, rather than needing to lean forward to reach water controls.
Sporadic water temperature	• Heat-sensitive safety valve installed in hot water line. *Note: Especially important for individuals with sensory deficits, those who live alone, or those who bathe unattended.
Family members want to use regular shower head	• Use diverter valve, available in hardware stores; attaches hand-held shower hose to showerhead, allowing dual use of regular shower head and hand-held shower hose.
Unable to stand or walk into shower or bathtub; unable to transfer onto bathtub bench	• Recommend rolling shower chair; usually high-backed, waterproof chair with large back wheels; can be used independently by some clients (i.e., paraplegics); must have roll-in shower.
Unable to use bathtub	• Utilize roll-in shower (no threshold); normally built by contractor according to American National Standards Institute specifications (ANSI, 1992)
Slippery bathroom scatter rugs	• Remove scatter rugs to prevent slipping. If patient prefers rugs, stabilize them with carpet tape or substitute rugs with a rubber tub mat on the floor.
Unable to see mirror	• Install mirror on wall at appropriate height. Install flexible mirror extenders or prop a mirror behind the faucets.

Reprinted from **Guidelines for Occupational Therapy Practice in Home Health,** *page 37, AOTA, 1995, Used with permission of American Occupational Therapy Association.*

Box 3-12   Kitchen Barriers and Adaptations

Problem	Solutions
Unable to reach sink from wheelchair	• Remove sink doors • Remove cabinet threshold • Pad drain pipe with insulated rubber. • Open sink doors and put feet on the inside shelf or threshold • Place overturned dishpan in sink and wash dishes on top of it to raise height of the bottom. • Use tilted mirror above sink to assist visual contact with dishes
Unable to reach stove from wheelchair	• Put tilted mirror above stove. • Use long-handled utensils. • Ideally, stove knobs should be located in front of stove. *Note: If stove knobs are in back, patient can use long-handled reacher or alternatives (i.e., potato masher) • Discourage wearing long, flowing sleeves.
Unstable standing balance	• May want to disconnect front burners to prevent patient from being burned. • Use high stools with rubber feet. • Movable high stools can be made by hammering nylon glides with spikes to bottom of stool legs, although make sure patient has good balance and cognitive awareness before recommending them.
Difficulty reaching into kitchen cabinets	• Pull-out storage units. • Turntables • Rearrange shelves so that frequently used items are on low shelves and special occasion items are on higher shelves. • Reachers. *Note: Can make reacher bag for walker/wheelchair by sewing two

	pieces of material together to form long tube; tie tube to walker or wheelchair. Reacher with locking lever effective for those with limited grasp. • Use regular kitchen or spaghetti tongs to reach items. • Lower shelves.
Unable to transport items	• Use two- or three-tiered wheeled cart; ideal with handles and feet with ball bearing casters that swivel 360°. • Apron with large pockets. • Wheelchair bags under or on back of wheelchair • Walker/crutch bags or baskets (beware of instability caused by too much weight in bags). • Walker bags with pockets, ideally hung inside walker, to reduce chance of walker falling forward. • Carry spillable (i.e., cup of coffee) in small dishpan • Place lids on all items that could spill, and on hot items.
Cannot reach/use countertop	• Pull out medium height drawer and over top with breadboard, cookie sheet, or tray. *Note: Can cut large circle in center of breadboard to stabilize mixing bowls.

*Reprinted from **Guidelines for Occupational Therapy Practice in Home Health,** page 38, AOTA, 1995, Used with permission of American Occupational Therapy Association.*

Box 3-13   Home Access Barriers and Adaptations

Problem	Solutions
Door too narrow for wheelchair	• Remove door. • Remove doorstops. • Substitute a curtain for the door. • Use alternate room. • Replace door with an offset door hinge, available from hardware stores
Unable to maneuver over door threshold (sill)	• Remove door threshold (sill). • Place thin mat over door threshold to eliminate the threshold hump.
Unable to turn door knobs or faucets	• Replace with levers. • Provide knob turner
Carpeting too thick for easy maneuvering (i.e., shag)	• Remove or replace carpeting; using indoor-outdoor carpeting is ideal for wheelchair and/or walking. • Replace with tile floors.
Steps	• Place handrails on both sides. *Note: If possible, extend railing beyond top and bottom step to allow individuals to continue holding on once they reach the top/bottom. • Attach a door pull (i.e., U-shaped handle or sturdy knob) to doorframe to give individuals a sturdy handhold to grab. • Install portable or permanent ramps • Use motorized stair glides - usually require at least a 22" stair width, although 28" stair width is recommended. Usually available for two levels of stairs. Consultation with a medical equipment dealer is highly recommended to assist in choosing and installing appropriate stair glide for the patient. • Motorized porch lifts - require a firm foundation (cement pad), access to home entrance, and a safety gate to

	prevent falling off lift. Consultation with a medical equipment dealer is highly recommended to provide installation assistance and specific model and safety features needed for the patient.
Stair climbing	• If patient cannot transport walker aids independently, a second walker, cane, or wheelchair may be needed on the second floor.
Floor surfaces	• Eliminate throw rugs. • Tape rug edges down with rug tape. • Use larger rugs. • Instruct patient to observe changes between floor coverings (i.e., rugs versus linoleum).
Electrical cords	• Place around room perimeter. • Tape to floor.
Furniture crowding	• Discuss repositioning furniture with patient and family.
Doorbell ringing/access	• Assess entranceway accessibility, ability to open/close door, ability to use door locks. • Use flashing light system (or other visual identification) for hearing impaired.

*Reprinted from **Guidelines for Occupational Therapy Practice in Home Health,** page 39, AOTA, 1995, Used with permission of American Occupational Therapy Association.*

ADDITIONAL RESOURCES FOR OCCUPATIONAL THERAPY

Excerpts from *Standards of Practice for Occupational Therapy*, (1998) American Occupational Therapy Association, Bethesda, MD. Used with permission of the American Occupational Therapy Association.

Standards of Practice for Occupational Therapy

Preface

The Standards of Practice for Occupational Therapy are requirements for the occupational therapy practitioner (registered occupational therapist and certified occupational therapy assistant) for the delivery of occupational therapy services that are client centered and interactive in nature (American Occupational Therapy Association [AOTA], 1995). The registered occupational therapist supervises the certified occupational therapy assistant, and both work together in a collaborative manner to meet the needs of the client. However, the registered occupational therapist is ultimately responsible and accountable for the delivery of occupational therapy services. This document identifies minimum standards for occupational therapy practice.

The minimum educational requirements for the registered occupational therapists are described in the current *Essentials and Guidelines of an Accredited Educational Program for the Occupational Therapist* (AOTA, 1991). The minimum educational requirements for the certified occupational therapy assistant are described in the current *Essentials and Guidelines of an Accredited Educational Program for the Occupational Therapy Assistant* (AOTA, 1991).

Referral

1. A registered occupational therapist accepts and responds to referrals in accordance with AOTA's *Statement of Occupational Therapy Referral* (AOTA, 1994) and in compliance with laws or regulations.
2. A registered occupational therapist accepts and responds to referrals for evaluation or evaluation with intervention in performance areas, performance components, or performance contexts when clients may have a functional limitation or disability or may be at risk for a disabling condition.
3. A registered occupational therapist refers clients to appropriate resources when the needs of the client can best be served by the expertise of other professionals or services.
4. An occupational therapy practitioner educates current and potential referral sources about the scope of occupational therapy services and the process of initiating occupational therapy services.

Screening

1. A registered occupational therapist screens independently or as a member of a team in accordance with laws and regulations. A certified occupational therapy assistant may contribute to the screening process under the supervision of a registered occupational therapist.

2. A registered occupational therapist selects screening methods appropriate to the client's performance context.

3. A registered occupational therapist communicates screening results and recommendations to the appropriate person, group, or organization. A certified occupational therapy assistant may contribute to this process under the supervision of a registered occupational therapist.

Evaluation

1. A registered occupational therapist evaluates performance areas, performance components, and performance contexts. A certified occupational therapy assistant may contribute to the evaluation process under the supervision of a registered occupational therapist.

2. An occupational therapy practitioner educates clients and appropriate others about the purposes and procedures of the occupational therapy evaluation.

3. A registered occupational therapist selects assessments to evaluate the client's level of function related to performance areas, performance components, and performance contexts.

4. An occupational therapy practitioner follows defined protocols when standardized assessments are used.

5. A registered occupational therapist analyzes, interprets, and summarizes assessment data to determine the client's current functional status and to develop an appropriate intervention plan. The certified occupational therapy assistant may contribute to this process under the supervision of a registered occupational therapist.

6. A registered occupational therapist completes and documents occupational therapy evaluation results within the time frames, formats, and standards established by practice settings, government agencies, external accreditation programs, and payers. A certified occupational therapy assistant may contribute to documentation of

evaluation results under the supervision of a registered occupational therapist and in accordance with laws or regulations.

7. A registered occupational therapist communicates evaluation results, within the boundaries of client confidentiality, to the appropriate person, group, or organization. A certified occupational therapy assistant may contribute to this process under the supervision of a registered occupational therapist.

8. A registered occupational therapist recommends additional consultations when the results of the evaluation indicate that intervention by other professionals would be beneficial.

Intervention Plan

1. A registered occupational therapist develops and documents an intervention plan that is based on the results of the occupational therapy evaluation and the desires and expectations of the client and appropriate others about the outcome of service. A certified occupational therapy assistant may contribute to the intervention plan under the supervision of a registered occupational therapist.

2. A registered occupational therapist ensures that the intervention plan is documented within time frames, formats, and standards established by the practice settings, agencies, external accreditation programs, and payers.

3. A registered occupational therapist includes in the intervention plan client-centered goals that are clear, measurable, behavioral, functional, contextually relevant, and appropriate to the client's needs, desire, and expected outcomes. A certified occupational therapy assistant may contribute to this process.

4. A registered occupational therapist includes in the intervention plan the scope, frequency, duration of services, and the needs of the client.

5. A registered occupational therapist reviews the intervention plan with the client and appropriate others. A certified occupational therapy assistant may contribute to this process.

Intervention

1. A registered occupational therapist implements the intervention plan through the use of specified purposeful activities or therapeutic methods that are meaningful to the client and are effective methods for enhancing occupational performance. A certified occupational

therapy assistant may implement the intervention plan under the supervision of a registered occupational therapist.

2. An occupational therapy practitioner informs clients and appropriate others regarding the relative benefits and risks of the intervention.

3. An occupational therapy practitioner maintains or seeks current information on resources relevant to the client's needs.

4. A registered occupational therapist reevaluates during the intervention process and documents changes in the client's goals, performance and needs. A certified occupational therapy assistant may contribute to the reevaluation process.

5. A registered occupational therapist modifies the intervention process to reflect changes in client status, desires, and response to intervention. A certified occupational therapy assistant may identify the need for modifications and may contribute to the intervention modifications under the supervision of a registered occupational therapist.

6. An occupational therapy practitioner documents the occupational therapy services provided within the time frames, formats, and standards established by the practice settings, agencies, external accreditation programs, and payers.

Transition Services

1. A registered occupational therapist prepares a formal transition plan that is based on identified needs. A certified occupational therapy assistant may contribute to the preparation of a formal transition plan.

2. An occupational therapy practitioner facilitates the transition process in cooperation with the client, family members, significant others, team, and community resources and individuals, when appropriate.

Discontinuation

1. A registered occupational therapist discontinues services when the client has achieved predetermined goals, has achieved maximum benefit from occupational therapy services, or does not desire to continue services. A certified occupational therapy assistant may recommend discontinuation of occupational therapy services to the supervising registered occupational therapist.

2. A registered occupational therapist prepares and implements a discontinuation plan that addresses appropriate follow-up resources. A certified occupational therapy assistant may contribute to the implementation of a discontinuation plan under the supervision of a registered occupational therapist.

3. A registered occupational therapist documents changes in the client's status between the initial evaluation and discontinuation of services. A certified occupational therapy assistant may contribute to the process under the supervision of a registered occupational therapist.

4. A registered occupational therapist documents recommendations for follow-up or reevaluation, when applicable.

American Occupational Therapy Association References:

(AOTA, 4720 Montgomery Lane, Bethesda, MD 20814-3425, 1-301-652-2682.)

The Guide to Occupational Therapy Practice. American Journal of Occupational Therapy, (1999), Vol. 53, No. 3.

Standards of Practice for Occupational Therapy, (1998), Linda K. Thomson, MOT, OT(C) , FAOTA, Chairperson-Commission on Practice/American Occupational Therapy Association.

Guidelines for Occupational Therapy Practice in Home Health, (1995), publication order #1134.

Occupational therapy roles. *American Journal of Occupational Therapy*, (1993), Vol. 47, pp 1087-1099.

Statement of Occupational Therapy Referral, *The American Journal of Occupational Therapy*, (1994), Vol. 48, No. 11, p. 1034.

Definition of Occupational Therapy Practice for State Regulation, (1994, July) *The American Occupational Therapy Association, Inc. Policy Manual* (Association Policy 5.3.1).

Position Paper: Purposeful Activity, *The American Journal of Occupational Therapy*, (1993), Vol. 47, No. 12, pp 1081-1082.

PART FOUR
Assessment: The Process

The assessment is the organized process of reviewing and verifying existing data and collecting additional data demonstrating the patient's current status in order to determine patient problems and care needs.

Referral

The therapy assessment process begins upon receipt of referral information. Prior to the assessment visit, the therapist reviews the referral information to ensure that the information is legible and complete. The agency and therapist should work together to ensure that an efficient referral process is in place, allowing consistent and timely communication of all information necessary to allow thorough evaluation and care planning activities. It goes without saying that there must be physician's orders prior to the provision of any care, including the assessment or evaluation visit.

Referral information should include:
- Patient demographic information
  - Primary caregiver information
  - Alternate contact information
  - Agency identification number
  - Date of birth
- Medical information
  - Primary and/or therapy diagnoses with onset dates
  - Secondary diagnoses with onset dates
  - Surgical procedures with dates
  - Significant medical information or conditions affecting rehabilitation potential
  - Prior level of function
  - Precautions and contraindications
  - Recent facility admission(s) with length of stay and discharge date(s)
  - Copy of facility continuity of care
- Physician / referral information
  - Physician's name and contact information
  - Therapy orders
  - Additional services ordered
  - Known restrictions or contraindications
  - DNR orders or advanced directives

- Payer Information
  - Payer source with contact information
  - Covered benefits
  - Authorization/reauthorization status and requirements
  - Identification numbers

Whenever possible, any incomplete or ambiguous information (i.e., weight bearing status, specific activity restrictions) should be clarified through contact with the home health agency, referring facility, or physician's office prior to the assessment visit.

Scheduling the Assessment

Upon completion of the referral information review, the therapist should make initial phone contact with the patient to schedule the assessment visit. The assessment visit should be scheduled in a timely manner, consistent with time requirements prescribed by the physician, payer, regulatory or accreditation bodies, or agency policy, and the patient's needs. The therapist should introduce him/herself and the home care agency, and identify the physician responsible for the therapy referral. The general purpose for the therapy referral should be discussed (i.e., "Dr. Jones recommended you have a speech therapy evaluation after your nurse reported that you were having difficulty swallowing.") Upon agreement by the patient to receive the service, a visit time should be set. Depending on the individual situation, additional determinations may need to be made to facilitate assessment activities (i.e., Has the case been opened? Has necessary equipment been delivered? Will a caregiver be available for necessary instruction? Does the patient have other scheduled visits or activities that will interfere with the scheduled time?) Answers to these or other questions will aid in determining an appropriate assessment time. The therapist should verify the address, and inquire about any special instructions (i.e., finding the home, entering the home or secured residence, parking considerations, etc.)

The Assessment Visit

The therapist should arrive at the patient's home at or near the predetermined appointment time, prepared with all tools and materials necessary for assessment, intervention, documentation, and patient teaching activities. Assessment data collection begins as the therapist approaches the patient's home, observing the environmental conditions and evaluating their potential impact on the patient's health, safety and function.

In most cases, the initial visit begins with a social phase, in which the therapist, patient, and caregiver(s) begin to build rapport. The therapist may immediately begin to demonstrate a respect for the patient's rights by allowing the patient to determine where the initial discussions will occur, where the therapist could sit, etc. Even during the social phase, the therapist is collecting assessment information (i.e., Is the patient able to get to the front door? Are they in pain? Are any deficits in functional communication apparent?)

The therapist reviews the referral information with the patient and caregiver and collects additional information through patient or caregiver report, observation, and physical assessment activities. In addition to collecting information dealing with the patient's physical functional status, a safety assessment is completed, identifying environmental (i.e. throw rugs, loose railings) or behavioral or performance issues (i.e. inadequate airway protection with eating/swallowing, poor compliance with precautions) that pose immediate, or potential future risk. The patient's homebound status is also assessed. Readers are referred to the homebound discussion in Part One for more information. As patient problems are identified through the assessment, the therapist begins to develop the patient care plan. The therapist should share the identified problems with the patient, and discuss potential goals and interventions. Care should be taken that understanding and agreement exists between the therapist and the patient and caregiver(s) regarding the desired outcomes and necessary interventions, including the anticipated visit frequency and duration. Patient understanding and acceptance with the plan of care is crucial in achieving outcomes, and is necessary for compliance with Medicare and accreditation requirements.

Documentation or data collection forms are a very important component to a successful patient assessment. Examples of a PT, SLP and OT Evaluation, follow respectively in (Figures 4-1, 4-2, and 4-3) for your review.

After the assessment activities and any skilled therapy interventions are completed, the therapist completes any necessary communication and documentation activities and the next therapy visit is scheduled. The patient should be given a means of contacting the therapist for issues related to the therapy plan or to reschedule visits.

Figure 4-1

PHYSICAL THERAPY EVALUATION

DATE OF SERVICE _____ / _____ / _____

OBJECTIVE DATA TESTS AND SCALES PRINTED ON REVERSE.

TIME IN _____ OUT _____

HOMEBOUND REASON: ☐ Needs assistance for all activities ☐ Residual weakness
☐ Requires assistance to ambulate ☐ Confusion, unable to go out of home alone
☐ Unable to safely leave home unassisted ☐ Severe SOB, SOB upon exertion
☐ Dependent upon adaptive device(s) ☐ Medical restrictions
☐ Other (specify) _____

TYPE OF EVALUATION
☐ Initial   ☐ Interim   ☐ Final
SOC DATE _____ / _____ / _____
(If Initial Evaluation, complete Physical Therapy Care Plan)

PT ORDERS: ☐ Evaluation ☐ Therapeutic Exercise ☐ Transfer Training ☐ Home Program Instruction ☐ Gait Training ☐ Chest PT
☐ Ultrasound ☐ Electrotherapy ☐ Prosthetic Training ☐ Muscle Re-education ☐ Other: _____

PERTINENT BACKGROUND INFORMATION

TREATMENT DIAGNOSIS/PROBLEM _____

_____ ONSET _____ / _____ / _____

MEDICAL HISTORY

☐ Hypertension   ☐ Fractures
☐ Cardiac   ☐ Cancer
☐ Diabetes   ☐ Infection
☐ Respiratory   ☐ Immunosuppressed
☐ Osteoporosis   ☐ Open wound
☐ Other (specify) _____

PRIOR LEVEL OF FUNCTION

ADLs:
☐ Independent   ☐ Needed assistance   ☐ Unable
Equipment used: _____

IN-HOME MOBILITY (gait or wheelchair/scooter):
☐ Independent   ☐ Needed assistance   ☐ Unable
Equipment used: _____

LIVING SITUATION

☐ Capable ☐ Able ☐ Willing caregiver available
☐ Limited caregiver support (ability/willingness)
☐ No caregiver available

COMMUNITY MOBILITY (gait or wheelchair/scooter):
☐ Independent   ☐ Needed assistance   ☐ Unable
Equipment used: _____

HOME SAFETY BARRIERS:
☐ Clutter   ☐ Throw rugs
☐ Needs grab bars   ☐ Needs railings
☐ Steps (number/condition) _____
☐ Other (specify) _____

PERTINENT MEDICAL/SOCIAL HISTORY AND/OR PREVIOUS THERAPY RECEIVED AND OUTCOMES

BEHAVIOR/MENTAL STATUS

☐ Alert   ☐ Oriented   ☐ Cooperative
☐ Confused   ☐ Memory deficits   ☐ Impaired Judgement
☐ Other (specify) _____

PAIN

INTENSITY: 0 1 2 3 4 5 6 7 8 9 10
LOCATION: _____
AGGRAVATING/RELIEVING FACTORS: _____

VITAL SIGNS/CURRENT STATUS

BP: _____ T.P.R.: _____ Edema: _____ Sensation: _____
Skin Condition: _____ Muscle Tone: _____ Posture: _____
Communication: _____ Vision: _____ Hearing: _____
Endurance: _____ Orthotic/Prosthetic Devices: _____

PART 1 — Clinical Record   **PART 2 — Therapist**

PATIENT/CLIENT NAME — Last, First, Middle Initial

ID#

Figure 4-1

PHYSICAL THERAPY EVALUATION (cont'd)

	AREA	STRENGTH Right	STRENGTH Left	ACTION	ROM Right	ROM Left		TASK	ASSIST SCORE	ASSISTIVE DEVICES/COMMENTS
UPPER EXTREMITIES	Shoulder			Flex/Extend			**BED MOBILITY**	Roll/Turn		
				Abd./Add.				Sit/Supine		
				Int. rot./Ext. rot.				Scoot/Bridge		
							TRANSFERS	Sit/Stand		
	Elbow			Flex/Extend				Bed/Wheelchair		
	Forearm			Sup./Pron.				Toilet		
	Wrist			Flex/Extend				Floor		
	Fingers			Flex/Extend				Auto		
LOWER EXTREMITIES	Hip			Flex/Extend			**BALANCE**	Static Sitting		
				Abd./Add.				Dynamic Sitting		
				Int. rot./Ext. rot.				Static Standing		
	Knee			Flex/Extend				Dynamic Standing		
	Ankle			Plant/Dors			**W/C SKILLS**	Propulsion		
	Foot			Inver/Ever				Pressure Reliefs		
								Foot Rests		
								Locks		

OBJECTIVE DATA TESTS AND SCALES

MANUAL MUSCLE TEST (MMT) MUSCLE STRENGTH

GRADE	DESCRIPTION
5	Normal functional strength - against gravity - full resistance.
4	Good strength - against gravity with some resistance.
3	Fair strength - against gravity - no resistance - safety compromise.
2	Poor strength - unable to move against gravity.
1	Trace strength - slight muscle contraction - no motion.
0	Zero - no active muscle contraction.

FUNCTIONAL RANGE OF MOTION (ROM) SCALE

GRADE	DESCRIPTION
5	100% active functional motion.
4	75% active functional motion.
3	50% active functional motion.
2	25% active functional motion.
1	Less than 25%.

FUNCTIONAL INDEPENDENCE SCALE (bed mobility, transfers, W/C skills)

GRADE	DESCRIPTION
5	Physically able and does task independently.
4	Verbal cue (VC) only needed.
3	Stand-by assist (SBA)—100% patient/client effort.
2	Minimum assist (Min A)—75% patient/client effort.
1	Maximum assist (Max A)—25% - 50% patient/client effort.
0	Totally dependent—total care/support.

BALANCE SCALE (sitting - standing)

GRADE	DESCRIPTION
5	Independent
4	Verbal cue (VC) only needed.
3	Stand-by assist (SBA)—100% patient/client effort.
2	Minimum assist (Min A)—75% patient/client effort.
1	Maximum assist (Max A)—25% patient/client effort.
0	Totally dependent for support.

NORMATIVE DATA FOR JOINT MOTION (ROM)

AREA	ACTION/MOVEMENT			
Shoulder	Flex	158°	Extend	55°
	Abd.	170°	Add.	50°
	Int. rot.	70°	Ext. rot.	90°
Elbow	Flex	145°	Ext.	0°
Forearm	Sup.	85°	Pron.	70°
Wrist	Flex	73°	Ext.	70°
Fingers	Flex all	90°	Ext.	0°
Hip	Flex	90°-115°	Ext.	25°
	Abd.	45°	Add.	30°
	Int. rot.	45°	Ext. rot.	45°
Knee	Flex	135°	Ext.	10°
Ankle	Plant.	50°	Dors.	20°
Foot	Inv.	30°	Ever.	20°

GAIT

ASSISTANCE: ☐ Independent   ☐ SBA   ☐ Min. assist   ☐ Mod. assist   ☐ Max. assist   ☐ Unable

SURFACES: ☐ Level   ☐ Uneven   ☐ Stairs (number/condition)_____ DISTANCE: _____

WEIGHT BEARING STATUS: ☐ FWB   ☐ WBAT   ☐ PWB   ☐ TDWB   ☐ NWB

ASSISTIVE DEVICE(S):   ☐ Cane   ☐ Quad cane   ☐ Crutches   ☐ Hemi-walker   ☐ Walker   ☐ Wheeled walker
☐ Other (specify)_____

QUALITY/DEVIATIONS:_____

EQUIPMENT

HAS: _____

NEEDS: _____

PATIENT/CLIENT SIGNATURE
(if applicable)_____ DATE ___/___/___

Complete TIME OUT (on front) prior to signing here →   THERAPIST'S SIGNATURE/TITLE_____ DATE ___/___/___

Reprinted with permission from Briggs Health Care Products, Des Moines, Iowa, 1999.

Figure 4-2

SPEECH THERAPY EVALUATION

DATE OF SERVICE ____ / ____ / ____

TIME IN ____   OUT ____

HOMEBOUND REASON: ☐ Needs assistance for all activities   ☐ Residual weakness
☐ Requires assistance to ambulate   ☐ Confusion, unable to go out of home alone
☐ Unable to safely leave home unassisted   ☐ Severe SOB, SOB upon exertion
☐ Dependent upon adaptive device(s)   ☐ Medical restrictions
☐ Other (specify) ____

TYPE OF EVALUATION
☐ Initial   ☐ Interim   ☐ Final
SOC DATE ____ / ____ / ____
(If Initial Evaluation, complete Speech Therapy Care Plan, for 3580/3P)

ORDERS FOR EVALUATION ONLY? ☐ Yes   ☐ No   If no, orders are ____

PERTINENT BACKGROUND INFORMATION

MEDICAL DX/TREATMENT DX ____ ONSET ____ / ____ / ____

MEDICAL PRECAUTIONS ____

PRIOR LEVEL OF FUNCTION ____

LIVING SITUATION/SUPPORT SYSTEM ____

DESCRIBE PERTINENT MEDICAL/SOCIAL HISTORY AND/OR PREVIOUS THERAPY PROVIDED ____

SAFE SWALLOWING EVALUATION? ☐ No ☐ Yes; specify date, facility and M.D. ____

VIDEO FLUOROSCOPY? ☐ No ☐ Yes; specify date, facility and M.D. ____

CURRENT DIET TEXTURE ____

LIQUIDS: ☐ Thin ☐ Thickened (Specify) ____ ☐ Other (Specify) ____

SPEECH/LANGUAGE EVALUATION

4 — WFL (within functional limits)   3 — Mild impairment   2 — Moderate impairment   1 — Severe impairment   0 — Unable to do/did not test

FUNCTION EVALUATED	SCORE	COMMENTS		FUNCTION EVALUATED	SCORE	COMMENTS
COGNITION Orientation (Person/Place/Time)			**VERBAL EXPRESSION**	Augmentative methods		
Attention span				Naming		
Short-term memory				Appropriate Yes / No		
Long-term memory				Complex sentences		
Judgment				Conversation		
Problem solving			**AUDITORY COMPREHENSION**	Word discrimination		
Organization				1 step directions		
Other:				2 step directions		
				Complex directions		
SPEECH/VOICE Oral/facial exam				Conversation		
Articulation				Speech reading		
Prosody			**READING**	Letters/Numbers		
Voice/Respiration				Words		
Speech intelligibility				Simple sentences		
Other:				Complex sentences		
				Paragraph		
SWALLOWING Chewing ability			**WRITING**	Letters/Numbers		
Oral stage management				Words		
Pharyngeal stage management				Sentences		
Reflex time				Spelling		
Other:				Formulation		
				Simple addition/subtraction		

REFERRAL FOR: ☐ Vision   ☐ Hearing   ☐ Swallowing   ☐ Other (Specify) ____

Complete **TIME OUT** (above) prior to signing below.

THERAPIST SIGNATURE/TITLE ____ DATE ____ / ____ / ____

PART 1 — Clinical Record	**PART 2 — Therapist**	**PART 3 — Physician**

PATIENT/CLIENT NAME — Last, First, Middle Initial   ID#

Reprinted with permission from Briggs Health Care Products, Des Moines, Iowa, 1999.

Figure 4-3

OCCUPATIONAL THERAPY EVALUATION

DATE OF SERVICE _____ / _____ / _____

OBJECTIVE DATA TESTS AND SCALES PRINTED ON REVERSE.

TIME IN _____ OUT _____

HOMEBOUND REASON: ☐ Needs assistance for all activities ☐ Residual weakness	TYPE OF EVALUATION
☐ Requires assistance to ambulate ☐ Confusion, unable to go out of home alone ☐ Unable to safely leave home unassisted ☐ Severe SOB, SOB upon exertion ☐ Dependent upon adaptive device(s) ☐ Medical restrictions ☐ Other (specify) _____	☐ Initial ☐ Interim ☐ Final SOC DATE _____ / _____ / _____ (If Initial Evaluation, complete Occupational Therapy Care Plan, form 3594/3P or 3594/3TP)

ORDERS FOR EVALUATION ONLY?   ☐ Yes   ☐ No   If No, orders are_____

PERTINENT BACKGROUND INFORMATION

TREATMENT DIAGNOSIS/PROBLEM_____

_____ ONSET _____ / _____ / _____

MEDICAL PRECAUTIONS _____

PRIOR LEVEL OF FUNCTION/WORK HISTORY _____

LIVING SITUATION/SUPPORT SYSTEM _____

ENVIRONMENTAL BARRIERS _____

PERTINENT MEDICAL/SOCIAL HISTORY AND/OR PREVIOUS THERAPY PROVIDED _____

KEY: I - Intact, MIN - Minimally Impaired, MOD - Moderately Impaired, S - Severely Impaired, U - Untested/Unable to Test

SENSORY/PERCEPTUAL MOTOR SKILLS

Area	Sharp/Dull		Light/Firm Touch		Proprioception		VISUAL TRACKING:
	Right	Left	Right	Left	Right	Left	R/L DISCRIMINATION:
							MOTOR PLANNING PRAXIS:
							Do sensory/perceptual impairments affect safety? ☐ Yes ☐ No
							If Yes, recommendations:
							COMMENTS:

COGNITIVE STATUS/COMPREHENSION

Area	I	MIN	MOD	S	U	ABILITY TO EXPRESS NEEDS
MEMORY: Short term						ATTENTION SPAN
Long term						ORIENTED: ☐ Person ☐ Place ☐ Time ☐ Reason for Therapy
SAFETY AWARENESS						**PSYCHOSOCIAL WELL-BEING**
JUDGMENT						INITIATION OF ACTIVITY
Visual Comprehension						COPING SKILLS ☐ Evaluate Further
Auditory Comprehension						SELF-CONTROL

MOTOR COMPONENTS (Enter Appropriate Response)

	I	MIN	MOD	S	U		I	MIN	MOD	S	U
FINE MOTOR COORDINATION (R)						GROSS MOTOR COORDINATION (R)					
FINE MOTOR COORDINATION (L)						GROSS MOTOR COORDINATION (L)					
PRIOR TO INJURY: ☐ Right Handed ☐ Left Handed				ORTHOSIS: ☐ Used ☐ Needed (Specify):							

MUSCLE STRENGTH/FUNCTIONAL ROM EVALUATION (Enter Appropriate Response)

PROBLEM AREA	STRENGTH		ROM		ROM TYPE			TONICITY		OTHER DESCRIPTIONS
	Right	Left	Right	Left	P	AA	A	Hyper	Hypo	

COMMENTS: _____

PART 1 — Clinical Record   PART 2 — Therapist *

PATIENT/CLIENT NAME — Last, First, Middle Initial	ID #

Figure 4-3

OCCUPATIONAL THERAPY EVALUATION (cont'd)

TASK	SCORE	COMMENTS	TASK	SCORE	COMMENTS
FUNCTIONAL MOBILITY/BALANCE EVALUATION					
BED MOBILITY			DYNAMIC SITTING BALANCE		
BED/WHEELCHAIR TRANSFER			STATIC SITTING BALANCE		
TOILET TRANSFER			STATIC STANDING BALANCE		
TUB/SHOWER TRANSFER			DYNAMIC STANDING BALANCE		
SELF CARE SKILLS					
FEEDING			TOILETING		
SWALLOWING			BATHING		
FOOD TO MOUTH			UE DRESSING		
ORAL HYGIENE			LE DRESSING		
GROOMING			MANIPULATION OF FASTENERS		
INSTRUMENTAL ADL'S					
LIGHT HOUSEKEEPING			USE OF TELEPHONE		
LIGHT MEAL PREPARATION			MONEY MANAGEMENT		
CLOTHING CARE			MEDICATION MANAGEMENT		

PATIENT GOALS:

PATIENT SIGNATURE VERIFYING VISIT:

Complete **TIME OUT** (on front) prior to signing here → THERAPIST SIGNATURE/TITLE _____ DATE ___/___/___

OBJECTIVE DATA TESTS AND SCALES

MANUAL MUSCLE TEST (MMT) MUSCLE STRENGTH

GRADE	DESCRIPTION
5	Normal functional strength - against gravity - full resistance.
4	Good strength - against gravity with some resistance.
3	Fair strength - against gravity - no resistance - safety compromise.
2	Poor strength - unable to move against gravity.
1	Trace strength - slight muscle contraction - no motion.
0	Zero - no active muscle contraction.

FUNCTIONAL RANGE OF MOTION (ROM) SCALE

GRADE	DESCRIPTION
5	100% active functional motion.
4	75% active functional motion.
3	50% active functional motion.
2	25% active functional motion.
1	Less than 25%.

FUNCTIONAL INDEPENDENCE, SELF-CARE SKILLS AND INSTRUMENTAL ADL SCALE

GRADE	DESCRIPTION
5	Physically able and does task independently.
4	Verbal cue (VC) only needed.
3	Stand-by assist (SBA) — 100% patient/client effort.
2	Minimum assist (Min A) — 75% patient/client effort.
1	Maximum assist (Max A) — 25% - 50% patient/client effort.
0	Totally dependent — total care.

AVERAGE RANGES OF JOINT MOTION (ROM)

AREA	ACTION/MOVEMENT			
Shoulder	Flex	158°	Extend	55°
	Abd.	170°	Add.	50°
	Int. rot.	70°	Ext. rot.	90°
Elbow	Flex	145°	Ext.	0°
Forearm	Sup.	85°	Pron.	70°
Wrist	Flex	73°	Ext.	70°
Fingers	Flex all	90°	Ext.	0°
Thumb	Abduction	50%		
Cervical	Flex	35°	Ext.	35°
Spine	Rotation	45°		

BALANCE SCALE (sitting - standing)

GRADE	DESCRIPTION
5	Independent
4	Verbal cue (VC) only needed.
3	Stand-by assist (SBA) — 100% patient/client effort.
2	Minimum assist (Min A) — 75% patient/client effort.
1	Maximum assist (Max A) — 25% patient/client effort.
0	Totally dependent for support.

"Therapy-Only" Case Admissions: Operational Challenge

For home health patients not requiring nursing services, and where allowed by state law, agency policy may designate one of the therapy providers the duties associated with the admission to home care services. For Medicare home health patients, the home care admission may be performed by any of the primary/ initial qualifying services—nursing, physical therapy, or speech-language pathology. Refer to Medicare coverage discussion in Part One. Beyond the tasks associated with the specific clinical assessment previously described, the home care admission is the process of determining the appropriateness of accepting a patient for agency services, and collecting and providing additional information to meet regulatory and accreditation requirements. The admitting clinician should be familiar with the agency's admission policy and/or admission criteria, and should have some familiarity with the ethical, legal, and reimbursement issues associated with inappropriate acceptance for home care admission.

Admission Activities Include:
- the process of reviewing and obtaining written patient consent for services
- reviewing the patient rights and responsibilities
- determining advanced directive status
- determining financial responsibility and/or obtaining assignment of benefits
- providing notice of non-coverage for Medicare patients
- completion of Medicare secondary payer form
- completion of a home safety assessment
- determination of emergency contacts, checklists, and plan
- completion of home health aide care plan; if appropriate
- completion of the comprehensive assessment (per agency policy) which includes:
  - identification of the patient's continuing need for home care
  - meeting the patient's medical, nursing, rehabilitative, social, and discharge planning needs
  - verification of eligibility for coverage (including homebound status determination for Medicare patients)
  - completion of drug regimen review
  - collection of the OASIS data elements
- completion of home care treatment plan/physician's orders (HCFA Form 485)

The HCFA Form 485

The Health Care Financing Administration requires home health agencies to collect and retain uniform physician's treatment plans on a mandatory form designed specifically for home care use: HCFA Form 485. The HCFA Form 485 is the home health certification and plan of care, and contains data necessary to meet regulatory and national survey requirements. The HCFA Form 485 is required at admission and at recertification for every patient receiving services from a Medicare-certified agency. Though organizations have varying policies regarding the process for HCFA Form 485 completion, all professional home care providers should be familiar with the form, its data elements and its intended use as a physician-approved treatment plan. A HCFA Form 485 (Figure 4-4) follows for review. ICD-9 codes, the data elements numbered 11, 12, and 13 on the HCFA Form 485, have important quality and reimbursement functions. A listing of common ICD-9 codes seen in home care therapy follow for review in Box 4-1.

Figure 4-4   HCFA Form 485

Department of Health and Human Services
Health Care Financing Administration

Form Approved
OMB No. 0938-0357

HOME HEALTH CERTIFICATION AND PLAN OF CARE

1. Patient's HI Claim No.	2. Start Of Care Date	3. Certification Period		4. Medical Record No.	5. Provider No.
		From:	To:		

6. Patient's Name and Address	7. Provider's Name, Address and Telephone Number

8. Date of Birth		9. Sex	☐ M ☐ F	10. Medications: Dose/Frequency/Route (N)ew (C)hanged
11. ICD-9-CM	Principal Diagnosis		Date	
12. ICD-9-CM	Surgical Procedure		Date	
13. ICD-9-CM	Other Pertinent Diagnoses		Date	

14. DME and Supplies	15. Safety Measures:
16. Nutritional Req.	17. Allergies:

18.A. Functional Limitations

1 ☐ Amputation	5 ☐ Paralysis	9 ☐ Legally Blind						
2 ☐ Bowel/Bladder (Incontinence)	6 ☐ Endurance	A ☐ Dyspnea With Minimal Exertion						
3 ☐ Contracture	7 ☐ Ambulation	B ☐ Other (Specify)						
4 ☐ Hearing	8 ☐ Speech							

18.B. Activities Permitted

1 ☐ Complete Bedrest	6 ☐ Partial Weight Bearing	A ☐ Wheelchair			
2 ☐ Bedrest BRP	7 ☐ Independent At Home	B ☐ Walker			
3 ☐ Up As Tolerated	8 ☐ Crutches	C ☐ No Restrictions			
4 ☐ Transfer Bed/Chair	9 ☐ Cane	D ☐ Other (Specify)			
5 ☐ Exercises Prescribed					

19. Mental Status:	1 ☐ Oriented	3 ☐ Forgetful	5 ☐ Disoriented	7 ☐ Agitated
	2 ☐ Comatose	4 ☐ Depressed	6 ☐ Lethargic	8 ☐ Other

20. Prognosis:	1 ☐ Poor	2 ☐ Guarded	3 ☐ Fair	4 ☐ Good	5 ☐ Excellent

21. Orders for Discipline and Treatments (Specify Amount/Frequency/Duration)

22. Goals/Rehabilitation Potential/Discharge Plans

23. Nurse's Signature and Date of Verbal SOC Where Applicable:	25. Date HHA Received Signed POT

24. Physician's Name and Address	26. I certify/recertify that this patient is confined to his/her home and needs intermittent skilled nursing care, physical therapy and/or speech therapy or continues to need occupational therapy. The patient is under my care, and I have authorized the services on this plan of care and will periodically review the plan.
27. Attending Physician's Signature and Date Signed	28. Anyone who misrepresents, falsifies, or conceals essential information required for payment of Federal funds may be subject to fine, imprisonment, or civil penalty under applicable Federal laws.

Form 3485R/4P BRIGGS, Des Moines, IA 50306 (800) 247-2343
PRINTED IN U.S.A.

PROVIDER

Form HCFA-485 (C-4) (02-94) (Print Aligned)

Reprinted with permission from Briggs Health Care Products, Des Moines, Iowa, 1999.

Box 4-1   Common ICD-9 Codes in Therapy Care

Abnormality of gait	781.2
Acquired immune deficiency syndrome	042
Amyotrophic lateral sclerosis	335.20
Alzheimer's disease	331.0
Ankylosing spondylitis	720.0
Angina	413.9
Aphasia	784.3
Amputation/surgical, above elbow	V49.66
Amputation/surgical, above knee	V49.76
Amputation/surgical, ankle	V49.74
Amputation/surgical, below elbow	V49.65
Amputation/surgical, below knee	V49.75
Amputation/surgical, hand	V49.63
Amputation/surgical, hip	V49.77
Amputation/surgical, foot	V 49.73
Amputation/surgical, shoulder	V49.67
Amputation/surgical, wrist	V49.64
Asthma	493.9
Ataxia	781.3
Bowel incontinence	787.6
Cancer, (see specific neoplasm)	
Cellulitis	682.9
Cerebrovascular accident	436
Cervicalgia	723.1
Chronic obstructive pulmonary disease	496
Collagen disease	710.9
Congestive heart failure	428.0
Coordination, lack of	781.3
Decubitus ulcer	707.0
Depression	311
Diabetes mellitus	250
Dislocation, elbow	832
Dislocation, finger	834
Dislocation, hip	835
Dislocation, knee	836
Dislocation, ankle	837
Dislocation, shoulder	831
Dislocation, wrist	833
Dizziness	780.4

Dysphagia	787.2
Dysphasia	784.5
Fracture, ankle	824
Fracture, carpal bone(s)	814
Fracture, femur	821
Fracture, humerus	812
Fracture, metacarpal bone(s)	815
Fracture, tarsal(s)/metatarsal(s)	825
Fracture, tibia	823.80
Fractures, ulna and radius	813
Fracture, wrist; colles	813.41
Gait disorder/disturbance	781.2
Gastrostomy	V44.1
Head Injury	959.01
Hypertension	401.9
Hypotension	458.9
Internal derangement of knee	717
Intervertebral disc disorders	722
Intracerebral hemorrhage	431
Joint contracture	718.40
Joint crepitus	719.6
Joint effusion	719.0
Joint pain, ankle	719.47
Joint pain, elbow	719.42
Joint pain, foot	719.47
Joint pain, hand	719.44
Joint pain, hip	719.45
Joint pain, knee	719.46
Joint pain, multiple sites	719.49
Joint pain, shoulder	719.41
Joint pain, wrist	719.43
Joint replacement, ankle	V43.66
Joint replacement, elbow	V43.62
Joint replacement, hip	V43.64
Joint replacement, knee	V43.65
Joint replacement, shoulder	V43.61
Lumbago	724.2
Malaise and fatigue	780.7
Memory disturbance	780.9
Multiple sclerosis	340

Muscle atrophy	728.2
Muscle spasm	728.85
Muscle weakness	728.9
Myocardial infarction	410.90
Neoplasm	199.1
Neoplasm, bone	170.9
Neoplasm, brain	191.9
Neoplasm, breast	174.90
Neoplasm, colon	153.8
Neoplasm, lung	162.9
Neuropathy	355.9
Nonhealing surgical wound	998.83
Organic brain syndrome	310.9
Orthopedic devices, fitting/adjustment	V53.7
Orthostatic hypotension	458.0
Osteoarthritis, ankle/foot	715.97
Osteoarthritis, elbow	715.92
Osteoarthritis, hip/pelvis	715.95
Osteoarthritis, knee	715.96
Osteoarthritis, shoulder	715.91
Osteoarthritis, spine	715.98
Osteoarthritis, wrist	715.93
Osteoarthritis, unspecified	715.90
Osteomyelitis	730.20
Osteoporosis	733.00
Pain (see also, joint pain)	
Pain, cervical	723.1
Pain, low back	724.2
Pain, radicular	729.2
Pain, sacroiliac	724.6
Pain, sciatic	724.3
Pain, trigeminal	350.1
Paralysis, hemiplegia flaccid	342.0
Paralysis, hemiplegia spastic	342.1
Paralysis, diplegia	344.2
Paralysis, monoplegia	344.4
Paralysis, paraplegia	344.1
Paralysis, quadriplegia	344.0
Parkinson's disease	332.0
Peripheral neuropathy	356.9

Peripheral vascular disease	443.9
Post-operative wound infection	998.59
Pressure ulcer	707.0
Prosthetic device, fitting and adjustment	V52
Quadriplegia	334.00
Raynaud's syndrome	443.0
Reflex sympathetic dystrophy	337.2
Rheumatoid arthritis	714.0
Sciatica	724.3
Senile dementia	290.0
Speech disturbance	784.5
Spinal stenosis	724
Sprains/strains, shoulder/upper arm	840
Sprains/strains, elbow/forearm	841
Sprains/strains, wrist/hand	842
Sprains/strains, hip/thigh	843
Sprains/strains, knee/leg	844
Sprains/strains, ankle/foot	845
Sprains/strains, sacroiliac	846
Subarachnoid hemorrhage	430
Trachestomy	V44.0
Transient ischemic attacks	435.9
Urinary incontinence	788.30
Urinary tract infection	599.0
Venous stasis ulcer	454.0
Vision, blurred	368.8
Vision, disturbance	368.9
Vision, loss	369.9
Vision, low	369.20
Visual field limitation	z368.4
Voice disturbance	784.4
Walking, difficulty in	719.7
Wheelchair, fitting/adjustment	V53.8
Wound, open	879.8

Clinical staff should be aware that the intermediary uses the HCFA Form 485 as a basis for paying or denying claims. Effective and compliant completion of the HCFA Form 485 upon home care admission, as well as at recertification, will minimize the financial burden placed on the agency when Medicare payments are delayed due to unclear or incomplete treatment plans. When patient plan of treatment information is extensive and cannot be contained on the single HCFA Form 485, an addendum or secondary form (e.g., HCFA 487) may be used for additional information. The *HIM-11* provides detailed information about the HCFA Form 485, as well as item-by-item instructions for completion of the form. See Part Nine, (HCFA Pub.-11), for completion instructions.

Completing the HCFA Form 485- A Patient Example: Mrs. Nicholas

Mrs. Nicholas is an 80-year-old female who experienced a fall at home resulting in a right humeral fracture. Her dominant right arm is placed in an immobilizer sling to treat the humeral fracture, with orders to maintain immobilization for three weeks. After examination in the emergency room, she is admitted to the hospital with hemoglobin of 8g/dl, to determine the site of her internal bleeding. She was diagnosed with an upper GI bleed attributed to excessive use of anti-inflammatory drugs used to control her knee arthritis. After medication changes she is discharged home with home care services. Ordered services include PT for gait and safety assessment, OT for ADL assessment, and home health aide for assist with personal care.

Past Medical History: Mrs. Nicholas has a 14-year history of IDDM, for which she was independent in self-injecting prior to her injury. She also has marked osteoarthritis in the right knee, with reports of recent exacerbation.

Social History: Mrs. Nicholas was living alone in her one-floor home, driving her car, and independent in all self care, domestic chores, and instrumental activities of daily living. She has a nephew who lives nearby and is available for brief daily visits and to assist with shopping and errands.

Home Care Admission: Mrs. Nicholas' case is assigned for case management by the physical therapist. The admission visit is made the day after hospital discharge, with the patient's nephew present for instruction and support. The therapist completes the activities associated with the home care admission, the comprehensive assessment with collection of OASIS data.

Assessment Findings:

- Mrs. Nicholas is unable to draw up or inject her insulin and maintain mobility restrictions for her right arm. Patient is dependent in self care dressing and bathing, due to right arm restrictions.
- Patient has difficulty with bed mobility and chair transfers, due to knee arthritis and non-use of right arm.
- Patient with decreased activity tolerance and limited endurance resulting from anemia.

- Patient constipated, reports no bowel movement since hospital admission.
- Unsteady gait from weakness and right knee pain.
- Patient has personal emergency response system.

Through interview and observation the therapist determines that the patient's nephew is also a diabetic, and has administered Mrs. Nicholas' insulin injections during past illnesses. He reports he can be available each morning on his way to work, and reports willingness and ability to assist patient with her medications and shopping. He also states that for a limited time, he could visit in the evenings to help with preparations for bed. In addition to the discipline-specific activities of developing and communicating the physical therapy treatment plan, the therapist completes the case management duties including informing the patient and family of the scope of home care services to be provided, developing the care plan for the home health aide, and identifying the unmet interdisciplinary need of nursing services. The therapist would contact the physician to obtain orders and notify the agency of the patient's need for nursing services. Upon timely completion of assessment visits by the occupational therapist and nurse, the patient's interdisciplinary treatment plan is developed and the HCFA Form 485 is completed (Figure 4-5) and sent to the physician for signature. This patient scenario continues in Part Five with sample completion of a comprehensive assessment with OASIS data collection for Mrs. Nicholas.

Changes to the Conditions of Participation:
Impact on the Home Care Admission

In 1997, the Health Care Financing Administration (HCFA) proposed changes to the existing Conditions of Participation (COPs) for home health agencies participating in the Medicare program. "The proposed requirements focus on the actual care delivered to patients by home health agencies and the results of that care, reflect an interdisciplinary view of patient care, allow home health agencies greater flexibility in meeting quality standards, and eliminate unnecessary procedural requirements." (*Federal Register*, Vol. 62, No. 46, March 10, 1997, 42 CFR Part 484 [BPD-819-P]) The proposal represented a change to a focus on patient-centered, outcome-oriented performance expectations. HCFA recognized the lack of data supporting a correlation between structure and process require- ments and positive patient outcomes for home care services. To this end, the proposed COPs would shift the responsibility to monitor quality away from the HCFA (through the state survey agencies) to the individual home health agency. The process of evaluating quality, identifying problem areas, developing and implementing performance improvement plans, and evaluating effectiveness is now the sole obligation of the organization. HCFA's role will focus on the

Figure 4-5   Completed HCFA Form 485

Department of Health and Human Services Health Care Financing Administration		Form Approved OMB No. 0938-0357

HOME HEALTH CERTIFICATION AND PLAN OF CARE

1. Patient's HI Claim No.	2. Start of Care Date	3. Certification Period	4. Medical Record No.	5. Provider No.
123-45-6789-A	060199	From: 060199 To: 080199	001	21-1234

6. Patient's Name and Address	7. Provider's Name, Address and Telephone Number 999-1000
Angela P. Nicholas 867-5309 1234 Happy Home Road Smallsville, USA 54321	Perfect Home Care, Inc. 8888 Compliance Highway Successtown, USA 32323

8. Date of Birth 032619	9. Sex ☐ M ☒ F	10. Medications: Dose/Frequency/Route (N)ew (C)hanged

11. ICD-9-CM Principal Diagnosis	Date
812.20 (R) Humeral fracture	052699

12. ICD-9-CM Surgical Procedure	Date
N/A N/A	N/A

13. ICD-9-CM Other Pertinent Diagnoses	Date
578.9 GI Bleed, unsp.	052699
781.2 Abnormality of Gait	052699
716.6 Osteoarthritis	050199
250.9 IDDM	000085

Medications (box 10):
Humulin 70/30 15 units qam SC
Naprosyn 250 mg qd po (c)
Advil 400 mg TID po (N)
Milk of Magnesia 5ml c̄ H₂O QID po (N)
B-12 100 mcg Qmo SC (N)

14. DME and Supplies	15. Safety Measures: Personal Emergency Response System,
personal hygiene/grooming aids, NBQC, Immobilizer Sling, Tub bench, Toilet Safety Frame	Fall Precautions, Remove throw rugs, add nightlight

16. Nutritional Req. 1500 Cal ADA diabetic diet	17. Allergies: Paper tape, Betadine, Pineapple

18.A. Functional Limitations						18.B. Activities Permitted					
1	☐ Amputation	5	☐ Paralysis	9	☐ Legally Blind	1	☐ Complete Bedrest	6	☐ Partial Weight Bearing	A	☐ Wheelchair
2	☐ Bowel/Bladder (Incontinence)	6	☒ Endurance	A	☐ Dyspnea With Minimal Exertion	2	☐ Bedrest BRP	7	☐ Independent At Home	B	☐ Walker
3	☐ Contracture	7	☒ Ambulation	B	☒ Other (Specify)	3	☒ Up As Tolerated I Restrictions as noted	8	☐ Crutches	C	☐ No Restrictions
4	☐ Hearing	8	☐ Speech		(R)UE immobilized in sling x 3 wks	4	☐ Transfer Bed/Chair	9	☒ Cane NBQC	D	☒ Other (Specify) Activity limited by Knee pain and immobilized UE.
						5	☐ Exercises Prescribed				

19. Mental Status:	1	☒ Oriented	3	☐ Forgetful	5	☐ Disoriented	7	☐ Agitated
	2	☐ Comatose	4	☐ Depressed	6	☐ Lethargic	8	☐ Other

20. Prognosis:	1	☐ Poor	2	☐ Guarded	3	☒ Fair	4	☐ Good	5	☐ Excellent

21. Orders for Discipline and Treatments (Specify Amount/Frequency/Duration)

PT 3wk 3, 2wk 2 Home Safety Assessment, Gait & Transfer training, Eval., Home program for strengthening, mobility, & safety. Arrange Meals on Wheels.

OT 2wk2 3wk2 Eval, Safety Evaluation related to ADLs, ADL training c̄ recommendation for assistive/adaptive equipment. Progress to IADL training as tolerated.

SN 3wk3 + 2 prn visits for patient complaints - abdominal pain/bleeding. Eval, observation, assessment and teaching of patient on new medication assessment and management of bowel program, assessment & teaching related to nutrition, assess for orthostatic changes, support home safety program.

Aide 3wk3, 2wk2 Personal care, ADL assistance, support home safety program.

22. Goals/Rehabilitation Potential/Discharge Plans Implement home safety/fall prevention program with no reported falls during homecare admission. Increase muscle strength (R) Quads 1grade Demonstrated independent transfers and gait in home s̄ Loss of balance. Safe and independent ADLs. Resume self-care management at home. Demonstrated compliance with drug regimen. Good rehab potential for (I) self care at home. OT therapy referral.

23. Nurse's Signature and Date of Verbal SOC Where Applicable:	25. Date HHA Received Signed POT x 5 wks
Jerry Cloth, PT 060199	

24. Physician's Name and Address 555-1234	26. I certify/recertify that this patient is confined to his/her home and needs intermittent skilled nursing care, physical therapy and/or speech therapy or continues to need occupational therapy. The patient is under my care, and I have authorized the services on this plan of care and will periodically review the plan.
Dr. Dan DeLine 3131 Allergy Way Weedville, USA 39393	

27. Attending Physician's Signature and Date Signed (X)	28. Anyone who misrepresents, falsifies, or conceals essential information required for payment of Federal funds may be subject to fine, imprisonment, or civil penalty under applicable Federal laws.

outcomes of care generated by the performance improvement process or approaches the agency determines and operationalizes.

Patient Outcomes

The degree to which the patient's functional status changes between two or more time points is the patient outcome. Patient outcomes should be measured using standardized assessment methods repeated at various time intervals throughout the patient's care. At a minimum, patient status should be measured at initiation of service, and at discharge. There are a variety of standardized tools used to measure patient status and outcomes which are directly or indirectly related to physical rehabilitation. There are global or comprehensive assessment instruments which measure function in a variety of functional and health domains; and there are specific measures, which focus on assessment items within a specific patient domain. Examples of global assessment instruments and domain-specific measures are listed in Boxes 4-2 and 4-3.

Box 4-2   Global Assessment Instruments

Outcome and Assessment Information Set (OASIS)
Functional Independence Measure (FIM)
PULSES Profile
Short-Form 36 (SF-36)

Box 4-3   Domain-Specific Assessment Instruments

Domain Measured:	Examples of Standardized Instruments:
ADL/IADL	Barthel Index Katz Index of ADL
Behavior	Hamilton Rating Scale for Depression Self-rating Depression Scale (SDS)
Cognition	Mini-Mental State Examination (MMSE) Short Portable Mental Status Questionnaire (SPMSQ)
Functional Communication	Communicative Abilities in Daily Living Functional Assessment of Communication Skills for Adults (ASHA FACS)
Mobility and Balance	Berg Balance Assessment Functional Reach Test Get-up-and-Go Test Tinetti Gait and Balance Assessment
Sensorimotor	Fugl-Meyer Assessment Standardized Test of Patient Mobility
Social Function/Support	Geriatric Coping Inventory (GCI) High-Risk Placement Worksheet (HRPW) Older Adult Resources and Services Social Resource Scale (OARS)

Standardized instruments are available to assess a multitude of domains which may impact patient function or rehabilitation potential, including caregiver assistance scales, disability scales, emergent care utilization scales, falls history or risk scales, health-related quality of life scales, etc. For greater review of available scales, their development and use, readers are referred to *Functional Assessment and Outcome Measures for the Rehabilitation Health Professional* (Aspen Publishers, Inc., 1997), and *In-Home Assessment of Older Adults: An Interdisciplinary Approach* (Aspen Publishers, Inc., 1996).

The Comprehensive Assessment:
Identifying Patient Needs and Facilitating Outcome Measurement

In January 1999, HCFA published regulations finalizing portions of the proposed COP revisions related to the comprehensive assessment, and OASIS data collection. These COPs require as a core condition (§484.55) that each patient must receive, and a home health agency must provide, a patient-specific, comprehensive assessment that accurately reflects the patient's current health status and includes information that may be used to demonstrate the patient's progress toward achievement of desired outcomes. The comprehensive assessment must identify the patient's continuing need for home care and meet the patient's medical, nursing, rehabilitative, social and discharge planning needs. The comprehensive assessment must also verify eligibility for coverage, including identification of the patient's homebound status for Medicare patients. The comprehensive assessment must also incorporate the verbatim use of the OASIS items. (*Federal Register*, Vol. 64, No. 15, January 25, 1999, 42 CFR Part 484, p. 3784). (See Box 4-4).

For a case where therapy services are the only services ordered, the responsibility for completion of the home care comprehensive assessment with OASIS data collection will most likely be assigned to the therapist performing the home care admission. The standards associated with the comprehensive assessment requirement will be described, with a thorough discussion of the OASIS data set, data collection activities and therapy-related considerations in Part Five.

Under the core Condition requiring the comprehensive patient assessment are five standards: 1) the initial assessment visit, 2) the completion of the comprehensive assessment, 3) the drug regimen review, 4) the requirement for updating the comprehensive assessment, and 5) incorporation of OASIS data items.

The Initial Assessment Visit: Timely Initiation of Services

The first standard [§484.55(a)] outlines the requirements for the initial assessment visit. The initial assessment visit must be performed within 48 hours of

Box 4-4

3784   **Federal Register**/Vol. 64, No. 15/Monday, January 25, 1999/Rules and Regulations

Interested persons are invited to send comments regarding the burden or any other aspect of these collections of information requirements. However, as noted above, comments on these information collection and recordkeeping requirements must be mailed and/or faxed to the designees referenced below, within 15 working days from the date of this publication in the **Federal Register** to:

Health Care Financing Administration, Office of Information Services, Security and Standards Group, Division of HCFA Enterprise Standards, Room N2–14–26, 7500 Security Boulevard, Baltimore, MD 21244–1850, Attention: John Burke HCFA–3007–F, Fax number: 410–786–0262, and

Office of Information and Regulatory Affairs, Office of Management and Budget, Room 10235, New Executive Office Building, Washington, D.C. 20503, Attention: Allison Herron Eydt, HCFA Desk Officer, Fax number: 202–395–6974 or 202–395–5167

List of Subjects in 42 CFR Part 484

Health facilities, Health professions, Medicare, Reporting and recordkeeping requirements.

42 CFR chapter IV is amended as follows:

PART 484—CONDITIONS OF PARTICIPATION: HOME HEALTH AGENCIES

1. The authority citation for part 484 continues to read as follows:

Authority: Secs. 1102 and 1871 of the Social Security Act (42 U.S.C. 1302 and 1395(hh)).

Subpart B—Administration

2. Section 484.18 is amended by revising paragraph (c) to read as follows:

§ 484.18   Condition of participation: Acceptance of patients, plan of care, and medical supervision.

*   *   *   *   *

(c) *Standard: Conformance with physician orders.* Drugs and treatments are administered by agency staff only as ordered by the physician. Verbal orders are put in writing and signed and dated with the date of receipt by the registered nurse or qualified therapist (as defined in § 484.4 of this chapter) responsible for furnishing or supervising the ordered services. Verbal orders are only accepted by personnel authorized to do so by applicable State and Federal laws and regulations as well as by the HHA's internal policies.

Subpart C—Furnishing of Services

3. Section 484.55 is added to subpart C to read as follows:

§ 484.55   Condition of participation: Comprehensive assessment of patients.

Each patient must receive, and an HHA must provide, a patient-specific, comprehensive assessment that accurately reflects the patient's current health status and includes information that may be used to demonstrate the patient's progress toward achievement of desired outcomes. The comprehensive assessment must identify the patient's continuing need for home care and meet the patient's medical, nursing, rehabilitative, social, and discharge planning needs. For Medicare beneficiaries, the HHA must verify the patient's eligibility for the Medicare home health benefit including homebound status, both at the time of the initial assessment visit and at the time of the comprehensive assessment. The comprehensive assessment must also incorporate the use of the current version of the Outcome and Assessment Information Set (OASIS) items, using the language and groupings of the OASIS items, as specified by the Secretary.

(a) *Standard: Initial assessment visit.* (1) A registered nurse must conduct an initial assessment visit to determine the immediate care and support needs of the patient; and, for Medicare patients, to determine eligibility for the Medicare home health benefit, including homebound status. The initial assessment visit must be held either within 48 hours of referral, or within 48 hours of the patient's return home, or on the physician-ordered start of care date.

(2) When rehabilitation therapy service (speech language pathology, physical therapy, or occupational therapy) is the only service ordered by the physician, and if the need for that service establishes program eligibility, the initial assessment visit may be made by the appropriate rehabilitation skilled professional.

(b) *Standard: Completion of the comprehensive assessment.* (1) The comprehensive assessment must be completed in a timely manner, consistent with the patient's immediate needs, but no later than 5 calendar days after the start of care.

(2) Except as provided in paragraph (b)(3) of this section, a registered nurse must complete the comprehensive assessment and for Medicare patients, determine eligibility for the Medicare home health benefit, including homebound status.

(3) When physical therapy, speech-language pathology, or occupational therapy is the only service ordered by the physician, a physical therapist, speech-language pathologist or occupational therapist may complete the comprehensive assessment, and for Medicare patients, determine eligibility for the Medicare home health benefit, including homebound status. The occupational therapist may complete the comprehensive assessment if the need for occupational therapy establishes program eligibility.

(c) *Standard: Drug regimen review.* The comprehensive assessment must include a review of all medications the patient is currently using in order to identify any potential adverse effects and drug reactions, including ineffective drug therapy, significant side effects, significant drug interactions, duplicate drug therapy, and noncompliance with drug therapy.

(d) *Standard: Update of the comprehensive assessment.* The comprehensive assessment must be updated and revised (including the administration of the OASIS) as frequently as the patient's condition warrants due to a major decline or improvement in the patient's health status, but not less frequently than—

(1) Every second calendar month beginning with the start of care date;

(2) Within 48 hours of the patient's return to the home from a hospital admission of 24 hours or more for any reason other than diagnostic tests;

(3) At discharge.

(e) *Standard: Incorporation of OASIS data items.* The OASIS data items determined by the Secretary must be incorporated into the HHA's own assessment and must include: clinical record items, demographics and patient history, living arrangements, supportive assistance, sensory status, integumentary status, respiratory status, elimination status, neuro/emotional/behavioral status, activities of daily living, medications, equipment management, emergent care, and data items collected at inpatient facility admission or discharge only.

(Catalog of Federal Domestic Assistance Program No. 93.773, Medicare—Hospital Insurance; and Program No. 93.778, Medical Assistance Program)

Dated: November 3, 1998.

Nancy-Ann Min DeParle,

Administrator, Health Care Financing Administration.

Dated: December 15, 1998.

Donna E. Shalala,

Secretary.

[FR Doc. 99–1449 Filed 1–22–99; 8:45 am]

BILLING CODE 4120–01–P

referral or within 48 hours after the patient's return home, or on the physician-ordered start of care date. If nursing services are ordered, then the registered nurse must conduct the initial assessment visit to determine the immediate care and support needs of the patient. When physical therapy, speech-language pathology, or occupational therapy is the only service ordered, and if the need for that service establishes program eligibility, the initial assessment visit may be made by the PT, SLP, or OT. Note that initial orders for occupational therapy services only do not establish eligibility for the Medicare program, but may establish eligibility for Medicaid or private insurance programs, in which case the OT would be eligible to conduct the initial assessment.

Completion of the Comprehensive Assessment

The second standard §484.55(b) outlines the requirements in completing the comprehensive assessment. This must occur in a timely manner consistent with the patient's immediate needs, but no later than five calendar days after the start of care (SOC). The start of care is defined as the date of the first billable service, or the date of the first visit which meets the coverage requirements (as outlined in the HIM-11 for Medicare beneficiaries).

The Drug Regimen Review: Models for Meeting Regulatory Intent

The third standard [§484.55 (c)] requires that the comprehensive assessment include a drug regimen review. This is defined as a review of all medications the patient is currently using in order to identify any potential adverse effects and drug reactions, including ineffective drug therapy, significant side effects, significant drug interactions, duplicate drug therapy, and noncompliance with drug therapy.

The medication review includes information required for completion of the Home Health Certification and Plan of Treatment (HCFA Form 485), including a listing of all prescription and over-the-counter medications that a patient is using. The review should include reporting the new or changed dosages of medications, as well as times and routes of administration. The therapist may assess the patient's or caregiver's knowledge related to the purpose, dosage and timing of medication administration, and assess consistency with physician's orders. When knowledge deficits or compliance problems are identified, the therapist should notify the physician, and if appropriate, facilitate a nursing or social work referral, based on the patient's unique findings. If the non-compliance is due to the patient's poor understanding of the role of medications in their health care, or the unawareness of potential consequences of inadequate drug therapy, nursing services should be referred for the provision of patient teaching. If the non-compliance is due to inadequate finances, medical social services may be consulted to identify potential resources to assist the patient in obtaining necessary medications.

The drug regimen standard also requires that a review of the medications identifies any potential adverse effects and drug reactions, including ineffective drug therapy, significant side effects, significant drug interactions, duplicate drug therapy, and noncompliance with drug therapy. *The degree to which the therapist is involved in this process should be based on scope of practice as defined by state practice acts, state home care and therapy regulations, agency policies, and individual clinician competence.* The standard may be met by a physical therapist identifying the medications involved, assessing the patient response, and identifying potential drug interactions or duplicative therapies through review by nursing or pharmacy staff. The therapist might also perform a drug interaction screen using a computerized drug management software program, and notify the patient, the physician, and nursing staff of potential drug interactions or duplicative drug therapies. Readers are referred to Part Three for national therapy association practice standards and to the resource section for information about *Mosby's Home Care and Hospice Drug Handbook* (1999) for an indepth discussion of medications and care planning.

Updates to the Comprehensive Assessment:
Ongoing Assessment and Data Collection

The fourth standard §484.55(d) concerns updates to the comprehensive assessment, including OASIS data collection. The comprehensive assessment updates are to be conducted as frequently as the patient's condition warrants due to a major decline or improvement in the patient's health status, but not less frequently than at recertification (defined as every second calendar month beginning with the start of care date), at resumption of care after an inpatient admission of greater than or equal to 24 hours for any reason except diagnostic testing, and at discharge. At each of these update time points, the comprehensive assessment with OASIS data collection may be conducted by any of the allowable disciplines (SN, PT, SLP, OT).

Summary

It is important to clarify that performance of a comprehensive assessment does not mean performance of a multidisciplinary assessment, but rather an assessment of multidisciplinary needs. For instance, in assessing the patient's living arrangements, it is not intended that the speech-language pathologist provide interventions to remedy structural barriers, but to identify the need for further assessment and intervention by appropriate disciplines, in this example, triggering a referral to the occupational therapist.

In addition to the scope of the comprehensive assessment outlined by the Medicare COPs, organizations should ensure that therapy-only admissions are compliant with the additional accreditation or licensure requirements and standards related to the required contents of the medical record and required components of a comprehensive assessment (i.e., language barriers, abuse/neglect identification).

PART FIVE
OASIS: Quality, Reimbursement, and Documentation Considerations with Sample Forms

Outcome-Based Quality Improvement: The Big Picture

While home care clinicians and administrators seek to function in the ever-challenging and ever-changing home care arena, few, if any, will dispute the benefit of one long-overdue capability: the availability of valid and standardized health and functional outcomes. These outcomes (describing the outcomes available from collection and analysis of data using the OASIS data items) allow agencies, clinicians, payers, patients, and surveyors to begin to analyze the impact of home care services provided in a standardized way, enabling comparison between agencies, and within an agency from one year to the next.

OASIS data is intended to provide the necessary information to support outcome-based quality improvement (OBQI) activities. OBQI involves a two-step process of 1) outcome analysis and 2) outcome enhancement (reinforcing) or remediation (correction/improvement) of identified challenges. The collection of OASIS data merely represents the first step in the outcome analysis process. Outcome reports generated from OASIS information will allow organizations to identify outcome areas where performance is higher or lower than outcomes from a national reference sample or from the agency's previous year's performance. Based on the outcome report findings, specific target outcomes are selected. The care delivery associated with the target areas is then investigated and specific care behaviors which may be responsible for, or impact the outcome variance (positive or negative) are identified. A plan of action to reinforce positive outcomes (enhancement) or to improve substandard outcomes (remediation) is developed and implemented. Future outcome analysis activities will demonstrate if outcome achievement has been affected.

It is clear through the wording accompanying the COP publications that HCFA expects home health agencies to promote the benefit of an interdisciplinary team approach in achieving positive patient care outcomes. The home care therapists should be involved in the OBQI process beyond the initial level of data collection. Representation from the rehabilitation therapists in the review of outcome reports for target outcome selection, the care investigation process, the plan of action development and implementation, and ongoing OBQI activities will be necessary to optimally involve and impact the multidisciplinary health status outcomes which OASIS addresses.

OASIS: Linking Quality and Reimbursement

In order for HCFA to effectively evaluate and compare outcomes of care, standardized data items and collection processes are necessary. In the past, standardized data for home care was essentially limited to the information required on the Home Health Certification and Plan of Care (HCFA Form 485), and resource utilization collected from billing records. A method for directly identifying the results of the plan of care implementation and resource utilization has been noticeably absent. It has been said that OASIS is *this* critical link between quality and reimbursement. The OASIS has been identified in the new COPs as the data set which HCFA has mandated as part of the comprehensive patient assessment. With the availability of OASIS data, the organization can evaluate performance improvement efforts, thereby allowing comparison between the agency's current and past performance, and with geographic or "like-agency" reference groups for benchmarking purposes. OASIS data provides HCFA with a vehicle by which agency performance in meeting patient outcomes may be assessed and linked with resource utilization data. In fact, HCFA intends on utilizing OASIS data to develop a reliable case mix adjustment system, which will reflect the differences in the amount of services required by patients of different diagnoses and severity. This data will be used to develop specific payment rates for categories of patients, based on their expected resource use. This shift in Medicare home care reimbursement, from a system reimbursing for each qualified visit performed, to a system reimbursing a fixed dollar amount for a patient "episode of care" describes the prospective payment system (PPS) for home care services, as required by the Balanced Budget Act of 1997.

OASIS: The Newest Documentation and Quality Requirement

The OASIS data set is a group of core data elements expected to be collected on all adult (>18 years old), non-maternity home care patients, receiving health services from a Medicare certified home health agency. The data is to be collected at specific time points of the patient's home care admission, and reported to HCFA, through the state survey agency (e.g., state department of health) on at least a monthly basis. Refer to Figure 5-1 for details on data collection requirements and Appendix B for the full text of the *Federal Register* from June 18, 1999 related to OASIS and its mandatory use.

The data set was developed at the University of Colorado's Center for Health Policy Research (CHPR), under grants from HCFA and the Robert Wood Johnson Foundation. According to CHPR, the OASIS items are "discipline-neutral", simply stated, OASIS data collection is performed by home care clinicians (e.g., registered nurses, physical therapists, speech-language pathologists, and occupational therapists) without affecting reliability. This is not to say that there would never be a difference in response selection of a particular OASIS item by varying disciplines, but that the differences demonstrated are not statistically significant. Therefore, the OASIS may be appropriate for use by all home care professional team members who potentially could be the only or last skilled service provider to a home care patient. This process also supports the collection of the required data at all prescribed time points (e.g., start of care, transfer to an inpatient facility, resumption of care after inpatient stay, follow-up, and discharge) by the skilled clinician, generally in conjunction with a billable skilled visit. Agency policy or state regulation may limit the data collection personnel. For instance, a state mandating that all home care admissions be performed by nursing, would practically restrict the initial visit from ever being conducted by any of the therapy providers. Similarly, home health agencies may adopt a policy limiting performance of the comprehensive assessment and OASIS data collection to the nursing discipline. Restricting therapy providers from data collection responsibilities will likely require the agency to perform multiple nonbillable nursing visits to patients with no identified nursing need (such as those in therapy-only cases), in order to collect OASIS data at the necessary time points throughout care delivery.

Rules for OASIS Data Collection

The OASIS data is intended to be collected as an integrated part of the assessment process. The therapist conducts the assessment in a clinically meaningful sequence, gathering patient history, environment and support information, and progressing to clinical assessment and function in accordance with agency policies related to patient assessment. The home care therapist should have access to a documentation tool which meets the requirements of the comprehensive assessment, the OASIS data set, the discipline-specific assessment items, as well as additional requirements imposed by accreditation bodies. This documentation tool should be thoughtfully integrated and not a separate comprehensive tool, OASIS set, and therapy assessment tool stapled together. Poor integration of the assessment tool will result in an inefficient assessment, possibly resulting in insufficient data collection, or duplicative data collection. The full text of the OASIS data set is located in Appendix B, and an example of an OASIS-integrated comprehensive assessment tool for physical therapy is presented as Figure 5-2.

Patient information to complete the OASIS data items is collected using traditional assessment strategies of observation and assessment, with observation being the preferred method of data collection. Detailed instructions for data collection are supplied in the *HCFA Outcome and Assessment Information Set*

Figure 5-1   COMPREHENSIVE ASSESSMENT/OASIS GRID

HOME HEALTH CARE TIME POINTS	DEFINITION
Initial Visit	The date of the first home health agency in-home visit. Must determine the immediate care and support needs of the patient. For Medicare beneficiaries, must determine eligibility for the Medicare home health benefit, including homebound status.
Start of Care Visit	The date of the first billable service, or the date of the first visit which meets the coverage requirements (as outlined in the HIM 11 for Medicare beneficiaries).
Comprehensive Assessment with OASIS data collection -Start of Care (SOC)	The core condition requirement that each patient must receive a patient-specific, comprehensive assessment that accurately reflects the patient's current health status and includes information that may be used to demonstrate the patient's progress toward achievement of desired outcomes. Must identify the patient's need for home care, and meet the patient's medical, nursing, rehabilitative, social and discharge planning needs. Must verify eligibility for the Medicare home health benefit, including homebound status. Must include a drug regimen review and incorporation of the appropriate OASIS items.
OASIS data collection - Transfer to inpatient facility	OASIS data collection to be collected for a patient admitted to an inpatient facility for >24 hours for any reason other than diagnostic testing. No home visit required.
Comprehensive Assessment with OASIS data collection - Resumption of care (ROC)	Update of the Comprehensive Assessment with OASIS data collection, required at resumption of home health care after inpatient admission of >24 hours for any reason other than diagnostic testing.
Comprehensive Assessment with OASIS data collection - Recertification (follow- up)	Update of the Comprehensive Assessment with OASIS data collection performed at recertification.
Comprehensive Assessment with OASIS data collection - Follow-up (due to major decline or improvement in the patient's health status)	Update of the Comprehensive Assessment with OASIS data collection performed due to a major decline or improvement in the patient's health status at a time other than during another required assessment and data collection time point.
Comprehensive Assessment with OASIS data collection - Discharge (D/C)	Update of the Comprehensive Assessment with OASIS data collection performed upon discharge of the patient for home health services.
OASIS data collection - Death at home	OASIS data collection to be performed upon notification of the patient's death at home. No home visit required.

*Reprinted with permission from Krulish, L: **Home Therapy OASIS Assessment Forms,** Powell, Ohio, 1999, Home Therapy Services.*

Figure 5-1 (cont'd)

TIMELINESS REQUIREMENTS	ASSESSMENT / DATA COLLECTION PERSONNEL
Must be performed within 48 hours of referral or within 48 hours after the patient's return home, or on the physician ordered start of care date.	Must be performed by a registered nurse, unless only rehabilitation therapy services are ordered. When therapy service (PT, SLP, OT) is the only service ordered by the physician, and if the need for that service establishes program eligibility, the initial visit may be performed by the appropriate therapist (PT, SLP, or OT).
No specific language regarding the timeliness of the start of care visit.	Must be performed by a registered nurse, unless only rehabilitation therapy services are ordered. When therapy service (PT, SLP, OT) is the only service ordered by the physician, and if the need for that service establishes program eligibility, the start of care visit may be performed by the appropriate therapist (PT, SLP, or OT).
Must be completed in a timely manner consistent with the patient's immediate needs, but no later than 5 calendar days after the start of care.	The Comprehensive Assessment with OASIS data collection must be performed by a registered nurse, unless only rehabilitation therapy services are ordered. When therapy service (PT, SLP, OT) is the only service ordered by the physician, and if the need for that service establishes program eligibility, the Comprehensive assessment may be performed by the appropriate therapist (PT, SLP, or OT).
Completion required within 48 hours of knowledge to the home health agency of the inpatient admission.	May be performed by any of the allowed disciplines (SN, PT, SLP, OT).
Completion required within 48 hours of the patient's return to the home from an inpatient admission.	May be performed by any of the allowed disciplines (SN, PT, SLP, OT).
Completion required no less frequently than every second calendar month beginning with the start of care date.	May be performed by any of the allowed disciplines (SN, PT, SLP, OT).
Completion required within 48 hours of knowledge to the home health agency of the major decline or improvement in the patient's health status.	May be performed by any of the allowed disciplines (SN, PT, SLP, OT).
Completion required within 48 hours of discharge.	May be performed by any of the allowed disciplines (SN, PT, SLP, OT).
Completion required within 48 hours of notification to the home health agency of the patient's death at home.	May be performed by any of the allowed disciplines (SN, PT, SLP, OT).

Implementation Manual, which can be downloaded from HCFA's OASIS web-site: www.hcfa.gov/medicare/hsqb/oasis/oasishmp.htm. Excerpts from HCFA's OASIS manual related to data collection rules and common three digit ICD-9 codes for OASIS completion are presented in Boxes 5-1 and 5-2.

Box 5-1   General OASIS Data Collection Instructions

1. OASIS items can be completed by any clinician who performs the comprehensive assessment. Agency policy should determine who is responsible for completing the comprehensive assessment (and OASIS items) if individuals from more than one discipline (e.g., RN and PT) are seeing the patient concurrently.

2. All items refer to the patient's usual status or condition at the time period or visit under consideration — unless otherwise indicated. Though patient status can vary from day to day and during a given day, the response should be selected that describes the patient's status most of the time during the specific day under consideration.

3. Some items inquire about events occurring within the past 14 days or at a specified point (e.g., discharge from an inpatient facility, ADL status at 14 days prior to start of care, etc.). In these situations, the specific time interval included in the item should be followed exactly.

4. OASIS items that are scales (e.g., shortness of breath, transferring, etc.) are arranged in order from least impaired to most impaired. For example, higher values (further down the list of options) on the transferring scale refer to greater dependence in transferring. This is true whether the scale describes a functional, physiologic, or emotional health status attribute.

5. Collection of data through direct observation is preferred to that obtained through interview, but some items (e.g., frequency of primary caregiver assistance) are most often obtained through interview. When interview data are collected, the patient should be the primary source (or a caregiver residing in the home). An out-of-home caregiver can be an alternate source of information if neither of the others are available, but should be considered only in unusual circumstances. In many instances, a combined observation-interview approach is necessary. For example, by speaking with the patient or informal caregiver while conducting the assessment, the provider can determine whether the observed ability to ambulate is typical or atypical at that time. Such combined approaches of observation and interview occur frequently during most well-conducted assessments, but warrant mention here in order to clarify the meaning of OASIS items.

6. The OASIS items may be completed in any order. Since the data collection is integrated into the clinician's usual assessment process, the clinician actuallyperforming the patient assessment is responsible for determining the precise order in which the items are completed.

Box 5-1   General OASIS Data Collection Instructions (cont'd)

7. Unless a skip pattern is indicated (and followed) every OASIS item for the specific time point should be completed.
8. Unless the item is noted as "Mark all that apply," only one answer should be marked.
9. Minimize the selection of "Not Applicable" and "Unknown" answer options.
10. Each agency is responsible for monitoring the accuracy of the assessment data and the adequacy of the assessment process.

*Reprinted with permission from the **Outcome and Assessment Information Set Implementation Manual,** Health Care Financing Administration, 1998, PP 8.11-8.12.*

Box 5-2   Common Three-Digit ICD-9 Code Categories for OASIS Completion

COMMON ICD CODE CATEGORIES

Disease Conditions

042	Acquired Immune Deficiency Syndrome (AIDS)
303	Alcohol Dependence
331	Alzheimer's Disease
897	Amputation (Traumatic), Leg
335	Amyotrophic Lateral Sclerosis (ALS)
285	Anemia 2° Chemotherapy
413	Angina
441	Aortic Aneurysm
429	Arteriosclerotic Cardiovascular Disease (ASCVD)
414	Arteriosclerotic Heart Disease (ASHD)
493	Asthma
427	Atrial Fibrillation/Flutter
440	Atherosclerosis
351	Bell's Palsy
560	Bowel Obstruction
466	Bronchitis, Acute
491	Bronchitis, Chronic
490	Bronchitis, Unspecified
426	Cardiac Conduction Disorders
427	Cardiac Dysrhythmias
424	Cardiac Valve Disorders (Not Rheumatic)
425	Cardiomyopathy
366	Cataract
682	Cellulitis/Abscess (Other than Finger/Toe)
331	Cerebral Degeneration
434	Cerebral Embolism/Thrombosis
428	CHF
574	Cholelithiasis
575	Cholecystitis
571	Cirrhosis
850	Concussion
496	COPD
436	CVA
595	Cystitis
707	Decubitus Ulcer
715	Degenerative Joint Disease
290	Dementia, Senile/Presenile/Arteriosclerotic
250	Diabetes Mellitus
562	Diverticulitis, Diverticulosis
304	Drug Dependence
492	Emphysema
345	Epilepsy
824	Fracture, Ankle
810	Fracture, Clavicle

821	Fracture, Femur
820	Fracture, Hip/Neck of Femur
812	Fracture, Humerus
808	Fracture, Pelvis
813	Fracture, Radius/Ulna
807	Fracture, Ribs/Sternum
823	Fracture, Tibia/Fibula
805	Fracture, Vertebra w/o Spinal Cord Injury
806	Fracture, Vertebra with Spinal Cord Injury
814	Fracture, Wrist
785	Gangrene
535	Gastritis
578	GI Bleeding/Hemorrhage
365	Glaucoma
274	Gout
342	Hemiplegia
455	Hemorrhoids
553	Hernia (Except Inguinal) w/o Obstruction or Gangrene
053	Herpes Zoster
275	Hypercalcemia
401	Hypertension
402	Hypertensive Heart Disease
458	Hypotension
244	Hypothyroidism
550	Inguinal Hernia
722	Intervertebral Disc Degeneration/Disorder
280	Iron-Deficiency Anemia
173	Kaposi's Sarcoma
571	Liver Disease, Chronic
340	Multiple Sclerosis
410	Myocardial Infarction
149- 239	Neoplasms (Dependent on Type and Site)
151	Neoplasm, Stomach
153	Neoplasm, Colon
155	Neoplasm, Liver and Intrahepatic Bile Ducts
157	Neoplasm, Pancreas
161	Neoplasm, Larynx
162	Neoplasm, Lung
172	Neoplasm, Melanoma of Skin
172	Neoplasm, Female Breast
180	Neoplasm, Cervix
188	Neoplasm, Bladder

Box 5-2   Common Three-Digit ICD-9 Code Categories for OASIS Completion (cont'd)

191	Neoplasm, Brain
344	Neurogenic Bladder
294	Organic Psychotic Conditions (Chronic)
715	Osteoarthritis
730	Osteomyelitis
733	Osteoporosis
382	Otitis Media
344	Paralysis, Single Limb
344	Paraplegia
332	Parkinson's Disease
443	Peripheral Vascular Disease
567	Peritonitis
281	Pernicious Anemia
451	Phlebitis
511	Pleural Effusion
136	Pneumocystis Carinii
482	Pneumonia, Bacterial (Other Than Pneumococcal)
483	Pneumonia, Other Organism
481	Pneumonia, Pneumococcal
480	Pneumonia, Viral
707	Pressure Ulcer
600	Prostatic Hypertrophy
415	Pulmonary Embolism
416	Pulmonary Hypertension
344	Quadriplegia
584	Renal Failure, Acute
585	Renal Failure, Chronic
586	Renal Failure, Unspecified
714	Rheumatoid Arthritis
295	Schizophrenic Disorders
724	Sciatica
290	Senile Dementia
038	Sepsis, Septicemia
711	Septic Joint
454	Stasis Ulcer
436	Stroke
451	Thrombophlebitis
245	Thyroiditis
435	TIAs
012	Tuberculosis, Other Respiratory
011	Tuberculosis, Pulmonary
532	Ulcer, Duodenal
531	Ulcer, Gastric
533	Ulcer, Peptic-Site Unspecified
599	Urinary Tract Infection
870-884, 890-894	Wound, Open (Category Dependent on Location)

Symptoms, Signs, and Ill-Defined Conditions

789	Abdominal Distension
789	Abdominal Tenderness/Pain
783	Anorexia
784	Aphasia
789	Ascites, Abdominal
786	Chest Pain
569	Colostomy/Enterostomy Malfunction
780	Coma/Stupor
564	Constipation
782	Cyanosis
799	Debilitation (Unspecified)
276	Dehydration
558	Diarrhea (Chronic)
780	Dizziness
784	Dysphasia/Dysarthria
787	Dysphagia
782	Edema
780	Fever
736	Foot Drop
310	Forgetfulness/Memory Loss
780	Hallucinations (w/o Psychosis)
790	Hyperglycemia
728	Immobility
560	Impaction (Bowel)
788	Incontinence (Urinary)
487	Influenza
780	Malaise and Fatigue
783	Malnutrition
787	Nausea/Vomiting
785	Necrosis (Skin and Subq. Tissue)
278	Obesity
724	Pain (Back)
729	Pain (Legs)
276	Potassium Deficiency/Excess
786	Respiratory Distress
780	Seizure Disorder/Convulsion NOS
797	Senility (w/o Psychosis)/Infirmity of Old Age
276	Sodium Deficiency/Excess
780	Syncope and Collapse (Blackout, Fainting)
785	Tachycardia
788	Urinary Retention
728	Weakness (Unspecified Disorder of Muscle/Fascia)

*Reprinted with permission from the **Outcome and Assessment Information Set Implementation Manual,** Health Care Financing Administration, 1998, PP E. 1-2.*

Documenting the Comprehensive Assessment and
OASIS Data Collection - Patient Example Revisited

In Part Four we developed a patient scenario in efforts to illustrate issues related to completion of the HCFA Form 485. In Part Five we continue with Mrs. Nicholas' scenario to demonstrate the scope of medical, nursing, rehabilitative, social and discharge planning issues that are addressed in the comprehensive assessment process. The comprehensive assessment completed by the physical therapist is demonstrated using a comprehensive assessment tool developed specifically for use by physical therapy at the start of care (Figure 5-2).

Figure 5-2   Comprehensive Assessment Example Based on Patient Scenario

PHYSICAL THERAPY START OF CARE ASSESSMENT (Also used for Resumption of Care Following Inpatient Stay) (page 1 of 15)	Client Name: Angela P Nichols Client Record No: CO I

(M0010) Agency Medicare Provider Number: 2 1 1 2 3 4

Branch Identification (Optional, for Agency Use)

(M0012) Agency Medicaid Provider Number:

(M0014) Branch State: __ __

(M0016) Branch ID Number: ___ ___ ___ ___ ___ ___ ___   (Agency-assigned)

(M0020) Patient ID Number: OO I ___ ___ ___ ___ ___

(M0030) Start of Care Date: O 6 / O 1 / 1 9 9 9
month day   year

(M0032) Resumption of Care Date: __ __/__ __/__ __ __ __   ☒ NA – Not Applicable
month day   year

(M0040) Patient Name: Angela ___ ___ ___   P   Nicholas ___ ___ ___ ___ ___ ___ ___ ___   ___ ___ ___
(First)   (MI) (Last)   (Suffix)

(M0050) Patient State of Residence: NY

(M0060) Patient Zip Code: 5 4 3 2 1 ___ ___ ___ ___

(M0063) Medicare Number: 1 2 3 4 5 6 7 8 9 A ___ ___   ☐ NA– No Medicare
(including suffix)

(M0064) Social Security Number: 1 2 3 - 4 5 - 6 7 8 9   ☐ UK– Unknown or Not Available

(M0065) Medicaid Number: ___ ___ ___ ___ ___ ___ ___ ___ ___ ___ ___ ___ ___ ___   ☒ NA–No Medicaid

(M0066) Birth Date: 0 3 / 2 6 / 1 9 1 9
month day   year

(M0069) Gender: ☐ 1-Male   ☒ 2-Female

Referring Physician: Dr. Dan DeLine

(M0072) Primary Referring Physician ID: 2 4 2 4 2 4 ___ ___   ☐ UK–Unknown or Not Available

(M0080) Discipline of Person Completing Assessment: ☐ 1-RN   ☒ 2-PT   ☐ 3-SLP/ST   ☐ 4-OT

(M0090) Date Assessment Completed: 0 6 / O 1 / 1 9 9 9
month day   year

(M0100) This Assessment is Currently Being Completed for the Following Reason:

Start/Resumption of Care
☒ 1– Start of care—further visits planned
☐ 2– Start of care—no further visits planned
☐ 3– Resumption of care (after inpatient stay)

Follow-Up
☐ 4–Recertification (follow-up) reassessment
☐ 5–Other follow-up

Transfer to an Inpatient Facility
☐ 6–Transferred to an inpatient facility— patient not discharged from agency
☐ 7–Transferred to an inpatient facility— patient discharged from agency
Discharge from Agency — Not to an Inpatient Facility
☐ 8 –Death at home
☐ 9 –Discharge from agency
☐ 10–Discharge from agency—no visits completed after start/resumption of care assessment

THERAPY DIAGNOSIS/ONSET (R) humeral fx - nonoperative s/p fall in home 052699, Exacerbation (R) Knee OA sx5, unsteady gait, dependent ADLs

PRIOR TREATMENTS/SERVICES: No prior home care or therapy services reported.

Response to previous services: ☐ Achieved outcomes ☐ Partial benefit ☐ No benefit

PATIENT HISTORY: ☐ Cancer ☐ Choking/Aspiration ☐ Congestive Heart Failure ☐ COPD ☐ CVA ☒ Diabetes IDDM 1985
☒ Fractures 052699 ☒ History of Falls x 1 ☐ Hypertension ☐ Infection ☐ Myocardial Infarction ☐ Osteoporosis
☐ Psychiatric History ☐ Recent Weight Gain/Loss ☐ History of Patient Abuse/Neglect
☒ Other: Osteoarthritis (R) Knee 050199, GI Bleed 052699, Anemia 052699
Are needs identified for further assessment, treatment, or instruction of above conditions? ☐ No ☒ Yes, (describe)
Pt currently unable to self inject insulin 2° to (R) UE immobilization in Sling x 3 wks

PHYSICAL THERAPY START OF CARE ASSESSMENT (Also used for Resumption of Care Following Inpatient Stay) (page 2 of 15)	Client Name: A. Nicholas Client Record No: 001

HOMEBOUND STATUS: (mark all that apply) ☒Requires considerable and taxing effort ☐Medically contraindicated
☒Dependent upon assistive/adaptive device(s) ☐Requires special transportation ☒Unable to safely leave home unassisted
☐Other: (specify) Supporting detail:
Does the patient meet the eligibility criteria for the Medicare home health benefit? ☒Yes ☐No ☐N/A

(M0140) Race/Ethnicity (as identified by patient): **(Mark all that apply.)**

☐1-American Indian or Alaska Native ☐3-Black or African-American ☐5-Native Hawaiian or Pacific Islander
☐2-Asian ☐4-Hispanic or Latino ☒6-White ☐UK-Unknown

(M0150) Current Payment Sources for Home Care: (Mark all that apply.)

☐0 -None; no charge for current services
☒1 -Medicare (traditional fee-for-service)
☐2 -Medicare (HMO/managed care)
☐3 -Medicaid (traditional fee-for-service)
☐4 -Medicaid (HMO/managed care)
☐5 -Workers' compensation

☐6 -Title programs (e.g., Title III, V, or XX)
☐7 -Other government (e.g., CHAMPUS, VA, etc.)
☐8 -Private insurance
☐9 -Private HMO/managed care
☐10 -Self-pay
☐11 -Other (specify)_____
☐UK -Unknown

(M0160) Financial Factors limiting the ability of the patient/family to meet basic health needs: **(Mark all that apply.)**

☒0 - None
☐1 -Unable to afford medicine or medical supplies
☐2 -Unable to afford medical expenses that are not covered by insurance/Medicare (e.g., copayments)
☐3 -Unable to afford rent/utility bills
☐4 -Unable to afford food
☐5 -Other (specify)

(M0170) From which of the following **Inpatient Facilities** was the patient discharged during the past 14 days? **(Mark all that apply.)**

☒ 1 - Hospital
☐ 2 - Rehabilitation facility
☐ 3 - Nursing home
☐ 4 - Other (specify) _____
☐ NA - Patient was not discharged from an inpatient facility **[If NA, go to M0200]**

(M0180) Inpatient Discharge Date (most recent):
0 5 / 3 1 / 1 9 9 9   ☐ UK - Unknown
month day year

(M0190) Inpatient Diagnoses and ICD code categories (three digits required; five digits optional) for only those conditions treated during an inpatient facility stay within the last 14 days (no surgical or V-codes):

Inpatient Facility Diagnosis   ICD
a. (R) Humeral fx   (8 1 2 . 2 0)
b. GI Bleed   (5 7 8 . 9 0)

(M0200) Medical or Treatment Regimen Change Within Past 14 Days: Has this patient experienced a change in medical or treatment regimen (e.g., medication, treatment, or service change due to new or additional diagnosis, etc.) within the last 14 days?

☐ 0 - No **[If No, go to M0220]**
☒ 1 - Yes

(M0210) List the patient's **Medical Diagnoses** and ICD code categories (three digits required; five digits optional) for those conditions requiring changed medical or treatment regimen (no surgical or V-codes):

Changed Medical Regimen Diagnosis   ICD
a. (R) Humeral fx   (8 1 2 . 2 0)
b. GI Bleed   (5 7 8 . 9 0)
c. Anemia   (2 8 5 . 1 0)
d. Osteoarthritis   (7 1 6 . 6 0)

(M0220) Conditions Prior to Medical or Treatment Regimen Change or Inpatient Stay Within Past 14 Days: If this patient experienced an inpatient facility discharge or change in medical or treatment regimen within the past 14 days, indicate any conditions which existed prior to the inpatient stay or change in medical or treatment regimen. **(Mark all that apply.)**

☐ 1 - Urinary incontinence
☐ 2 - Indwelling/suprapubic catheter
☐ 3 - Intractable pain
☐ 4 - Impaired decision-making
☐ 5 - Disruptive or socially inappropriate behavior

☐ 6 - Memory loss to the extent that supervision required
☒ 7 - None of the above
☐ NA - No inpatient facility discharge and no change in medical or treatment regimen in past 14 days
☐ UK - Unknown

PHYSICAL THERAPY START OF CARE ASSESSMENT (Also used for Resumption of Care Following Inpatient Stay) (page 3 of 15)	Client Name: A. Nicholas Client Record No: 001

| MEDICALLY PRESCRIBED DIET: ☐No ☒Yes, 1500 Cal ADA Diabetic diet | ALLERGIES: ☐No Known Allergies ☒Yes | Drug Allergies: Betadine Pineapple
Non-Drug Allergies: Paper Tape |

(M0230/M0240) **Diagnoses and Severity Index**: List each medical diagnosis or problem for which the patient is receiving home care and ICD code category (three digits required; five digits optional – no surgical or V-codes) and rate them using the following severity index. (Choose one value that represents the most severe rating appropriate for each diagnosis.)

    0   - Asymptomatic, no treatment needed at this time
    1   - Symptoms well controlled with current therapy
    2   - Symptoms controlled with difficulty, affecting daily functioning; patient needs ongoing monitoring
    3   - Symptoms poorly controlled, patient needs frequent adjustment in treatment and dose monitoring
    4   - Symptoms poorly controlled, history of rehospitalizations

(M0230) Primary Diagnosis   ICD   Severity Rating

a. ⓇHumeral fracture (812.20)   ☐0 ☐1 ☒2 ☐3 ☐4

(M0240) Other Diagnoses   ICD   Severity Rating

b. Osteoarthritis (716.60)   ☐0 ☐1 ☒2 ☐3 ☐4

c. Anemia (285.10)   ☐0 ☒1 ☐2 ☐3 ☐4

d. _____ (___.__)   ☐0 ☐1 ☐2 ☐3 ☐4

e. _____ (___.__)   ☐0 ☐1 ☐2 ☐3 ☐4

f. _____ (___.__)   ☐0 ☐1 ☐2 ☐3 ☐4

(M0250) **Therapies** the patient receives <u>at home</u>: **(Mark all that apply.)**	(M0260) **Overall Prognosis:** BEST description of patient's overall prognosis for <u>recovery from this episode of illness</u>.
☐ 1 - Intravenous or infusion therapy (excludes TPN) ☐ 2 - Parenteral nutrition (TPN or lipids) ☐ 3 - Enteral nutrition (nasogastric, gastrostomy, jejunostomy, or any other artificial entry into the alimentary canal) ☒ 4 - None of the above	☐ 0 - Poor: little or no recovery is expected and/or further decline is imminent ☒ 1 - Good/Fair: partial to full recovery is expected ☐ UK - Unknown

(M0270) **Rehabilitative Prognosis:** BEST description of patient's prognosis for <u>functional status</u>.	(M0280) **Life Expectancy:** (Physician documentation is not required.)
☐ 0 - Guarded: minimal improvement in functional status is expected; decline is possible ☒ 1 - Good: marked improvement in functional status is expected ☐ UK - Unknown	☒ 0 - Life expectancy is greater than 6 months ☐ 1 - Life expectancy is 6 months or fewer

(M0290) **High Risk Factors** characterizing this patient: **(Mark all that apply.)**	**LIVING ARRANGEMENTS / SUPPORTIVE ASSISTANCE** (M0300) **Current Residence:**
☐ 1 - Heavy smoking ☐ 2 - Obesity ☐ 3 - Alcohol dependency ☐ 4 - Drug dependency ☒ 5 - None of the above ☐ UK - Unknown	☒ 1 - Patient's owned or rented residence (house, apartment, or mobile home owned or rented by patient/couple/significant other) ☐ 2 - Family member's residence ☐ 3 - Boarding home or rented room ☐ 4 - Board and care or assisted living facility ☐ 5 - Other (specify) _____

PHYSICAL THERAPY START OF CARE ASSESSMENT (Also used for Resumption of Care Following Inpatient Stay) (page 4 of 15)	Client Name: A. Nicholas
	Client Record No: 001

HOME ENVIRONMENT:
Safety recommendations made? ☐No ☒Yes

Mobility Pathways:
☐ Adequate
☐ Cluttered
☐ Obstructed
☒ Throw Rugs Removed & Consent
☒ Other: Add Night Light - Hall

Steps in Home:
☒No
☐Yes, Number?
Railing?
Frequency of use?

Home Entry:
Steps ☐No
☒Yes, Number? 3
Railing? East
Walkway condition? Side
uneven stone

(M0310) Structural Barriers in the patient's environment limiting independent mobility: (Mark all that apply.)

☐ 0 - None
☐ 1 - Stairs inside home which must be used by the patient (e.g., to get to toileting, sleeping, eating areas)
☐ 2 - Stairs inside home which are used optionally (e.g., to get to laundry facilities)
☒ 3 - Stairs leading from inside house to outside
☐ 4 - Narrow or obstructed doorways

(M0320) Safety Hazards found in the patient's current place of residence: (Mark all that apply.)

☐ 0 - None
☐ 1 - Inadequate floor, roof, or windows
☒ 2 - Inadequate lighting
☐ 3 - Unsafe gas/electric appliance
☐ 4 - Inadequate heating
☐ 5 - Inadequate cooling
☐ 6 - Lack of fire safety devices
☐ 7 - Unsafe floor coverings
☐ 8 - Inadequate stair railings
☐ 9 - Improperly stored hazardous materials
☐ 10 - Lead-based paint
☐ 11 - Other (specify) _____

(M0330) Sanitation Hazards found in the patient's current place of residence: (Mark all that apply.)

☒ 0 - None
☐ 1 - No running water
☐ 2 - Contaminated water
☐ 3 - No toileting facilities
☐ 4 - Outdoor toileting facilities only
☐ 5 - Inadequate sewage disposal
☐ 6 - Inadequate/improper food storage
☐ 7 - No food refrigeration
☐ 8 - No cooking facilities
☐ 9 - Insects/rodents present
☐ 10 - No scheduled trash pickup
☐ 11 - Cluttered/soiled living area
☐ 12 - Other (specify) _____

(M0340) Patient Lives With: (Mark all that apply.)

☒ 1 - Lives alone
☐ 2 - With spouse or significant other
☐ 3 - With other family member
☐ 4 - With a friend
☐ 5 - With paid help (other than home care agency staff)
☐ 6 - With other than above

SUPPORTIVE ASSISTANCE:

☐ Caregiver willing and able to assist in care
☒ Caregiver with limited willingness or ability to assist in care
☐ No Caregiver available
Nephew is diabetic, available each am for insulin injection & evening for bed prep.

(M0350) Assisting Person(s) Other than Home Care Agency Staff: (Mark all that apply.)

☒ 1 - Relatives, friends, or neighbors living outside the home
☐ 2 - Person residing in the home (EXCLUDING paid help)
☐ 3 - Paid help
☐ 4 - None of the above [If None of the above, go to M0390]
☐ UK - Unknown [If Unknown, go to M0390]

(M0360) Primary Caregiver taking lead responsibility for providing or managing the patient's care, providing the most frequent assistance, etc. (other than home care agency staff):

☐ 0 - No one person [If No one person, go to M0390]
☐ 1 - Spouse or significant other
☐ 2 - Daughter or son   John Nicholas
☒ 3 - Other family member Nephew 339-0615
☐ 4 - Friend or neighbor or community or church member
☐ 5 - Paid help
☐ UK - Unknown [If Unknown, go to M0390]

(M0370) How Often does the patient receive assistance from the primary caregiver?

☐ 1 - Several times during day and night
☒ 2 - Several times during day am x 1 pm x 1
☐ 3 - Once daily
☐ 4 - Three or more times per week
☐ 5 - One to two times per week
☐ 6 - Less often than weekly
☐ UK - Unknown

PHYSICAL THERAPY START OF CARE ASSESSMENT	Client Name: A. Nicholas
(Also used for Resumption of Care Following Inpatient Stay) (page 5 of 15)	Client Record No: 001

(M0380) Type of Primary Caregiver Assistance: (Mark all that apply.)

- ☒ 1 - ADL assistance (e.g., bathing (dressing) toileting, bowel/bladder, eating/feeding)
- ☒ 2 - IADL assistance (e.g. (meds) (meals) (housekeeping, laundry) telephone (shopping,) finances)
- ☐ 3 - Environmental support (housing, home maintenance)
- ☒ 4 - Psychosocial support ((socialization) companionship) recreation)
- ☐ 5 - Advocates or facilitates patient's participation in appropriate medical care
- ☐ 6 - Financial agent, power of attorney, or conservator of finance
- ☐ 7 - Health care agent, conservator of person, or medical power of attorney
- ☐ UK - Unknown

SENSORY STATUS

(M0390) Vision with corrective lenses if the patient usually wears them:

- ☒ 0 - Normal vision: sees adequately in most situations; can see medication labels, newsprint.
- ☐ 1 - Partially impaired: cannot see medication labels or newsprint, but can see obstacles in path, and the surrounding layout; can count fingers at arm's length.
- ☐ 2 - Severely impaired: cannot locate objects without hearing or touching them or patient nonresponsive.

(M0400) Hearing and Ability to Understand Spoken Language in patient's own language (with hearing aids if the patient usually uses them):

- ☒ 0 - No observable impairment. Able to hear and understand complex or detailed instructions and extended or abstract conversation.
- ☐ 1 - With minimal difficulty, able to hear and understand most multi-step instructions and ordinary conversation. May need occasional repetition, extra time, or louder voice.
- ☐ 2 - Has moderate difficulty hearing and understanding simple, one-step instructions and brief conversation; needs frequent prompting or assistance.
- ☐ 3 - Has severe difficulty hearing and understanding simple greetings and short comments. Requires multiple repetitions, restatements, demonstrations, additional time.
- ☐ 4 - Unable to hear and understand familiar words or common expressions consistently, or patient nonresponsive.

(M0410) Speech and Oral (Verbal) Expression of Language (in patient's own language):

- ☒ 0 - Expresses complex ideas, feelings, and needs clearly, completely, and easily in all situations with no observable impairment.
- ☐ 1 - Minimal difficulty in expressing ideas and needs (may take extra time; makes occasional errors in word choice, grammar or speech intelligibility; needs minimal prompting or assistance).
- ☐ 2 - Expresses simple ideas or needs with moderate difficulty (needs prompting or assistance, errors in word choice, organization or speech intelligibility). Speaks in phrases or short sentences.
- ☐ 3 - Has severe difficulty expressing basic ideas or needs and requires maximal assistance or guessing by listener. Speech limited to single words or short phrases.
- ☐ 4 - Unable to express basic needs even with maximal prompting or assistance but is not comatose or unresponsive (e.g., speech is nonsensical or unintelligible).
- ☐ 5 - Patient nonresponsive or unable to speak.

☒ Corrective Lenses   ☐ Hearing Aid(s)   ☒ Dentures

(M0420) Frequency of Pain interfering with patient's activity or movement:	**(M0430) Intractable Pain:** Is the patient experiencing pain that is not easily relieved, occurs at least daily, and affects the patient's sleep, appetite, physical or emotional energy, concentration, personal relationships, emotions, or ability or desire to perform physical activity?
☐ 0 - Patient has no pain or pain does not interfere with activity or movement ☐ 1 - Less often than daily ☒ 2 - Daily, but not constantly ☐ 3 - All of the time	☒ 0 - No ☐ 1 - Yes

PAIN: Intensity 0 1 2 3 ④ 5 ⑥ ⑦ 8 9 10
                    R Knee R UE
Location/Characteristics:
Ⓡ Knee Ache   Ⓡ shoulder, upper arm frequent
                                            ache
Aggravating/Relieving Factors:
Ⓡ Knee worse c̄ transfers, steps
	SENSATION:
	intact to light touch, pressure,
	hot/cold × 4 extremities

PHYSICAL THERAPY START OF CARE ASSESSMENT (Also used for Resumption of Care Following Inpatient Stay) (page 6 of 15)	Client Name: A. Nicholas
	Client Record No: 001

EDEMA/SWELLING:
Mild edema (R) hand; Mod edema (B) upper arm (Mid humeral girth 33cm (R), 29 cm (L))
Mod edema (R) Knee (Mid Patellar Girth 42cm (R), 38 cm (L))

HEART RATE:	**BLOOD PRESSURE:**	**RESPIRATION:**	**TEMPERATURE:**	**HEIGHT:**	**WEIGHT:**
68 rest 84 peak	124/90 sit 116/78 stand	16	98.6°	5'4"	138#

INTEGUMENT:	Skin Lesion	Pressure Ulcer	Stasis Ulcer	Surgical Wound	Bruise	Rash	Other:
Location					(B) upper arm - posterior		
Size					10cm x 8cm		
Description					dark purple, uneven edges		

(M0440) Does this patient have a **Skin Lesion** or an **Open Wound?** This excludes "OSTOMIES."

☐ 0 - No [If No, go to *M0490*]
☒ 1 - Yes

(M0445) Does this patient have a **Pressure Ulcer?**

☒ 0 - No [If No, go to *M0468*]
☐ 1 - Yes

(M0450)	Pressure Ulcer Stages		Number of Pressure Ulcers				
Current Number of Pressure Ulcers at Each Stage: (Circle one response for each stage.)	a)Stage 1: Nonblanchable erythema of intact skin; the heralding of skin ulceration. In darker-pigmented skin, warmth, edema, hardness, or discolored skin may be indicators.		0	1	2	3	4 or more
	b)Stage 2: Partial thickness skin loss involving epidermis and/or dermis. The ulcer is superficial and presents clinically as an abrasion, blister, or shallow crater.		0	1	2	3	4 or more
	c)Stage 3: Full-thickness skin loss involving damage or necrosis of subcutaneous tissue which may extend down to, but not through, underlying fascia. The ulcer presents clinically as a deep crater with or without undermining of adjacent tissue.		0	1	2	3	4 or more
	d)Stage 4: Full-thickness skin loss with extensive destruction, tissue necrosis, or damage to muscle, bone, or supporting structures (e.g., tendon, joint capsule, etc.)		0	1	2	3	4 or more
	e)In addition to the above, is there at least one pressure ulcer that cannot be observed due to the presence of eschar or a nonremovable dressing, including casts? ☐ 0 - No ☐ 1 - Yes						

(M0460) Stage of Most Problematic (Observable) Pressure Ulcer:

☐ 1 - Stage 1
☐ 2 - Stage 2
☐ 3 - Stage 3
☐ 4 - Stage 4
☐ NA - No observable pressure ulcer

(M0464) Status of Most Problematic (Observable) Pressure Ulcer:

☐ 1 - Fully granulating
☐ 2 - Early/partial granulation
☐ 3 - Not healing
☐ NA - No observable pressure ulcer

(M0468) Does this patient have a **Stasis Ulcer?**

☒ 0 - No [If No, go to *M0482*]
☐ 1 - Yes

(M0470) Current Number of Observable Stasis Ulcer(s):

☐ 0 - Zero
☐ 1 - One
☐ 2 - Two
☐ 3 - Three
☐ 4 - Four or more

(M0474) Does this patient have at least one **Stasis Ulcer that Cannot be Observed** due to the presence of a nonremovable dressing?

☐ 0 - No
☐ 1 - Yes

(M0476) Status of Most Problematic (Observable) Stasis Ulcer:

☐ 1 - Fully granulating
☐ 2 - Early/partial granulation
☐ 3 - Not healing
☐ NA - No observable stasis ulcer

PHYSICAL THERAPY START OF CARE ASSESSMENT (Also used for Resumption of Care Following Inpatient Stay) (page 7 of 15)	Client Name: A. Nicholas Client Record No: 001

(M0482) Does this patient have a **Surgical Wound**? ☒ 0 - No **[If No, go to M0490]** ☐ 1 - Yes	(M0484) **Current Number of (Observable) Surgical Wounds:** (If a wound is partially closed but has more than one opening, consider each opening as a separate wound.) ☐ 0 - Zero ☐ 1 - One ☐ 2 - Two ☐ 3 - Three ☐ 4 - Four or more
(M0486) Does this patient have at least one **Surgical Wound that Cannot be Observed** due to the presence of a nonremovable dressing? ☐ 0 - No ☐ 1 - Yes	(M0488) **Status of Most Problematic (Observable) Surgical Wound:** ☐ 1 - Fully granulating ☐ 2 - Early/partial granulation ☐ 3 - Not healing ☐ NA - No observable surgical wound

RESPIRATORY STATUS

(M0490) When is the patient dyspneic or noticeably **Short of Breath**? ☐ 0 -Never, patient is not short of breath ☐ 1 -When walking more than 20 feet, climbing stairs ☐ 2 -With moderate exertion (e.g., while dressing, using commode or bedpan, walking distances less than 20 feet) ☒ 3 -With minimal exertion (e.g., while eating, talking, or performing other ADLs) or with agitation ☐ 4 -At rest (during day or night)	(M0500) **Respiratory Treatments** utilized at home: **(Mark all that apply.)** ☐ 1 - Oxygen (intermittent or continuous) ☐ 2 - Ventilator (continually or at night) ☐ 3 - Continuous positive airway pressure ☒ 4 - None of the above Endurance: Poor endurance with minimal activity - SOB and rapid fatigue limit in home mobility and function.

ELIMINATION STATUS

(M0510) Has this patient been treated for a **Urinary Tract Infection** in the past 14 days? ☒ 0 - No ☐ 1 - Yes ☐ NA - Patient on prophylactic treatment ☐ UK - Unknown	(M0520) **Urinary Incontinence or Urinary Catheter Presence:** ☒ 0 - No incontinence or catheter (includes anuria or ostomy for urinary drainage) **[If No, go to M0540]** ☐ 1 - Patient is incontinent ☐ 2 - Patient requires a urinary catheter (i.e., external, indwelling, intermittent, suprapubic) **[Go to M0540]**
(M0530) When does **Urinary Incontinence** occur? ☐ 0 - Timed-voiding defers incontinence ☐ 1 - During the night only ☐ 2 - During the day and night	(M0540) **Bowel Incontinence Frequency:** ☒ 0 -Very rarely or never has bowel incontinence ☐ 1 -Less than once weekly ☐ 2 -One to three times weekly ☐ 3 -Four to six times weekly ☐ 4 -On a daily basis ☐ 5 -More often than once daily ☐ NA -Patient has ostomy for bowel elimination ☐ UK -Unknown

(M0550) **Ostomy for Bowel Elimination:** Does this patient have an ostomy for bowel elimination that (within the last 14 days): a) was related to an inpatient facility stay, or b) necessitated a change in medical or treatment regimen?

☒ 0 - Patient does not have an ostomy for bowel elimination.

☐ 1 - Patient's ostomy was not related to an inpatient stay and did not necessitate change in medical or treatment regimen.

☐ 2 - The ostomy was related to an inpatient stay or did necessitate change in medical or treatment regimen.

PHYSICAL THERAPY START OF CARE ASSESSMENT (Also used for Resumption of Care Following Inpatient Stay) (page 8 of 15)	Client Name: A. Nicholas Client Record No: 001

NEURO/EMOTIONAL/BEHAVIORAL STATUS

BEHAVIOR/MENTAL STATUS: (mark all that apply) ☑Alert ☒Oriented ☐Confused ☐Memory Deficits ☒Cooperative

☐Impaired Judgement ☒Motivated ☒Receptive to Therapy Services ☐Other:

(M0560) Cognitive Functioning: (Patient's current level of alertness, orientation, comprehension, concentration, and immediate memory for simple commands.)

- ☒ 0 - Alert/oriented, able to focus and shift attention, comprehends and recalls task directions independently.
- ☐ 1 - Requires prompting (cuing, repetition, reminders) only under stressful or unfamiliar conditions.
- ☐ 2 - Requires assistance and some direction in specific situations (e.g., on all tasks involving shifting of attention), or consistently requires low stimulus environment due to distractibility.
- ☐ 3 - Requires considerable assistance in routine situations. Is not alert and oriented or is unable to shift attention and recall directions more than half the time.
- ☐ 4 - Totally dependent due to disturbances such as constant disorientation, coma, persistent vegetative state, or delirium.

(M0570) When Confused (Reported or Observed):	**(M0580) When Anxious (Reported or Observed):**
☐ 0 - Never ☒ 1 - In new or complex situations only ☐ 2 - On awakening or at night only ☐ 3 - During the day and evening, but not constantly ☐ 4 - Constantly ☐ NA - Patient nonresponsive	☐ 0 - None of the time ☒ 1 - Less often than daily ☐ 2 - Daily, but not constantly ☐ 3 - All of the time ☐ NA - Patient nonresponsive

(M0590) Depressive Feelings Reported or Observed in Patient: (Mark all that apply.)	**(M0600) Patient Behaviors (Reported or Observed): (Mark all that apply.)**
☐ 1 - Depressed mood (e.g., feeling sad, tearful) ☐ 2 - Sense of failure or self reproach ☐ 3 - Hopelessness ☐ 4 - Recurrent thoughts of death ☐ 5 - Thoughts of suicide ☒ 6 - None of the above feelings observed or reported	☐ 1 -Indecisiveness, lack of concentration ☐ 2 -Diminished interest in most activities ☐ 3 -Sleep disturbances ☐ 4 -Recent change in appetite or weight ☐ 5 -Agitation ☐ 6 -A suicide attempt ☒ 7 -None of the above behaviors observed or reported

(M0610) Behaviors Demonstrated at Least Once a Week (Reported or Observed): (Mark all that apply.)

- ☐ 1 - Memory deficit: failure to recognize familiar persons/places, inability to recall events of past 24 hours, significant memory loss so that supervision is required
- ☐ 2 - Impaired decision-making: failure to perform usual ADLs or IADLs, inability to appropriately stop activities, jeopardizes safety through actions
- ☐ 3 - Verbal disruption: yelling, threatening, excessive profanity, sexual references, etc.
- ☐ 4 - Physical aggression: aggressive or combative to self and others (e.g., hits self, throws objects, punches, dangerous maneuvers with wheelchair or other objects)
- ☐ 5 - Disruptive, infantile, or socially inappropriate behavior (**excludes** verbal actions)
- ☐ 6 - Delusional, hallucinatory, or paranoid behavior
- ☒ 7 - None of the above behaviors demonstrated

(M0620) Frequency of Behavior Problems (Reported or Observed) (e.g., wandering episodes, self abuse, verbal disruption, physical aggression, etc.):	**(M0630)** Is this patient receiving **Psychiatric Nursing Services** at home provided by a qualified psychiatric nurse?
☒ 0 - Never ☐ 1 - Less than once a month ☐ 2 - Once a month ☐ 3 - Several times each month ☐ 4 - Several times a week ☐ 5 - At least daily	☒ 0 - No ☐ 1 - Yes **LANGUAGE BARRIER:** Note noted **LEARNING BARRIER:** Patient requests instructions IN WRITING

PHYSICAL THERAPY START OF CARE ASSESSMENT (Also used for Resumption of Care Following Inpatient Stay) (page 9 of 15)	Client Name: A. Nicholas Client Record No: 001

FUNCTIONAL ASSESSMENT

PRIOR FUNCTIONAL LEVEL:	Independent	Independent (using assistive / adaptive equipment)	Dependent	Comments:
ADLs	X			
IADLs	X			
Home Ambulation	X			↑ing Knee pain x 1 mo
Community Ambulation	X			up to 2 blocks
Wheelchair Mobility	N/A			
Functional Communication	X			

MUSCULOSKELETAL STATUS:	Range of Motion		Strength		Comments: (posture, tone, crepitus, effusion)
	Left	Right	Left	Right	
Shoulder	90% AROM	IMMOBILIZED	4+/5	N/T	
Elbow	WFL	IN SLING	5/5	N/T	
Wrist	WFL	WFL	5/5	4-/5	
Grip	WFL	WFL	5/5	4/5	
Hip	WFL	WFL	5/5	5/5	
Knee	WFL	-8° to 87°AROM	4+/5	3+/5	(R) Knee crepitus, 13° valgus
Ankle	WFL	WFL	4+/5	4/5	deformity
Spine	WFL		WFL		↓'d Lumbar lordosis
Other:					pelvic obliquity, (R) low

ORTHOTIC/PROSTHETIC DEVICES: None

FUNCTIONAL MOBILITY:		Independent	Verbal Cues Supervision	SBA	CGA	Min Assist	Mod Assist	Max Assist	Unable	Not Tested N/A	Comments:
Bed Mobility	Turn/Roll	X									
	Scoot/Bridge	X									
	Sit to Supine		X								
	Supine to Sit				X						
Transfers	Sit to Stand				X						
	Stand Pivot				X						
	Toilet				X						
	Shower/Tub						X				
	Floor									X	
	Car									X	Mod (A) by pt. report
	Other:										
Wheelchair Mobility	Propulsion Level Surfaces								N/A		
	Propulsion Unlevel Surfaces										
	Safety Locks										
	Foot/Leg Rests										
Emergency Response Needs:		X									Has Personal Emerg. Response System

SITTING BALANCE: Static: ☒Good ☐Fair ☐Poor Dynamic: ☐Good ☒Fair ☐Poor	STANDING BALANCE: Static: ☐Good ☒Fair ☐Poor Dynamic: ☐Good ☒Fair–☐Poor

AMBULATION: Weight Bearing Status: ☐FWB ☐PWB ☐LLE ☐TDWB ☐R LE ☒NWB ☐L UE ☐WBAT ☒R UE	Ambulation Surfaces: ☒Level ☐Uneven ☒Stairs ☐Other:	Assistance: CGA + verbal cues Mod (A) x1	Distances: 15'- limited by endurance 3 steps	Assistive Devices: NBQC (L)UE handheld (A)

PHYSICAL THERAPY START OF CARE ASSESSMENT (Also used for Resumption of Care Following Inpatient Stay) (page 10 of 15)	Client Name: A. Nicholas Client Record No: 001

GAIT DEVIATIONS: Antalgic gait related to (R) Knee pain trunk asymmetry due to shortened (R) LE 2° valgus deformity

EQUIPMENT:

	Wheeled Walker	Walker	Quad Cane	Straight Cane	Crutches	Wheelchair	Electric Scooter	Tub Seat	Shower Bench	Bath Grab Bars	3-in-1 Commode	Elevated Toilet Seat	Commode Grab Bars / Arm rests	Gait Belt	Ramp	Other:
Has			NBQC													
Needs									X	X						

Comments: PT to coordinate equipment needs c̄ OT

For M0640-M0800, complete the "Current" column for all patients. For these same items, complete the "Prior" column only at start of care and at resumption of care; mark the level that corresponds to the patient's condition 14 days prior to start of care date (M0030) or resumption of care date (M0032). In all cases, record what the patient is *able to do.*

(M0640) Grooming: Ability to tend to personal hygiene needs (i.e., washing face and hands, hair care, shaving or make up, teeth or denture care, fingernail care).

Prior	Current			
☒	☐	0	-	Able to groom self unaided, with or without the use of assistive devices or adapted methods.
☐	☐	1	-	Grooming utensils must be placed within reach before able to complete grooming activities.
☐	☒	2	-	Someone must assist the patient to groom self.
☐	☐	3	-	Patient depends entirely upon someone else for grooming needs.
☐		UK	-	Unknown

(M0650) Ability to Dress Upper Body (with or without dressing aids) including undergarments, pullovers, front-opening shirts and blouses, managing zippers, buttons, and snaps:

Prior	Current			
☒	☐	0	-	Able to get clothes out of closets and drawers, put them on and remove them from the upper body without assistance.
☐	☐	1	-	Able to dress upper body without assistance if clothing is laid out or handed to the patient.
☐	☒	2	-	Someone must help the patient put on upper body clothing.
☐	☐	3	-	Patient depends entirely upon another person to dress the upper body.
☐		UK	-	Unknown

(M0660) Ability to Dress Lower Body (with or without dressing aids) including undergarments, slacks, socks or nylons, shoes:

Prior	Current			
☒	☐	0	-	Able to obtain, put on, and remove clothing and shoes without assistance.
☐	☐	1	-	Able to dress lower body without assistance if clothing and shoes are laid out or handed to the patient.
☐	☒	2	-	Someone must help the patient put on undergarments, slacks, socks or nylons, and shoes.
☐	☐	3	-	Patient depends entirely upon another person to dress lower body.
☐		UK	-	Unknown

(M0670) Bathing: Ability to wash entire body. Excludes grooming (washing face and hands only).

Prior	Current			
☒	☐	0	-	Able to bathe self in shower or tub independently.
☐	☐	1	-	With the use of devices, is able to bathe self in shower or tub independently.
☐	☒	2	-	Able to bathe in shower or tub with the assistance of another person: (a) for intermittent supervision or encouragement or reminders, OR (b) to get in and out of the shower or tub, OR (c) for washing difficult to reach areas.
☐	☐	3	-	Participates in bathing self in shower or tub, but requires presence of another person throughout the bath for assistance or supervision.
☐	☐	4	-	Unable to use the shower or tub and is bathed in bed or bedside chair.
☐	☐	5	-	Unable to effectively participate in bathing and is totally bathed by another person.
☐		UK	-	Unknown

PHYSICAL THERAPY START OF CARE ASSESSMENT (Also used for Resumption of Care Following Inpatient Stay) (page 11 of 15)	Client Name: A. Nicholas Client Record No: 001

(M0680) Toileting: Ability to get to and from the toilet or bedside commode.

Prior	Current			
☒	☒	0	-	Able to get to and from the toilet independently with or without a device.
☐	☐	1	-	When reminded, assisted, or supervised by another person, able to get to and from the toilet.
☐	☐	2	-	Unable to get to and from the toilet but is able to use a bedside commode (with or without assistance).
☐	☐	3	-	Unable to get to and from the toilet or bedside commode but is able to use a bedpan/urinal independently.
☐	☐	4	-	Is totally dependent in toileting.
☐		UK	-	Unknown

(M0690) Transferring: Ability to move from bed to chair, on and off toilet or commode, into and out of tub or shower, and ability to turn and position self in bed if patient is bedfast.

Prior	Current			
☒	☐	0	-	Able to independently transfer.
☐	☒	1	-	Transfers with minimal human assistance or with use of an assistive device.
☐	☐	2	-	Unable to transfer self but is able to bear weight and pivot during the transfer process.
☐	☐	3	-	Unable to transfer self and is unable to bear weight or pivot when transferred by another person.
☐	☐	4	-	Bedfast, unable to transfer but is able to turn and position self in bed.
☐	☐	5	-	Bedfast, unable to transfer and is unable to turn and position self.
☐		UK	-	Unknown

(M0700) Ambulation/Locomotion: Ability to SAFELY walk, once in a standing position, or use a wheelchair, once in a seated position, on a variety of surfaces.

Prior	Current			
☒	☐	0	-	Able to independently walk on even and uneven surfaces and climb stairs with or without railings (i.e., needs no human assistance or assistive device).
☐	☒	1	-	Requires use of a device (e.g., cane, walker) to walk alone or requires human supervision or assistance to negotiate stairs or steps or uneven surfaces.
☐	☐	2	-	Able to walk only with the supervision or assistance of another person at all times.
☐	☐	3	-	Chairfast, unable to ambulate but is able to wheel self independently.
☐	☐	4	-	Chairfast, unable to ambulate and is unable to wheel self.
☐	☐	5	-	Bedfast, unable to ambulate or be up in a chair.
☐		UK	-	Unknown

(M0710) Feeding or Eating: Ability to feed self meals and snacks. **Note: This refers only to the process of eating, chewing, and swallowing, not preparing the food to be eaten.**

Prior	Current			
☒	☒	0	-	Able to independently feed self.
☐	☐	1	-	Able to feed self independently but requires: (a) meal set-up; OR (b) intermittent assistance or supervision from another person; OR (c) a liquid, pureed or ground meat diet.
☐	☐	2	-	Unable to feed self and must be assisted or supervised throughout the meal/snack.
☐	☐	3	-	Able to take in nutrients orally and receives supplemental nutrients through a nasogastric tube or gastrostomy.
☐	☐	4	-	Unable to take in nutrients orally and is fed nutrients through a nasogastric tube or gastrostomy.
☐	☐	5	-	Unable to take in nutrients orally or by tube feeding.
☐		UK	-	Unknown

(M0720) Planning and Preparing Light Meals (e.g., cereal, sandwich) or reheat delivered meals:

PT to arrange Meals on Wheels

Prior	Current			
☒	☒	0	-	(a) Able to independently plan and prepare all light meals for self or reheat delivered meals; OR (b) Is physically, cognitively, and mentally able to prepare light meals on a regular basis but has not routinely performed light meal preparation in the past (i.e., prior to this home care admission).
☐	☐	1	-	Unable to prepare light meals on a regular basis due to physical, cognitive, or mental limitations.
☐	☐	2	-	Unable to prepare any light meals or reheat any delivered meals.
☐		UK	-	Unknown

PHYSICAL THERAPY START OF CARE ASSESSMENT (Also used for Resumption of Care Following Inpatient Stay) (page 12 of 15)	Client Name: A.Nicholas Client Record No: 001

(M0730) Transportation: Physical and mental ability to <u>safely</u> use a car, taxi, or public transportation (bus, train, subway).

Prior Current
- ☒ ☐ 0 - Able to independently drive a regular or adapted car; <u>OR</u> uses a regular or handicap-accessible public bus.
- ☐ ☒ 1 - Able to ride in a car only when driven by another person; <u>OR</u> able to use a bus or handicap van only when assisted or accompanied by another person.
- ☐ ☐ 2 - <u>Unable</u> to ride in a car, taxi, bus, or van, and requires transportation by ambulance.
- ☐   UK - Unknown

(M0740) Laundry: Ability to do own laundry -- to carry laundry to and from washing machine, to use washer and dryer, to wash small items by hand.

Prior Current
- ☒ ☐ 0 - (a) Able to independently take care of all laundry tasks; <u>OR</u>
    (b) Physically, cognitively, and mentally able to do laundry and access facilities, <u>but</u> has not routinely performed laundry tasks in the past (i.e., prior to this home care admission).
- ☐ ☐ 1 - Able to do only light laundry, such as minor hand wash or light washer loads. Due to physical, cognitive, or mental limitations, needs assistance with heavy laundry such as carrying large loads of laundry.
- ☐ ☒ 2 - <u>Unable</u> to do any laundry due to physical limitation or needs continual supervision and assistance due to cognitive or mental limitation.
- ☐   UK - Unknown

(M0750) Housekeeping: Ability to safely and effectively perform light housekeeping and heavier cleaning tasks.

Prior Current
- ☒ ☐ 0 - (a) Able to independently perform all housekeeping tasks; <u>OR</u>
    (b) Physically, cognitively, and mentally able to perform <u>all</u> housekeeping tasks but has not routinely participated in housekeeping tasks in the past (i.e., prior to this home care admission).
- ☐ ☐ 1 - Able to perform only <u>light</u> housekeeping (e.g., dusting, wiping kitchen counters) tasks independently.
- ☐ ☒ 2 - Able to perform housekeeping tasks with intermittent assistance or supervision from another person.
- ☐ ☐ 3 - <u>Unable</u> to consistently perform any housekeeping tasks unless assisted by another person throughout the process.
- ☐ ☐ 4 - Unable to effectively participate in any housekeeping tasks.
- ☐   UK - Unknown

(M0760) Shopping: Ability to plan for, select, and purchase items in a store and to carry them home or arrange delivery.

Prior Current
- ☒ ☐ 0 - (a) Able to plan for shopping needs and independently perform shopping tasks, including carrying packages; <u>OR</u>
    (b) Physically, cognitively, and mentally able to take care of shopping, but has not done shopping in the past (i.e., prior to this home care admission).
- ☐ ☐ 1 - Able to go shopping, but needs some assistance:
    (a) By self is able to do only light shopping and carry small packages, but needs someone to do occasional major shopping; <u>OR</u>
    (b) <u>Unable</u> to go shopping alone, but can go with someone to assist.
- ☐ ☒ 2 - <u>Unable</u> to go shopping, but is able to identify items needed, place orders, and arrange home delivery.
- ☐ ☐ 3 - Needs someone to do all shopping and errands.
- ☐   UK - Unknown

(M0770) Ability to Use Telephone: Ability to answer the phone, dial numbers, and <u>effectively</u> use the telephone to communicate.

Prior Current
- ☒ ☒ 0 - Able to dial numbers and answer calls appropriately and as desired.
- ☐ ☐ 1 - Able to use a specially adapted telephone (i.e., large numbers on the dial, teletype phone for the deaf) and call essential numbers.
- ☐ ☐ 2 - Able to answer the telephone and carry on a normal conversation but has difficulty with placing calls.
- ☐ ☐ 3 - Able to answer the telephone only some of the time or is able to carry on only a limited conversation.
- ☐ ☐ 4 - <u>Unable</u> to answer the telephone at all but can listen if assisted with equipment.
- ☐ ☐ 5 - Totally unable to use the telephone.
- ☐ ☐ NA - Patient does not have a telephone.
- ☐   UK - Unknown

PHYSICAL THERAPY START OF CARE ASSESSMENT (Also used for Resumption of Care Following Inpatient Stay) (page 13 of 15)	Client Name: A. Nicholas Client Record No: 001

MEDICATION ADMINISTRATION/DRUG REGIMEN REVIEW

Medications: Dose / Frequency /Route (N) ew (C)hanged

Humulin 70/30 15 units qam SC

Naprosyn 250 mg qd PO (C)

Advil 400 mg TID PO (N)

Milk of Magnesia 5 mL c̄ H₂O QID po (N)

B/12 100 mcg Qmo SC (N)

Note: Naprosyn dose ↓'d during hospitalization, from 250mg Q 8° to 250mg qd. B/12 injection to be given @ MD appt. 062899.

(M0780) Management of Oral Medications: Patient's ability to prepare and take all prescribed oral medications reliably and safely, including administration of the correct dosage at the appropriate times/intervals. **Excludes injectable and IV medications. (NOTE: This refers to ability, not compliance or willingness.)**

Does the patient report any side effects or reactions to current medications? ☐No ☒Yes
Does the patient and/or caregiver demonstrate a knowledge deficit related to current medication use? ☐No ☒Yes
Does the patient demonstrate noncompliance with medication use, as prescribed by physician? ☒No ☐Yes
Does patient and/or caregiver have any questions related to current medications, including purpose, dosage, or administration? ☐No ☒Yes
(describe problem and action for any "yes" responses)

Patient reports no bowel movement X 4 days c̄ abdominal cramping. "Could my medicine be causing this?"

Prior	Current		
☒	☒	0 -	Able to independently take the correct oral medication(s) and proper dosage(s) at the correct times.
☐	☐	1 -	Able to take medication(s) at the correct times if: (a) individual dosages are prepared in advance by another person; OR (b) given daily reminders; OR (c) someone develops a drug diary or chart.
☐	☐	2 -	Unable to take medication unless administered by someone else.
☐	☐ NA -		No oral medications prescribed.
☐	UK -		Unknown

(M0790) Management of Inhalant/Mist Medications: Patient's ability to prepare and take all prescribed inhalant/mist medications (nebulizers, metered dose devices) reliably and safely, including administration of the correct dosage at the appropriate times/intervals. **Excludes all other forms of medication (oral tablets, injectable and IV medications).**

Prior	Current		
☐	☐	0 -	Able to independently take the correct medication and proper dosage at the correct times.
☐	☐	1 -	Able to take medication at the correct times if: (a) individual dosages are prepared in advance by another person, OR (b) given daily reminders.
☐	☐	2 -	Unable to take medication unless administered by someone else.
☒	☒ NA -		No inhalant/mist medications prescribed.
☐	UK -		Unknown

(M0800) Management of Injectable Medications: Patient's ability to prepare and take all prescribed injectable medications reliably and safely, including administration of correct dosage at the appropriate times/intervals. **Excludes IV medications.**

Prior	Current		
☒	☐	0 -	Able to independently take the correct medication and proper dosage at the correct times.
☐	☐	1 -	Able to take injectable medication at correct times if: (a) individual syringes are prepared in advance by another person, OR (b) given daily reminders.
☐	☒	2 -	Unable to take injectable medications unless administered by someone else.
☐	☐ NA -		No injectable medications prescribed.
☐	UK -		Unknown

- Nephew to administer until patient self care restored.

Drug Interaction Review:
☐ Drug interaction review performed by assessing therapist   ☒ Drug interaction review to be performed by agency, per policy

Drug interaction review completed on: 060199 (date) by Nancy Nurse, RN (signature)
☐ Potential adverse effects identified? ☐No ☒Yes, (describe potential problem and/or action)

Potential for GI irritation 2° Naprosyn - Pt. to report GI sxs to RN or MD
Constipation/Abdominal Cramping - ↑ mobility, bowel & nutrition mgmt.

| PHYSICAL THERAPY START OF CARE ASSESSMENT
(Also used for Resumption of Care Following Inpatient Stay)
(page 14 of 15) | Client Name: A. Nicholas

Client Record No: 001 |

EQUIPMENT MANAGEMENT

(M0810) Patient Management of Equipment (includes ONLY oxygen, IV/infusion therapy, enteral/parenteral nutrition equipment or supplies): Patient's ability to set up, monitor and change equipment reliably and safely, add appropriate fluids or medication, clean/store/dispose of equipment or supplies using proper technique. **(NOTE: This refers to ability, not compliance or willingness.)**

- ☐ 0 - Patient manages all tasks related to equipment completely independently.
- ☐ 1 - If someone else sets up equipment (i.e., fills portable oxygen tank, provides patient with prepared solutions), patient is able to manage all other aspects of equipment.
- ☐ 2 - Patient requires considerable assistance from another person to manage equipment, but independently completes portions of the task.
- ☐ 3 - Patient is only able to monitor equipment (e.g., liter flow, fluid in bag) and must call someone else to manage the equipment.
- ☐ 4 - Patient is completely dependent on someone else to manage all equipment.
- ☒ NA - No equipment of this type used in care **[If NA, skip M0820]**

(M0820) Caregiver Management of Equipment (includes ONLY oxygen, IV/infusion equipment, enteral/parenteral nutrition, ventilator therapy equipment or supplies): Caregiver's ability to set up, monitor, and change equipment reliably and safely, add appropriate fluids or medication, clean/store/dispose of equipment or supplies using proper technique. **(NOTE: This refers to ability, not compliance or willingness.)**

- ☐ 0 - Caregiver manages all tasks related to equipment completely independently.
- ☐ 1 - If someone else sets up equipment, caregiver is able to manage all other aspects.
- ☐ 2 - Caregiver requires considerable assistance from another person to manage equipment, but independently completes significant portions of task.
- ☐ 3 - Caregiver is only able to complete small portions of task (e.g., administer nebulizer treatment, clean/store/dispose of equipment or supplies).
- ☐ 4 - Caregiver is completely dependent on someone else to manage all equipment.
- ☐ NA - No caregiver
- ☐ UK - Unknown

SKILLED INTERVENTIONS PERFORMED THIS VISIT / PATIENT/CAREGIVER RESPONSE TO TREATMENT/TEACHING:

☒ Safety Instruction throw rugs, lighting, use of pers. emerg. response, 911 for emerg.

☒ Home Program Instruction Isometric ex prog ⒷLEs; distal AROM & edema reduction for Ⓡ UE

☒ Activity Precautions Immobilizer sling ⒷUE x 3wks - No wt. bearing Ⓡ UE

☒ Therapeutic Exercise AROM all major jts ⒷLEs x 10 reps seated & supine c̄ demonstration & verbal cues

☒ Transfer Training Bed Mobility, sit ⇄ stand training from bed, chair, commode c̄ NWB ⒷUE

☒ Gait Training Instructed in 3 pt gait pattern c̄ NBQC ⒻUE

☒ Patient/Caregiver Education pain/edema management, Instruction in fall precautions and fall prevention protocol

☐ Other:

PHYSICAL THERAPY START OF CARE ASSESSMENT (Also used for Resumption of Care Following Inpatient Stay) (page 15 of 15)	Client Name: A. Nicholas
	Client Record No: 001

PHYSICAL THERAPY CARE PLAN (last page of assessment may be used as PT Plan of Care/Physician's Orders)

CLINICAL ASSESSMENT:

Unsteady gait 2° to:
- localized ℝ Quad weakness
- arthritic pain ℝ Knee
- ↓'d endurance, weakness 2° to anemia S/P GI bleed.

dependent ADL/IADL and limited functional mobility 2° to immobilized ℝ UE.

Problem List:	Interventions:	Amount/Frequency/ Duration:	Goals: (Short term/Long term)
ℝ Quad weakness	Ther. Ex - progressive strengthening program, isometrics, home program	3wk3, 2wk2 c̄ PT; daily home program	↑ ℝ Quad strength 1 grade in 3 weeks
Hx fall	Pt. education in fall precautions/ Fall prevention protocol		No reported falls during home care admission.
ℝ UE edema	Pt. education distal AROM & edema reduction measures		Resolution of ℝ UE edema in 10 days.
↓ endurance/ Weakness	Instruct in h.e.p. for strengthening/ endurance		Safe and Ⓘ transfers and amb'n c̄ NBQC in home & ↑↓ stairs in 5 weeks.
↓'d transfers/gait	Gait/Transfer training		**REHAB POTENTIAL** (for achievement of above stated goals) ☒ Good ☐ Fair ☐ Poor

NEED FOR INTERDISCIPLINARY REFERRAL?
☐ No ☒ Yes, (explain) Nursing for assessment re: medication & bowel 5x5.
Verbal order received? ☒ Yes ☐ No, (explain)

PATIENT/CAREGIVER AWARE OF AND AGREEABLE TO TREATMENT PLAN/SCHEDULE? ☒ Yes ☐ No,

DISCHARGE PLAN: When goals met, maximum function achieved, or at request of patient or physician...
☐ Discharge to self care with home program   ☐ Discharge to care of caregiver
☐ Other:
☒ Transition to Outpatient services
anticipate 5 weeks

DATE: 060199	TIME IN: 9.35 am	TIME OUT: 11:45 am
THERAPIST SIGNATURE: *Terry Cloth, PT*	PATIENT SIGNATURE: (if applicable) X John Nicholas (Nephew) patient unable to sign 2° to sling	
PHYSICIAN SIGNATURE: (if applicable)	DATE:	

*Reprinted with permission from Krulish, L: **Home Therapy OASIS Assessment Forms**, Powell, Ohio, 1999, Home Therapy Services.*

Intent of OASIS Data Collection

Many of the OASIS items are intended to identify the patient's physical and cognitive status as it relates to performance of various tasks. The OASIS items related to medication (M0780, M0790, M0800) and equipment management (M0810, M0820) are intended, in part, to be used to address the patient's (or caregiver's) physical and cognitive status as it relates to administration of medications or management of equipment. Questions to elicit accurate scoring for the OASIS items include:

- Do they have sufficient strength and coordination to retrieve and open the pill bottles?
- Can they swallow the pills effectively?
- Can they describe the ordered dosages and administration schedule?
- Do they remember to take the medications as ordered?

For example, OASIS assessment of administration of injectable medications includes evaluation of the patient's cognitive function, and gross and fine motor skills necessary to perform the necessary associated tasks, including filling syringes and injecting the medication as ordered. All skilled disciplines are eligible to perform the preliminary screening of patient needs (the OASIS item M0800), with identification of problem areas (e.g., fine motor deficits) resulting in an appropriate interdisciplinary referral (e.g,. occupational therapy consult).

Similarly, all the skilled disciplines are eligible to perform the preliminary screening of patient needs (the OASIS item M0700) to determine whether the patient can demonstrate safe ambulation on a variety of surfaces. Questions to elicit accurate item scoring may include:

- Does the patient walk without assistive devices or railings without losing balance or appearing unsteady?
- Does the patient report, or do observations suggest a history of falls?

Although all skilled disciplines could perform the general screen, identification of functional deficits, safety concerns, or questionable gait techniques should result in an interdisciplinary referral for physical therapy. In addition to use for outcome analysis, OASIS data should present opportunities to benefit each individual patient through promoting a comprehensive assessment of a broad range of pertinent functional and health-related domains, and when identified, timely referral to appropriate disciplines to allow the greatest opportunity for impacting positive outcome achievement.

While the specificity of the information collected by some OASIS data elements may be more detailed than that routinely found in documentation resulting from a therapy admission, the scopes of clinical practice for the therapy disciplines, as available from the American Physical Therapy Association, the American Speech-Language-Hearing Association, and the American Occupational Therapy Association (see Part Three) do not restrict the participation of the therapy providers in any activities required by the comprehensive assessment requirement. In fact documents and comments from the associations support the involvement of these specialized therapists in the performance of a comprehensive assessment. Therefore, with appropriate training, the OASIS and comprehensive assessment requirements will not only result in standardized data, and hopefully standardized care and care processes, but will likely yield a more thorough assessment of an individual patient's status and individualized care needs.

Competency Assessment: Key to Success for OASIS

While OASIS data collection activities are within the scopes of practice of the therapy disciplines, the OASIS items do cover several specific clinical and health-related domains which may not have been routinely addressed by all therapists in the past. Competence in assessing the domains related to OASIS and the comprehensive assessment of the patient should be established for all disciplines involved in data collection, and become a part of the organization's policies and procedures.

Use of competency assessment tools, such as those presented in Figures 5-3 through 5-8, allow individual clinicians, peers, and clinical supervisors a means of identifying knowledge or skill deficits that may affect OASIS data-integrity and patient outcomes. The areas of the OASIS data collection appearing most problematic for therapists are those items assessing medication administration, equipment management, and integumentary assessment. Additionally, ICD-9 coding may present another area requiring inservicing for therapists completing the OASIS tool. Inservicing of therapy staff in these, and any other areas of identified weakness, is essential in achieving the cross-discipline reliability of the OASIS data set, as well as necessary in identifying the multi-disciplinary needs of the individual patient and facilitating appropriate care plan development and interdisciplinary referral.

SAMPLE OASIS COMPETENCY TOOLS

Figure 5-3   Competency Tool for OASIS Data Collection Rules

Competency: **OASIS DATA COLLECTION RULES**			
The therapist or nurse:	YES	NO	COMMENTS:
Lists the appropriate time points and situations which require OASIS data collection			
Identifies the appropriate OASIS items which must be collected at each specific time point			
Identifies the time requirements for data collection and submission at each specific time point			
Describes the rules related to skip patterns			
Describes the rules related to the use of "not applicable" or "unknown" responses			
Describes the rules related to collecting "usual status" data			
Describes the rules related to collection "prior status" data			

SAMPLE OASIS COMPETENCY TOOLS

Figure 5-4   Competency Assessment Tool for ICD-9 Coding for OASIS

Competency: **ICD-9 CODING FOR OASIS**			
The therapist or nurse: Identifies the appropriate OASIS items which require ICD-9 code categories	YES	NO	COMMENTS:
Describes the potential differences in the codes requested in M0190, M0210, M0230, and M0240			
Describes the rules related to the number of digits required, and the use of surgical or V-codes in OASIS collection			
Describes the agency policy for completion, verification, and reporting of the code categories for OASIS			

SAMPLE OASIS COMPETENCY TOOLS

Figure 5-5   Competency Assessment Tool for Sensory Assessment for OASIS

Competency: **SENSORY ASSESSMENT FOR OASIS**			
The therapist or nurse:	YES	NO	COMMENTS:
Describes the performance variances dividing the OASIS response options for Vision (M0390)			
Identifies assessment strategies to score Vision (M0390)			
Describes the performance variances dividing the OASIS response options for Hearing (M0400)			
Identifies assessment strategies to score Hearing (M0400)			
Describes the performance variances dividing the OASIS response options for Speech (M0410)			
Identifies assessment strategies to score Speech (M0410)			
Describes the performance variances dividing the OASIS response options for Pain (M0420, M0430)			
Identifies assessment strategies to score Pain (M0420, M0430)			

SAMPLE OASIS COMPETENCY TOOLS

Figure 5-6   Competency Assessment Tool for Integumentary Assessment for OASIS

Competency: **INTEGUMENTARY ASSESSMENT FOR OASIS**			
The therapist or nurse:	YES	NO	COMMENTS:
Demonstrates knowledge of definitions of "skin lesion" and "open wound" as related to OASIS data collection			
Describes physical characteristics of pressure ulcers			
Describes pressure ulcer staging criteria, as derived from the National Pressure Ulcer Advisory Panel			
Describes the physical characteristics of stasis ulcers			
Identifies the criteria for classification and numbering of surgical wounds as related to OASIS data collection			
Describes clinical manifestations of wound healing necessary to score OASIS items (M0464, M0476, and M0488)			
Describes characteristics which could assist in the determination of the "most problematic" ulcer or wound (M0460, M0464, M0476, M0488)			

SAMPLE OASIS COMPETENCY TOOLS

**Figure 5-7   Competency Assessment Tool for
ADL/IADL Assessment for OASIS**

Competency: **ADL/IADL ASSESSMENT FOR OASIS**			
The therapist or nurse:	YES	NO	COMMENTS:
Describes the time points and rules for collecting current and prior OASIS information			
Describes the performance variances dividing the OASIS response options for Grooming (M0640)			
Identifies assessment strategies to score Grooming (M0640)			
Describes the performance variances dividing the OASIS response options for Dressing (M0650, M0660)			
Identify assessment strategies to score Dressing (M0650, M0660)			
Describes the performance variances dividing the OASIS response options for Bathing (M0670)			
Identifies assessment strategies to score Bathing (M0670)			
Describes the performance variances dividing the OASIS response options for Toileting (M0680)			
Identifies assessment strategies to score Toileting (M0680)			
Describes the performance variances dividing the OASIS response options for Transferring (M0690)			
Identifies assessment strategies to score Transferring (M0690)			
Describes the performance variances dividing the OASIS response options for Ambulation/Locomotion (M0700)			

SAMPLE OASIS COMPETENCY TOOLS

Figure 5-7   Competency Assessment Tool for
ADL/IADL Assessment for OASIS (cont'd)

The therapist or nurse:	YES	NO	COMMENTS:
Identifies assessment strategies to score Ambulation/Locomotion (M0700)			
Describes the performance variances dividing the OASIS response options for Eating (M0710)			
Identifies assessment strategies to score Eating (M0710)			
Describes the performance variances dividing the OASIS response options for Meal Preparation (M0720)			
Identifies assessment strategies to score Meal Preparation (M0720)			
Describes the performance variances dividing the OASIS response options for Laundry (M0740)			
Identify assessment strategies to score Laundry (M0740)			
Describes the performance variances dividing the OASIS response options for Housekeeping (M0750)			
Identifies assessment strategies to score Housekeeping (M0750)			
Describes the performance variances dividing the OASIS response options for Shopping (M0760)			
Identifies assessment strategies to score Shopping (M0760)			
Describes the performance variances dividing the OASIS response options for Telephone use (M0770)			
Identifies assessment strategies to score Telephone use (M0770)			

SAMPLE OASIS COMPETENCY TOOLS

Figure 5-8   Competency Assessment Tool for Medications Assessment and Equipment Management for OASIS

Competency: **MEDICATIONS ASSESSMENT AND EQUIPMENT MANAGEMENT FOR OASIS**			
The therapist or nurse:	YES	NO	COMMENTS:
Describes the intended assessments of physical and cognitive function as it relates to Medication Administration and Equipment Management OASIS items			
Describes the performance variances dividing the OASIS response options for Oral Medications (M0780)			
Identifies assessment strategies to score Oral Medication (M0780)			
Describes the performance variances dividing the OASIS response options for Inhalant/Mist Medications (M0790)			
Identifies assessment strategies to score Inhalant/Mist Medications (M0790)			
Describes the performance variances dividing the OASIS response options for Injectable Medications (M0800)			
Identifies assessment strategies to score Injectable Medications (M0800)			
Describes the performance variances dividing the OASIS response options for Patient Management of Equipment (M0810)			

SAMPLE OASIS COMPETENCY TOOLS

Figure 5-8   Competency Assessment Tool for Medications Assessment and Equipment Management for OASIS (cont'd)

The therapist or nurse:	YES	NO	COMMENTS:
Identifies assessment strategies to score Patient Management of Equipment (M0810)			
Describes the performance variances dividing the OASIS response options for Caregiver Management of Equipment (M0820)			
Identifies assessment strategies to score Caregiver Management of Equipment (M0820)			

Summary

With OASIS comes increased opportunity for the interdisciplinary team to work collaboratively, sharing the unique and specialized knowledge that each discipline possesses for the benefit of maximizing patient outcomes. Interdisciplinary teams should discuss assessment strategies and develop necessary skills to improve the validity and reliability of the OASIS data collected. As the data collection practices become more consistent within and between team members, the value of the OASIS data for outcome purposes is enhanced, with associated benefits to patients, providers, and payers.

PART SIX
Therapy Care Guides: Focus on Function

This chapter presents interdisciplinary therapy care guides related to a variety of functional limitations experienced by patients receiving home care services. The care guides are organized using a disablement model focusing on the functional impact of the patient's condition, as opposed to a medical model, which organizes patients solely by medical diagnosis.

The premise on which the care guides are based include an assumption that treatment plans and interventions will be based on the individual patient and their unique medical, rehabilitative, social, and discharge planning needs. Therefore, the interventions, goals, and outcome measures outlined in the care guides may not be appropriate for every patient with a given functional limitation. Additionally, not every intervention suggested may be a covered service for every payer. Readers are referred to Part One to review overall coverage considerations, and to Part Nine for excerpts from the Home Health Agency Manual (HCFA-Pub-11). Readers are encouraged to contact agency supervisors with individual coverage questions, as coverage varies based on the specific insurance.

Focus on the patient's functional abilities, limitations, and potential may more effectively identify appropriate referrals, compared with the model of identifying rehabilitation referrals based on medical diagnosis or ICD-9 codes. For instance, a patient with a medical diagnosis of CVA, a diagnosis common for rehabilitation referral, may have no resulting functional limitations and not necessarily be an appropriate candidate for a rehabilitation referral. Compare this with a patient with the diagnosis of anemia exhibiting functional limitations of activity intolerance and dependent mobility due to weakness and poor endurance. Whatever the patient's specific findings and function, all team members must involve or access other disciplines when appropriate.

The intention in supplying care guides is to encourage investment in the patient assessment process; to determine not only the functional limitations, but the concomitant factors which should be considered in care plan development to maximize outcomes through the achievement of optimal function. If a patient demonstrates restricted performance in bathing; in addition to addressing issues of transfers, strength, range of motion, balance, and endurance, it may also be necessary to address wound management, and the affects of the bathing activities on issues of infection, healing, wound/dressing precautions, positioning, pressure, etc.

If a functional limitation in toileting is present, thorough assessment may reveal that dependency in transfers (physical limitation) and inability to effectively communicate the need for assistance in a timely manner (functional communication deficit) are both areas in need of remediation to affect the desired outcome (continence). If the assessment is not thorough, then the mobility goals (decreasing transfer assistance from maximum assistance to minimum assistance) may be achieved, but because the patient is still unable to communicate need for assistance, the incontinence continues (no change in outcome).

In order to facilitate a comprehensive assessment of factors which could affect patient function, a listing of general functional limitations with possible general functional goals and therapeutic interventions by discipline are detailed. (See General Care Guide Summary). Following this general care guide summary are eighteen specific care guides organized by functional limitation, providing therapists with a format for reviewing, identifying, and addressing patient problems in a standardized manner. The specific functional care guides present the restricted performance area (i.e., the functional limitation), the related OASIS data item(s), and provide lists of 1) identified/assessed problems/restricted performance areas, 2) a safety checklist, 3) actions/interventions/activities, and 4) specific functional goals related to the specific functional limitation.

In the context of these care guides, functional limitation is defined as restriction of the ability to perform a physical action, activity, or task in an efficient, typically expected, or competent manner.

The functional limitations present with a below-knee amputation could vary dramatically between patients. These differences are affected by a variety of factors including co-morbidities, general health/strength, motivation, pain, etc. Therefore, through comprehensive assessment and analysis of individual patient findings, functional limitations exhibited by a patient can be identified and addressed.

A healthy patient with a below-knee amputation due to trauma may likely initially demonstrate performance limitations in several functional areas/tasks (i.e., ambulation, transfers, bed mobility, wheelchair function). Through identification of problem performance areas and rehabilitation potential, an appropriate care plan could be developed to restore the patient's independence. An elderly patient with a below-knee amputation due to vascular insufficiency may have additional co-morbidities (i.e., significant cardiac or respiratory history, pain, depression,) which would likely result in identification of a different listing of problem performance areas and poorer rehabilitation potential. Therefore, when utilizing the therapy care guides, it is imperative that the guides selected (i.e., actions/interventions/activities, or specific functional goals) are individualized, and based on specific functional limitations and rehabilitation potential exhibited by the patient.

The care guides are in no way intended to be an exhaustive list of the possible functional limitations that may be identified in the home care patient, nor do the proposed interventions and goals represent the boundaries of all available care options or opportunities. It is expected that in addition to the listed interventions, all skilled home care providers are able to identify interdisciplinary needs, make appropriate referrals throughout the patient's home care admission, and develop and implement an appropriate discharge plan.

Increasing the uniformity of care provided through use of tools such as the functional care guides referred to in this chapter will facilitate identification of "best practices" in home care provision. Provision of care using a standardized and outcome-focused approach increases the predictability of both patient outcomes and the associated resource utilization; two key factors in surviving in a prospective payment environment.

GENERAL CARE GUIDE SUMMARY

Functional Limitations:
Restricted Performance in: ◆ **Ambulation** ◆ **Bathing-Tub/Shower Transfers** ◆ **Bed Mobility** ◆ **Car Transfers** ◆ **Dressing** ◆ **Eating/Self-Feeding** ◆ **Emergency Response Needs** ◆ **Functional Communication** ◆ **Grooming** ◆ **Homemaking** ◆ **Kitchen Functioning** ◆ **Laundry** ◆ **Medication Management** ◆ **Money Management** ◆ **Pain Management** ◆ **Toileting** ◆ **Transfers** ◆ **Wheelchair Function**

Provider:	Therapeutic Interventions:	Functional Goals:
PT	• Airway clearance techniques	• Improve functional or health status through minimizing or preventing consequences of acute and chronic lung diseases and impairment
	• Coordination, communication, and documentation	• Improve functional or health status through effective care coordination and communication
	• Electrotherapeutic modalities	• Improve functional or health status through pain, swelling, inflammation, or restriction reduction; maintenance of post-injury/surgery strength, assist in muscle contraction for functional training or facilitation of wound healing
	• Functional training in self-care and home management, including ADL and IADL	• Improve functional or health status measured by decreased intensity of care or level of supervision, decreased need for assistive equipment or environmental adaptations, improved safety, improved ability to perform ADL (toileting, bathing, dressing, eating, transferring, and gait) and/or IADL tasks (housework, meal preparation, cooking, laundry, and community access)
	• Functional training in community and work(job/school/play) integration or reintegration, including IADL, work hardening, and work conditioning	• Improve functional or health status measured by decreased intensity of care or level of supervision; improved safety and tolerance of positions and activities

	• Manual therapy techniques, including mobilization and manipulation	• Improve functional or health status (or reduce or prevent disability) through decreased pain, swelling and/or inflammation, and increased joint range of motion (ROM), circulation and/or relaxation
	• Patient/client-related instruction	• Improve functional or health status through increased patient or caregiver knowledge relative to the diagnosis, prognosis, interventions, goals, and outcomes; increased awareness and utilization of community resources, increased knowledge of personal and environmental factors associated with the condition; or increased self-management and safety
	• Physical agents and mechanical modalities	• Improve functional or health status through increased connective tissue extensibility, decreased pain, reduced soft tissue swelling, inflammation or restriction; facilitation of wound healing
		• Improve functional or health status through decreased pain, provision of temporary support, increased range of motion (ROM), or improved tissue perfusion and oxygenation
	• Prescription, application, and fabrication of assistive, adaptive, orthotic, protective, supportive, or prosthetic devices and equipment	• Improve functional or health status through increasing joint stability and/or mobility, safety, or tolerance to positions or weight bearing; decreased risk for deformity, decreased edema, effusion, pain, or pressure areas; achievement of optimal joint alignment

	• Therapeutic exercise, including aerobic conditioning	• Improve functional or health status (or reduce or prevent disability) through improved strength, balance, aerobic capacity, endurance, joint and/or soft tissue swelling, inflammation or restriction; or decreased energy expenditure or need for manual or equipment assistance
	• Wound management	• Improve functional or health status through debridement of nonviable tissue, reduced risk factors for infection, progression, or secondary impairment, improved tissue perfusion and oxygenation, decreased wound size
SLP	• Augmentative and Alternative Communication (ACC) System and/or Device Treatment/ Orientation	• Improved functional communication or health status through enhanced communication in presence of expressive and/or receptive communication disorders through use of alternative communication components (ACC) (aids, techniques, symbols, strategies)
	• Cognitive-Communication Treatment	• Improved functional or health status through remediation of deficits related to cognitive factors (attention, memory, problem solving) and related language components (semantics and pragmatics)

	• Fluency Treatment	• Improved functional communication or health status through remediation of frequency, severity, or affects of fluency disorders
	• Orofacial Myofunctional Treatment	• Improved functional communication or health status through improvement or correction of orofacial myofunctional patterns and related speech patterns
	• Prosthetic/ Adaptive Device Treatment/ Orientation	• Improved functional or health status through enhanced functional communication using prosthetic/adaptive devices
	• Swallowing Function Treatment	• Improve functional or health status through improved swallowing and feeding function, improved respiratory function with swallowing activities, improved effectiveness of bolus clearance, decreased pulmonary complications of aspiration
	• Treatment of Central Auditory Processing Disorders (CAPD) in Adults	• Improve function or health status through enhanced auditory processing, listening, spoken language processing and overall communication processing
	• Voice Treatment	• Improve functional communication or health status through enhanced voice production, coordination or respiration and laryngeal valving, and/or acquisition of alaryngeal speech sufficient to allow for functional communication

OT	• Activities of daily living (ADLs) interventions	• Improve functional or health status measured by decreased intensity of care or level of supervision, decreased need for assistive equipment or environmental adaptations, improved safety, improved ability to perform ADL tasks (toileting, bathing, transferring, dressing, and eating)
	• Cognitive status interventions	• Improved functional or health status through enhanced alertness, orientation, memory skills, attention span and/or problem-solving abilities • Improved functional or health status through the planning, implementation and supervision of individualized therapeutic activity programs as part of an overall active treatment program for a patient with a diagnosed psychiatric illness
	• Environmental adaptation	• Improved functional or health status through decreased intensity of care or level of supervision, improved safety, and enhanced mobility through environmental modification or equipment use
	• Functional communication interventions	• Improved functional communication or health status through achievement of practical telephone use, writing skills, and/or effective emergency response mechanism(s)

	• Functional mobility interventions	• Improve functional or health status measured by decreased intensity of care or level of supervision, decreased need for assistive equipment or environmental adaptations, improved energy conservation, and improved safety
	• Instrumental activities of daily living (IADLs) interventions	• Improve functional or health status measured by decreased intensity of care or level of supervision, decreased need for assistive equipment or environmental adaptations, improved safety, improved ability to perform IADL tasks (housework, meal preparation, cooking, laundry, money management and community access)
	• Medication administration	• Improved functional or health status through improved medication self-administration through remediation of cognitive or motoric deficits
	• Perceptual processing interventions	• Improved functional or health status through improved body scheme, right-left discrimination, depth perception, spatial relations, eye/hand coordination, and figure ground awareness
	• Sensory status interventions	• Improved functional or health status through enhanced sensory awareness and processing abilities
	• Splinting interventions	• Improved functional or health status through decreased pain, decreased actual or risk of deformity, and/or enhanced joint support through splinting techniques

Performance Area: AMBULATION
Corresponding OASIS Component: (M0700)
(See also Assistive Devices for Gait in Part Seven, and Home Access Barriers and Adaptations -Box 3-13).
1. **Identified/Assessed Problems/Restricted Performance Areas**
    ◆ Balance deficits
    ◆ Endurance limitations
    ◆ Impaired communication with caregiver related to assistance needs
    ◆ Joint precautions
    ◆ Lower extremity weakness
    ◆ Pain
    ◆ Range of motion limitations
    ◆ Tonal abnormalities
    ◆ Transfer limitations
    ◆ Upper extremity weakness
    ◆ Weight bearing limitations/precautions
    ◆ Other problems, based on the patient's unique medical history and environment

2. **Safety Checklist**
    ◆ Caregiver availability, capability and willingness to provide care
    ◆ Compliance with assistive device use
    ◆ Compliance with joint precautions
    ◆ Compliance with weight bearing precautions/limitations
    ◆ History of falls
    ◆ Home layout, structure, and environment
    ◆ Home safety assessment completed, including disaster evacuation plan
    ◆ Identified safety concerns documented and communicated to case manager
    ◆ Impaired judgment
    ◆ Lack of caregiver (specify, e.g., in daytime, at nighttime)
    ◆ Medication profile, history and side effects (e.g., orthostatic hypotension)
    ◆ Patient behaviors (e.g., wandering)
    ◆ Patient lives alone
    ◆ Other safety issues, based on the patient's unique medical history, environment, and support

3. Actions/Interventions/Activities

PT:
◆ Teach home exercise to increase strength, range of motion, balance, etc.
◆ Increase independence and safety in transfers and ambulation through use of adaptive techniques and recommendations and instruction in use of assistive, orthotic, protective, supportive, or prosthetic devices.
◆ Provide recommendations on environment modification.
◆ Provide patient/caregiver fall prevention and home safety measures related to gait and transfers.
❧ Teach home care aide in repetitive exercise program and techniques to support gait and transfer safety.
◆ Provide home program and teach caregivers and home care aide in strategies to support patient's PT goals.
◆ Other interventions/activities based on the patient's unique needs.

SLP:
◆ Address communication needs related to ambulation activities (e.g., amount and type of assistance needed).
◆ Teach patient/caregiver in alternative communications (e.g., communication board, bell).
◆ Teach patient/caregiver compensatory memory strategies to increase patient's ability to carry out PT and/or OT instructions related to ambulation activities (e.g., weight bearing precautions, use of assistive device).
◆ Provide home program and teach caregivers and home care aide in strategies to support communication program and SLP goals.
◆ Other interventions/activities based on the patient's unique needs.

OT:
◆ Increase independence and safety in gait through use of adaptive techniques (e.g., energy conservation, diaphragmatic breathing, relaxation techniques), perceptual processing (e.g. depth perception, figure ground awareness), or splinting interventions (e.g., providing support for upper extremity to allow use of assistive device or support limb during gait activities).
◆ Teach in-home exercises to increase UE strength, ROM, balance for ambulation.
◆ Identify home modification needs (e.g., floor surfaces, door thresholds, steps).
◆ Provide home program and teach caregivers and home care aide in strategies to support patient's OT goals.
◆ Other interventions/activities based on the patient's unique needs.

4. Specific Functional Goals

PT:

◆ Patient will be (max/mod/min/no) assist for safe transfers required for ambulation by _____(date).

◆ Patient will be (max/mod/min/no) assist for safe gait in home on (level, unlevel) surfaces for _____ feet by _____(date).

◆ Patient will improve from (max/mod/min assist) to (mod/min/no assist) for gait by _____(date).

◆ Patient/ Family/Therapist/Social Worker will obtain equipment or arrange home modification needs by _____(date).

◆ Patient will demonstrate a decrease in fall frequency from ____falls per (day, week) to _____falls per (day, week) by _____(date).

◆ Patient/caregiver will demonstrate appropriate use of (assistive, adaptive, orthotic, protective, supporting, prosthetic devices) for gait by _____(date).

◆ Patient will demonstrate compliance with (prescribed device use, weight bearing status) by _____(date).

◆ Other functional goals based on the patient's unique needs.

SLP:

◆ Patient uses adaptive communication techniques to achieve ambulation goals by _____(date).

◆ Caregivers report improved communications related to ambulation needs by _____(date).

◆ Other functional communication goals based on the patient's unique needs.

OT:

◆ Patient/caregiver will demonstrate home program for therapeutic exercises for increased strength/ROM/coordination for ambulation with (max/mod/min/no) assist by _____(date).

◆ Patient/caregiver will be (max./mod/min/no assist) for safe, functional gait activities utilizing prescribed techniques or equipment by _____(date).

◆ Patient/Family/Therapist/Social Worker will obtain assistive devices for ambulation and/or home modification arrangements by _____(date).

◆ Patient/caregiver will demonstrate safety measures and fall prevention per instructions for ambulation by _____(date).

◆ Patient/caregiver will demonstrate home program for energy conservation/diaphragmatic breathing/relaxation techniques to reduce SOB by _____(date).

◆ Other functional goals based on the patient's unique needs.

Performance Area: BATHING-TUB/SHOWER TRANSFERS
Corresponding OASIS Components: (M0670, M0690)
(See also Bathroom Equipment in Part Seven, and Bathtub Barriers and Adaptations -Box 3-11).
1. **Identified/Assessed Problems/Restricted Performance Areas**
   ◆ Accessibility of tub/shower
   ◆ Balance deficits
   ◆ Endurance limitations
   ◆ Impaired communication with caregiver related to assistance and bathing/hygiene needs
   ◆ Joint precautions
   ◆ Lower extremity weakness
   ◆ Pain
   ◆ Range of motion limitations
   ◆ Tonal abnormalities
   ◆ Upper extremity weakness
   ◆ Weight bearing limitations/precautions
   ◆ Wounds, dressings, or casts requiring special attention during bathing
   ◆ Other problems, based on the patient's unique medical history and environment

2. **Safety Checklist**
   ◆ Bathroom layout, structure, and environment
   ◆ Caregiver availability, capability and willingness to provide care
   ◆ Compliance with equipment use
   ◆ Compliance with joint precautions
   ◆ Compliance with weight bearing precautions/limitations
   ◆ History of falls
   ◆ Home safety assessment completed, including disaster evacuation plan
   ◆ Identified safety concerns documented and communicated to case manager
   ◆ Impaired judgment
   ◆ Lack of caregiver (specify, e.g., in daytime, at nighttime)
   ◆ Medication profile, history and side effects (e.g., orthostatic hypotension)
   ◆ Patient lives alone
   ◆ Sensory status (e.g., intact to dangerous water temperatures)
   ◆ Other safety issues, based on the patient's unique medical history, environment, and support

3. Actions/Interventions/Activities

PT:

◆ Teach home exercise to increase strength/ROM/balance, to improve independence in tub/shower transfers and bathing activities.

◆ Increase independence and safety in tub/shower transfers through training and use of adaptive techniques and recommendation and instruction in use of assistive devices or equipment.

◆ Provide recommendations on environment modification.

◆ Teach fall prevention and bathroom safety measures.

◆ Teach home care aide repetitive exercise program and techniques to support bathing function and safety.

◆ Provide home program and teach caregivers and home care aide in strategies to support patient's PT goals.

◆ Other interventions/activities based on the patient's unique needs.

SLP:

◆ Address communication needs related to hygiene and bathing activities (e.g., amount and type of assistance needed).

◆ Teach patient/caregiver alternative communications (e.g., communication board).

◆ Teach patient/caregiver compensatory memory strategies to increase patient's ability to carry out multi-step bathing activities.

◆ Teach caregivers and home care aide strategies to support communication program and SLP goals.

◆ Other interventions/activities based on the patient's unique needs.

OT:

◆ Increase independence and safety in bathing through use of adaptive techniques (e.g., energy conservation) and equipment (e.g., tub/shower chair/bench,).

◆ Teach therapeutic exercises and provide home program to increase UE strength, ROM, and balance for bathing and related transfers.

◆ Teach energy conservation/diaphragmatic breathing/relaxation techniques to reduce SOB with bathing.

◆ Teach adaptive techniques for bathing tasks and transfers related to ROM restrictions/precautions (e.g., total hip precautions). Teach bathroom modification needs, including proper installation of grab bars, hand held shower head, removal of sliding tub doors, etc.

◆ Assist in obtaining assistive bathing devices and provide instruction on bathroom modification details.

◆ Teach caregivers and home care aide in strategies to support patient's OT goals.

◆ Other interventions/activities based on the patient's unique needs.

4. Specific Functional Goals
PT:
◆ Patient/caregiver will be (independent/max/mod/min. assist) in safe tub/shower transfers within _____ weeks/visits.
◆ Patient will improve from (max/ mod/ min. assist) to (mod./min. assist/independent) for tub/shower transfers by _____visit.
◆ Patient/ Family/Therapist/Social Worker will arrange for delivery of equipment or home modification needs.
◆ Patient/caregiver will demonstrate compliance with (prescribed device use, weight bearing status) during bathing activities with (max/mod/min/no assist) by _____(date).
◆ Other functional goals based on the patient's unique needs.

SLP:
◆ Patient uses adaptive communication techniques or compensatory memory strategies to achieve bathing goals by _____(date).
◆ Caregivers report improved communications related to bathing/ hygiene needs.
◆ Other functional communication goals based on the patient's unique needs.

OT:
◆ Patient/caregiver will demonstrate adaptive techniques for safe bathing with (max/mod/min/no assist) by _____(date).
◆ Patient/Family/Therapist/Social Worker will obtain equipment/complete bathroom modification by _____(date).
◆ Patient/caregiver will demonstrate proper use of assistive bathing devices by _____(date).
◆ Patient will demonstrate home program for energy conservation/ diaphragmatic breathing/relaxation techniques to reduce SOB during bathing by _____(date).
◆ Other functional goals based on the patient's unique needs.

Performance Area: BED MOBILITY
Corresponding OASIS Component: (M0690)
1. **Identified/Assessed Problems/Restricted Performance Areas**
   - ◆ Accessibility of bed
   - ◆ Balance deficits
   - ◆ Endurance limitations
   - ◆ Impaired communication with caregiver related to assistance and mobility needs
   - ◆ Joint precautions
   - ◆ Lower extremity weakness
   - ◆ Pain
   - ◆ Range of motion limitations
   - ◆ Tonal abnormalities
   - ◆ Upper extremity weakness
   - ◆ Weight bearing limitations/precautions
   - ◆ Other problems, based on the patient's unique medical history and environment

2. **Safety Checklist**
   - ◆ Bedroom layout, structure, and environment
   - ◆ Caregiver availability, capability and willingness to provide care
   - ◆ Compliance with joint precautions
   - ◆ Compliance with weight bearing precautions/limitations
   - ◆ History of falls from bed
   - ◆ Home safety assessment completed, including disaster evacuation plan
   - ◆ Identified safety concerns documented and communicated to case manager
   - ◆ Impaired judgment
   - ◆ Lack of caregiver (specify, e.g., in daytime, at nighttime)
   - ◆ Medication profile, history and side effects (e.g. orthostatic hypotension)
   - ◆ Patient lives alone
   - ◆ Sensory status (e.g., intact to prolonged pressure)
   - ◆ Other safety issues, based on the patient's unique medical history, environment, and support

3. Actions/Interventions/Activities
PT:
◆ Teach therapeutic exercise to increase strength/ROM/balance, to improve independence in bed mobility and related transfers.
◆ Increase independence and safety in bed mobility and transfers through training and use of adaptive techniques, recommendations and instructions in use of assistive devices or equipment (e.g., side railings, trapeze bar).
◆ Provide recommendations on environment modification (e.g., elevate bed on blocks, firmer mattress).
◆ Teach patient/caregiver fall prevention and home safety measures related to bed mobility.
◆ Teach home care aide repetitive exercise program and techniques to support bed mobility and transfer function and safety.
◆ Teach caregivers and home care aide strategies to support patient's PT goals.
◆ Other interventions/activities based on the patient's unique needs.

SLP:
◆ Address communication needs related to bed mobility and transfer activities (e.g., amount and type of assistance needed, desired position change).
◆ Teach patient/caregiver alternative communications (e.g., communication board, bell) to signal need for assistance.
◆ Teach patient/caregiver compensatory memory strategies to increase patient's ability to carry out multi-step transferring/positioning tasks.
◆ Teach caregivers and home care aide strategies to support communication program and SLP goals.
◆ Other interventions/activities based on the patient's unique needs.

OT:
◆ Teach adaptive techniques and use of assistive devices for increased independence in bed mobility.
◆ Teach therapeutic exercises and provide home program to increase UE strength/ROM/balance for bed mobility.
◆ Identify home modification needs (e.g., floor surfaces, bed height).
◆ Teach safety measures regarding bed mobility, including ROM and weight bearing restrictions, as needed.
◆ Teach functional positioning for proper body alignment and ROM restrictions.
◆ Teach caregivers and home care aide strategies to support patient's OT goals.
◆ Other interventions/activities based on the patient's unique needs.

4. Specific Functional Goals

PT:

◆ Patient/caregiver will demonstrate safe bed mobility and transfers with (max/mod/min/no) assist by _____(date).

◆ Patient/ Family/Therapist/Social Worker will obtain equipment/ complete home modifications by _____(date).

◆ Patient/caregiver will demonstrate compliance with (prescribed techniques/weight bearing status) during bed mobility activities by _____(date).

◆ Patient/caregiver will demonstrate prescribed home program with (max/mod/min/no) assist by _____(date).

◆ Other functional goals based on the patient's unique needs.

SLP:

◆ Patient/caregiver demonstrates use of adaptive communication techniques or compensatory memory strategies to achieve bed mobility goals by _____(date).

◆ Caregivers report improved communications related to bed mobility/ transfer needs by _____(date).

◆ Other functional communication goals based on the patient's unique needs.

OT:

◆ Patient/caregiver will demonstrate adaptive techniques for safe bed transfer with (max/mod/min/no) assist by _____(date).

◆ Patient/caregiver will demonstrate proper use of assistive devices for bed mobility by _____(date).

◆ Patient/Family/Therapist/Social Worker will obtain equipment/ complete home modification by _____(date).

◆ Patient/caregiver will demonstrate home program for therapeutic exercises for improved strength/ROM/coordination needed for bed mobility with (max/mod/min/no assist) by _____(date).

◆ Patient/caregiver will demonstrate home program for energy conservation/diaphragmatic breathing/relaxation techniques to reduce SOB by _____(date).

◆ Other functional goals based on the patient's unique needs.

Performance Area: CAR TRANSFERS
Corresponding OASIS Component: (no specific M0 item addresses car transfer)
1. **Identified/Assessed Problems/Restricted Performance Areas**
    ◆ Accessibility of car and car entrance
    ◆ Balance deficits
    ◆ Endurance limitations
    ◆ Impaired communication with caregiver related to assistance and mobility needs
    ◆ Joint precautions
    ◆ Lower extremity weakness
    ◆ Pain
    ◆ Range of motion limitations
    ◆ Tonal abnormalities
    ◆ Upper extremity weakness
    ◆ Weight bearing limitations/precautions
    ◆ Other problems, based on the patient's unique medical history and environment

2. **Safety Checklist**
    ◆ Caregiver availability, capability and willingness to provide care
    ◆ Compliance with prescribed equipment use
    ◆ Compliance with joint precautions
    ◆ Compliance with weight bearing precautions/limitations
    ◆ History of falls
    ◆ Identified safety concerns documented and communicated to case manager
    ◆ Impaired judgment
    ◆ Lack of caregiver
    ◆ Medication profile, history and side effects (e.g., orthostatic hypotension)
    ◆ Patient lives alone
    ◆ Safety assessment completed/ environmental safety hazards identified
    ◆ Other safety issues, based on the patient's unique medical history, environment, and support

3. **Actions/Interventions/Activities**
    PT:
    ◆ Teach home exercise to increase strength/ROM/balance, to improve independence in car transfer activities.
    ◆ Increase independence and safety in car transfers through training and use of adaptive techniques, recommendations and instructions in use of assistive devices or equipment (e.g., seat swivel disks, transfer board).
    ◆ Provide recommendations on environment modification (e.g., elevate car seat with cushion, slide car seat backwards).
    ◆ Teach patient/caregiver fall prevention and safety measures related to car transfers.
    ◆ Teach home care aide repetitive exercise program and techniques to support car transfer function and safety.
    ◆ Teach caregivers and home care aide strategies to support patient's PT goals.
    ◆ Other interventions/activities based on the patient's unique needs.
    SLP:
    ◆ Identify and teach communication needs related to car transfer activities (e.g., amount and type of assistance needed).
    ◆ Teach patient/caregivers compensatory memory strategies to increase patient's ability to carryout multi-step transferring activities.
    ◆ Teach caregivers and home care aide strategies to support communication program and SLP goals.
    ◆ Other interventions/activities based on the patient's unique needs.
    OT:
    ◆ Teach adaptive techniques and use of assistive devices for increased independence in car transfers.
    ◆ Teach safety measures regarding car transfers, including car modifications.
    ◆ Teach therapeutic exercises and provide home program to increase UE strength/ROM/balance/coordination for car transfers.
    ◆ Identify environmental modification needs (e.g., ramp, outdoor transfer surface alternatives for snowy conditions).
    ◆ Teach caregivers and home care aide strategies to support patient's OT goals.
    ◆ Other interventions/activities based on the patient's unique needs.

4. **Specific Functional Goals**
   PT:
   ◆ Patient/caregiver will demonstrate safe car transfers with (max/mod/min/no) assist by _____(date).
   ◆ Patient/ Family/Therapist/Social Worker will obtain equipment/ complete environmental modification by _____(date).
   ◆ Patient/caregiver will demonstrate compliance with (prescribed techniques/weight bearing status) during car transfer activities by _____(date).
   ◆ Other functional goals based on the patient's unique needs.
   SLP:
   ◆ Patient uses adaptive communication techniques or compensatory memory strategies to achieve car transfer by _____(date).
   ◆ Caregivers report improved communications related to car transfer needs by _____(date).
   ◆ Other functional communication goals based on the patient's unique needs.
   OT:
   ◆ Patient/caregiver will demonstrate adaptive techniques for safe car transfers with (max/mod/min/no) assist by _____(date).
   ◆ Patient/caregiver will demonstrate proper use of assistive devices for car transfers by _____(date).
   ◆ Patient/Family/Therapist/Social Worker will obtain equipment/ complete environmental/car modifications by _____(date).
   ◆ Patient/caregiver will demonstrate home program for therapeutic exercises for improved strength/ROM/balance/coordination needed for car transfers with (max/mod/min/no assist) by _____(date).
   ◆ Other functional goals based on the patient's unique needs.

Performance Area: DRESSING
Corresponding OASIS Components: (M0650, M0660)
(See also Equipment for Self-Care in Part Seven).
1. **Identified/Assessed Problems/Restricted Performance Areas**
   ◆ Accessibility of clothing
   ◆ Balance deficits
   ◆ Endurance limitations
   ◆ Impaired communication with caregiver related to assistance and dressing needs
   ◆ Joint precautions
   ◆ Lower extremity weakness
   ◆ Pain
   ◆ Range of motion limitations
   ◆ Tonal abnormalities
   ◆ Upper extremity weakness
   ◆ Weight bearing limitations/precautions
   ◆ Wounds, dressings, casts, splints, orthotics or prosthetics requiring special attention during dressing
   ◆ Other problems, based on the patient's unique medical history and environment

2. **Safety Checklist**
   ◆ Caregiver availability, capability and willingness to provide care
   ◆ Compliance with adaptive equipment use
   ◆ Compliance with joint precautions
   ◆ Compliance with weight bearing precautions/limitations
   ◆ History of falls
   ◆ Home layout, structure, and environment
   ◆ Identified safety concerns documented and communicated to case manager
   ◆ Impaired judgment
   ◆ Lack of caregiver (specify, e.g., in daytime, at nighttime)
   ◆ Medication profile, history and side effects (e.g., orthostatic hypotension)
   ◆ Patient lives alone
   ◆ Other safety issues, based on the patient's unique medical history, environment, and support

3. **Actions/Interventions/Activities**
   PT:
   ◆ Teach home exercise to increase strength/ROM/balance to improve independence in dressing activities.
   ◆ Teach environmental modification to improve safety and independent dressing.
   ◆ Teach fall prevention and safety measures related to dressing.
   ◆ Teach home care aide repetitive exercise program and techniques to support dressing function and safety.
   ◆ Provide home program and teach caregivers and home care aide in strategies to support patient's PT goals.
   ◆ Other interventions/activities based on the patient's unique needs.
   SLP:
   ◆ Address communication needs related to dressing activities (e.g., amount and type of assistance needed, clothing preferences, etc).
   ◆ Teach patient/caregiver alternative communications (e.g., communication board).
   ◆ Teach patient/caregiver compensatory memory strategies to increase patient's ability to carry out multi-step dressing activities.
   ◆ Teach caregivers and home care aide strategies to support communication program and SLP goals.
   ◆ Other interventions/activities based on the patient's unique needs.
   OT:
   ◆ Teach adaptive techniques and use of assistive devices for increased independence in dressing (including donning/doffing splints, etc.).
   ◆ Teach safety measures regarding dressing.
   ◆ Teach use of assistive devices for safe and independent dressing.
   ◆ Teach therapeutic exercises and provide home program to increase UE strength/ROM/balance/coordination for dressing.
   ◆ Teach adaptive techniques for dressing tasks related to ROM restrictions/precautions (e.g., total hip precautions).
   ◆ Teach energy conservation/diaphragmatic breathing/relaxation techniques to reduce SOB with dressing activities.
   ◆ Other interventions/activities based on the patient's unique needs.

4. Specific Functional Goals

PT:

◆ Patient/caregiver will demonstrate safe tub/shower transfers with (max/mod/min/no assist) by _____(date).

◆ Patient/ Family/Therapist/Social Worker will obtain equipment/ complete home modification by _____(date).

◆ Patient/caregiver will demonstrate compliance with (prescribed device use/weight bearing status) during dressing activities by _____(date).

◆ Other functional goals based on the patient's unique needs.

SLP:

◆ Patient/caregiver uses adaptive communication techniques or compensatory memory strategies to achieve dressing goals by _____(date).

◆ Caregivers report improved communications related to dressing needs by _____(date).

◆ Other functional communication goals based on the patient's unique needs.

OT:

◆ Patient/caregiver will demonstrate adaptive dressing techniques with (max/mod/min/no) assist by _____(date).

◆ Patient will demonstrate proper use of assistive devices for dressing by _____(date).

◆ Patient/Family/Therapist/Social Worker will obtain equipment/complete bathroom modification by _____(date).

◆ Patient/caregiver will demonstrate compliance with ROM restrictions/ joint precautions during dressing activities by __ __(date).

◆ Patient will demonstrate home program for energy conservation/ diaphragmatic breathing/relaxation techniques to reduce SOB during dressing activities by _____(date).

◆ Other functional goals based on the patient's unique needs.

Performance Area: EATING/SELF-FEEDING
Corresponding OASIS Components: (M0710)
(See also Equipment for Self-Care in Part Seven).

1. **Identified/Assessed Problems/Restricted Performance Areas**
   ◆ Accessibility of food/utensils/table
   ◆ Balance deficits
   ◆ Endurance limitations
   ◆ Impaired communication with caregiver related to assistance and related needs
   ◆ Joint precautions
   ◆ Pain
   ◆ Range of motion limitations
   ◆ Tonal abnormalities
   ◆ Trunk weakness
   ◆ Upper extremity weakness
   ◆ Weight bearing limitations/precautions
   ◆ Other problems, based on the patient's unique medical history and environment

2. **Safety Checklist**
   ◆ Caregiver availability, capability and willingness to provide care
   ◆ Compliance with adaptive equipment use
   ◆ Compliance with joint precautions/ROM restrictions
   ◆ Identified safety concerns documented and communicated to case manager
   ◆ Impaired judgment
   ◆ Lack of caregiver (specify, e.g., at meal times)
   ◆ Medication profile, history and side effects (e.g., food-related interactions)
   ◆ Patient lives alone
   ◆ Patient high risk for aspiration/choking
   ◆ Other safety issues, based on the patient's unique medical history, environment, and support

3. **Actions/Interventions/Activities**
   PT:
   ◆ Teach home exercise to increase endurance/ROM/balance/posture to improve independence in eating activities.
   ◆ Teach home care aide repetitive exercise program and techniques to support eating function, positioning and safety.

◆ Provide home program and teach caregivers and home care aide in strategies to support patient's PT goals.
◆ Other interventions/activities based on the patient's unique needs.

SLP:
◆ Address communication needs related to eating activities (e.g., amount and type of assistance needed, food preferences, when hungry, etc.)
◆ Teach patient/caregiver alternative communication methods (e.g., communication board, menu, schedule, etc.)
◆ Teach safe swallowing techniques.
◆ Teach safety precautions related to aspiration.
◆ Teach food texture recommendations.
◆ Teach patient/caregiver compensatory memory strategies to increase patient's ability to carry out multi-step eating activities.
◆ Teach caregivers and home care aide strategies to support communication program and SLP goals.
◆ Other interventions/activities based on the patient's unique needs.

OT:
◆ Teach adaptive techniques and use of assistive devices for increased independence in eating/feeding.
◆ Teach safety measures regarding eating/feeding/swallowing to prevent aspiration.
◆ Teach use of assistive devices for safe and independent eating/feeding.
◆ Teach environmental modification/seating to improve posture and promote independent/safe eating.
◆ Assist in obtaining assistive feeding devices.
◆ Teach therapeutic exercises and provide home program to increase UE fine motor skills/strength/ROM/coordination for self-feeding.
◆ Other interventions/activities based on the patient's unique needs.

4. **Specific Functional Goals**
   PT:
◆ Patient will demonstrate home program to improve endurance/ROM/balance/posture with (max/mod/min/no) assist by _____(date).
◆ Other functional goals based on the patient's unique needs.

   SLP:
◆ Patient/caregiver use adaptive communication techniques or compensatory memory strategies to achieve eating/self-feeding goals by _____(date).
◆ Caregivers report improved communications related to eating/self-feeding needs by _____(date).

tient/Family/Therapist/Social Worker will obtain assistive devices for ergency response/complete home modifications by _____(date).
tient/caregiver will demonstrate home program for energy nservation/diaphragmatic breathing/relaxation techniques to reduce B by _____(date).
er functional goals based on the patient's unique needs.

◆ Patient demonstrates safe swallowing techniques by _____(date).
◆ Patient/caregiver demonstrate compliance with food texture recommendations by _____(date).
◆ Other functional communication goals based on the patient's unique needs.

OT:

◆ Patient/caregiver will demonstrate adaptive techniques for eating/ feeding with (max/mod/min/no) assist by _____(date).
◆ Patient/caregiver will demonstrate safety precautions for swallowing with (min/no) coughing/choking by _____(date).
◆ Patient will demonstrate proper use of assistive devices for eating/ feeding by _____(date).
◆ Patient/caregiver will demonstrate proper positioning to prevent risk of aspiration by _____(date).
◆ Patient/Family/Therapist/Social Worker will obtain assistive devices for eating or positioning by _____(date).
◆ Patient/caregiver will demonstrate compliance with ROM restrictions/ joint precautions during eating activities by _____(date).
◆ Patient will demonstrate home program for therapeutic exercises for increased strength/ROM/coordination needed for self-feeding with (max/mod/min/no) assist by _____(date).
◆ Other functional goals based on the patient's unique needs.

Performance Area: EMERGENCY RESPONSE NEEDS
Corresponding OASIS Components: (M0770)

1. **Identified/Assessed Problems/Restricted Performance Areas**
   - Accessibility of phone/doorbell/personal emergency response alarm
   - Impaired communication with caregiver related to emergency needs
   - Impaired mobility
   - Impaired recognition of emergency situation/poor judgment
   - Other problems, based on the patient's unique medical history and environment

2. **Safety Checklist**
   - Caregiver availability, capability and willingness to provide care
   - Compliance with instructions to call for assistance
   - Identified safety concerns documented and communicated to case manager
   - Impaired judgment
   - Knowledge of symptoms to report via emergency response methods
   - Lack of caregiver (specify, e.g., at nighttime)
   - Medication profile, history and side effects (e.g., life threatening side effects or drug interactions)
   - Patient lives alone
   - Other safety issues, based on the patient's unique medical history, environment, and support

3. **Actions/Interventions/Activities**
   PT:
   - Teach home exercise to increase endurance/strength/ROM/balance/posture to improve functional mobility to facilitate exiting home, or access emergency assistance (e.g., phone, door, etc)
   - Teach home care aide repetitive exercise program and techniques to support emergency response mobility function.
   - Provide home program and teach caregivers and home care aide in strategies to support patient's PT goals.
   - Other interventions/activities based on the patient's unique needs.
   SLP:
   - Address communication needs related to emergency response activities (e.g., amount and type of assistance needed, methods to communicate significant symptoms to caregivers, methods to communicate emergency needs to community resources, etc.)
   - Teach patient /caregiver alternative communication methods (e.g., personal emergency response systems, siren, etc.)

   - Teach patient/caregiver compensatory memory patient's ability to carry out multi-step emerge
   - Teach caregivers and home care aide strategie communication program and SLP goals.
   - Other interventions/activities based on the pa
   OT:
   - Teach adaptive techniques and use of assisti independence in initiating emergency call.
   - Teach safety measures regarding functional access to initiate emergency call.
   - Assist in obtaining emergency response de instruction and home modification to opti
   - Teach therapeutic exercises and provide h UE strength/ROM/coordination for carry
   - Teach energy conservation/diaphragmati techniques to reduce SOB with emergen
   - Other interventions/activities based on t

4. **Specific Functional Goals**
   PT:
   - Patient/caregiver will demonstrate hor endurance/strength/ROM/balance/pos mobility to facilitate exiting home, o with (max/mod/min/no) assist by __
   - Other functional goals based on the
   SLP:
   - Patient/caregiver uses adaptive con compensatory memory strategies t by _____(date).
   - Caregivers report improved comn response needs by _____(date).
   - Other functional communication needs.
   OT:
   - Patient/caregiver will demonstr adaptive techniques for emerge
   - Caregiver/other will demonstr urgency call by _____(date).
   - Patient will demonstrate effec devices for assistive devices

   - P: er
   - Pa co SC
   - Ot

Performance Area: FUNCTIONAL COMMUNICATION
Corresponding OASIS Components: (M0400, M0410, M0770)
1. **Identified/Assessed Problems/Restricted Performance Areas**
    ◆ Accessibility of communication aids (e.g., phone, hearing aids, interpreter, communication board, etc.)
    ◆ Impaired communication with caregiver affecting patient function/ safety/quality of life
    ◆ Impaired mobility limiting communication (e.g., unable to get to phone/door)
    ◆ Other problems, based on the patient's unique medical history and environment

2. **Safety Checklist**
    ◆ Caregiver availability, capability and willingness to assist in communication needs
    ◆ Identified safety concerns documented and communicated to case manager
    ◆ Impaired judgment
    ◆ Knowledge of symptoms to report to caregivers/health care providers (e.g., pain, SOB, etc.)
    ◆ Lack of caregiver (specify, e.g., in daytime)
    ◆ Language barrier/Learning barrier due to communication deficits
    ◆ Medication profile, history and side effects (e.g., knowledge of side effects and symptoms to communicate to caregivers)
    ◆ Patient lives alone
    ◆ Other safety issues, based on the patient's unique medical history, environment, and support

3. **Actions/Interventions/Activities**
    PT:
    ◆ Teach home exercise to increase endurance/strength/ROM/balance/ posture to improve functional mobility to facilitate functional communication (e.g., phone, door, etc).
    ◆ Teach home care aide repetitive exercise program and techniques to support emergency response mobility function.
    ◆ Provide home program and teach caregivers and home care aide in strategies to support patient's PT goals.
    ◆ Other interventions/activities based on the patient's unique needs.

SLP:
- Address needs related to functional communication (e.g., hearing aids, interpreter, visual cues).
- Teach patient/caregiver alternative communication methods (e.g., communication board, bell, symbols, techniques, etc.)
- Teach caregivers and home care aide strategies to support communication program and SLP goals.
- Other interventions/activities based on the patient's unique needs.

OT:
- Teach adaptive techniques and use of assistive devices for increased independence in functional communication activities.
- Teach safety measures regarding functional mobility as needed for access to communication tools (e.g., phone/door).
- Assist in obtaining communication devices (e.g., adapted phones, or adaptive devices to improve reading or writing function) and provide instruction and home modification to optimize use.
- Teach therapeutic exercises and provide home program to increase UE strength/ROM/coordination for carrying out functional communication activities (e.g., reading/writing/phone use, etc).
- Teach energy conservation/diaphragmatic breathing/relaxation techniques to reduce SOB with communication activities.
- Other interventions/activities based on the patient's unique needs.

4. **Specific Functional Goals**
   PT:
   - Patient will demonstrate home program to improve endurance/ strength/ROM/balance/posture to improve functional mobility required for functional communication with (max/mod/min/no) assist by _____(date).
   - Other functional goals based on the patient's unique needs.

   SLP:
   - Patient/caregiver use adaptive communication techniques or compensatory memory strategies to achieve functional communication goals by _____(date).
   - Patient/caregiver demonstrate effective use of alternative communication systems or devices by _____(date).
   - Caregivers report improved communications positively affecting patient function by _____(date).
   - Other functional communication goals based on the patient's unique needs.

OT:

◆ Patient/caregiver will demonstrate effective and consistent use of adaptive communication techniques by _____(date).

◆ Patient/caregiver will demonstrate effective and consistent use of assistive devices for communication by _____(date).

◆ Patient/Family/Therapist/Social Worker will obtain assistive devices for functional communication by _____(date).

◆ Patient/caregiver will demonstrate home program to increase UE strength/ROM/coordination for carrying out functional communication activities (e.g., reading/writing/phone use, etc.) with (max/mod/min/no) assist by _____(date).

◆ Other functional goals based on the patient's unique needs.

Performance Area: GROOMING
Corresponding OASIS Component: (M0640)
(See also Equipment for Self-Care in Part Seven).
1. **Identified/Assessed Problems/Restricted Performance Areas**
    ◆ Accessibility of grooming aids/mirror/sink
    ◆ Balance deficits
    ◆ Endurance limitations
    ◆ Impaired communication with caregiver related to assistance and grooming needs
    ◆ Joint precautions
    ◆ Lower extremity weakness
    ◆ Pain
    ◆ Range of motion limitations
    ◆ Tonal abnormalities
    ◆ Upper extremity weakness
    ◆ Weight bearing limitations/precautions
    ◆ Wounds, dressings, or casts requiring special attention during grooming activities
    ◆ Other problems, based on the patient's unique medical history and environment

2. **Safety Checklist**
    ◆ Bathroom/home layout, structure, and environment
    ◆ Caregiver availability, capability and willingness to provide care
    ◆ Compliance with equipment use
    ◆ Compliance with joint precautions
    ◆ Compliance with weight bearing precautions/limitations
    ◆ History of falls
    ◆ Home safety assessment completed, including disaster evacuation plan
    ◆ Identified safety concerns documented and communicated to case manager
    ◆ Impaired judgment
    ◆ Lack of caregiver (specify, e.g., in daytime, at nighttime)
    ◆ Medication profile, history and side effects (e.g., bleeding precautions, orthostatic hypotension)
    ◆ Patient lives alone
    ◆ Sensory status (e.g., can perceive/feel dangerous water temperatures)
    ◆ Other safety issues, based on the patient's unique medical history, environment, and support

3. **Actions/Interventions/Activities**
   PT:
   ◆ Teach home exercise to increase strength/ROM/balance, to improve independence in grooming activities.
   ◆ Increase independence and safety in grooming activities through training and use of adaptive techniques and recommendation and instruction in use of assistive devices or equipment.
   ◆ Provide recommendations on environment modification.
   ◆ Provide education related to fall prevention and bathroom safety, and compliance with weight bearing/ROM restrictions during grooming activities.
   ◆ Teach home care aide repetitive exercise program and techniques to support bathing function and safety.
   ◆ Provide home program and teach caregivers and home care aide in strategies to support patient's PT goals
   ◆ Other interventions/activities based on the patient's unique needs.
   SLP:
   ◆ Address communication needs related to grooming activities (e.g., amount and type of assistance needed).
   ◆ Teach patient/caregiver alternative communications (e.g., communication board).
   ◆ Teach patient/caregiver compensatory memory strategies to increase patient's ability to carry out multi-step grooming activities.
   ◆ Teach caregivers and home care aide strategies to support communication program and SLP goals.
   ◆ Other interventions/activities based on the patient's unique needs.
   OT:
   ◆ Teach adaptive techniques and use of adapted/assistive devices for increased independence with grooming.
   ◆ Teach safety measures regarding grooming tasks (e.g., use of razor).
   ◆ Teach therapeutic exercises and provide home program to increase UE strength/ROM/coordination/balance for grooming tasks.
   ◆ Teach bathroom modification needs, including identification of safe/stable surface for grooming tasks, modification of mirror height, etc.
   ◆ Assist in obtaining assistive grooming devices and provide instruction on bathroom modification details.
   ◆ Teach caregivers and home care aide in strategies to support patient's OT goals.
   ◆ Other interventions/activities based on the patient's unique needs.

4. Specific Functional Goals
PT:

◆ Patient/caregiver will demonstrate functional mobility to allow safe and effective performance of grooming activities with (max/mod/min/no) assist by _____(date).

◆ Patient/ Family/Therapist/Social Worker will obtain equipment/complete home modifications by _____(date).

◆ Patient/caregiver will demonstrate compliance with (ROM restrictions, weight bearing status) during grooming activities by _____(date).

◆ Other functional goals based on the patient's unique needs.

SLP:

◆ Patient/caregiver use adaptive communication techniques or compensatory memory strategies to achieve grooming goals by _____(date).

◆ Caregivers report improved communications related to grooming needs.

◆ Other functional communication goals based on the patient's unique needs.

OT:

◆ Patient/caregiver will demonstrate adaptive techniques for grooming with (max/mod/min/no) assist by _____(date).

◆ Patient/Family/Therapist/Social Worker will obtain assistive devices/equipment /complete bathroom modification by _____(date).

◆ Patient/caregiver will demonstrate proper use of assistive devices for grooming by _____(date).

◆ Patient will demonstrate home program for energy conservation/diaphragmatic breathing/relaxation techniques to reduce SOB during grooming activities by _____(date).

◆ Other functional goals based on the patient's unique needs.

Performance Area: HOMEMAKING
Corresponding OASIS Component: (M0750)
(See also Equipment for Self-Care in Part Seven).
1. **Identified/Assessed Problems/Restricted Performance Areas**
   ◆ Balance deficits
   ◆ Endurance limitations
   ◆ Impaired communication with caregiver related to assistance needs
     with homemaking tasks
   ◆ Joint precautions
   ◆ Lower extremity weakness
   ◆ Pain
   ◆ Range of motion limitations
   ◆ Tonal abnormalities
   ◆ Upper extremity weakness
   ◆ Weight bearing limitations/precautions
   ◆ Other problems, based on the patient's unique medical history and
     environment

2. **Safety Checklist**
   ◆ Caregiver availability, capability and willingness to provide assistance
   ◆ Compliance with assistive device use during homemaking activities
   ◆ Compliance with joint precautions
   ◆ Compliance with weight bearing precautions/limitations
   ◆ History of falls
   ◆ Home layout, structure, and environment
   ◆ Home safety assessment completed, including disaster evacuation plan
   ◆ Identified safety concerns documented and communicated to case
     manager
   ◆ Impaired judgment
   ◆ Lack of caregiver (specify, e.g., in daytime)
   ◆ Medication profile, history and side effects (e.g., orthostatic
     hypotension)
   ◆ Patient lives alone
   ◆ Sanitation or safety hazards resulting from inadequate homemaking
     performance
   ◆ Other safety issues, based on the patient's unique medical history,
     environment, and support

3. **Actions/Interventions/Activities**
   PT:
   ◆ Teach home exercise to increase endurance/strength/ROM/balance/ posture for homemaking tasks.
   ◆ Increase independence and safety in homemaking tasks through use of adaptive techniques and use of assistive, protective, or supportive devices.
   ◆ Provide recommendations on environment modification to improve safe and effective homemaking performance.
   ◆ Provide patient/caregiver fall prevention and home safety measures related to homemaking tasks.
   ◆ Teach home care aide in repetitive exercise program and techniques to support safety and function.
   ◆ Provide home program and teach caregivers and home care aide in strategies to support patient's PT goals.
   ◆ Other interventions/activities based on the patient's unique needs.
   SLP:
   ◆ Address communication needs related to homemaking activities (e.g., amount and type of assistance needed, supplies needed).
   ◆ Teach patient/caregiver in alternative communications (e.g., preparing list of needed supplies, etc).
   ◆ Teach patient/caregiver in compensatory memory strategies to increase patient's ability to carry out homemaking activities (e.g., weight bearing precautions, use of assistive device, activity limitations).
   ◆ Provide home program and teach caregivers and home care aide in strategies to support communication program and SLP goals.
   ◆ Other interventions/activities based on the patient's unique needs.
   OT:
   ◆ Teach adaptive techniques and use of assistive devices for increased independence in homemaking tasks.
   ◆ Teach support or splinting interventions to protect impaired UE during homemaking activities.
   ◆ Teach safety measures regarding homemaking tasks, including home modification.
   ◆ Teach therapeutic exercises and provide home program to increase UE strength/ROM/balance for homemaking tasks.
   ◆ Teach energy conservation/diaphragmatic breathing/relaxation techniques to reduce SOB with homemaking tasks.
   ◆ Teach caregivers and home care aide in strategies to support patient's OT goals.
   ◆ Other interventions/activities based on the patient's unique needs.

4. **Specific Functional Goals**
   PT:
   - Patient/caregiver will demonstrate home exercise program to increase endurance/strength/ROM/balance/posture for homemaking tasks with (max/mod/min/no) assist by _____(date).
   - Patient/caregiver will demonstrate proper use of adaptive techniques and assistive, protective, or supportive devices during homemaking tasks by _____(date).
   - Patient/caregiver/therapist/social worker will obtain equipment/ complete home modifications to improve safe and effective homemaking performance by _____(date).
   - Patient/caregiver demonstrate compliance with fall prevention and home safety during homemaking tasks with (max/mod/min/no) assist by _____(date).
   - Teach home care aide in repetitive exercise program and techniques to support safety and function.
   - Patient will demonstrate performance of homemaking tasks with (max/mod/min/no) assist by _____(date).
   - Other functional goals based on the patient's unique needs.

   SLP:
   - Patient demonstrates effective communication needs related to homemaking activities by _____(date).
   - Patient/caregiver demonstrate effective use of alternative communications to facilitate homemaking tasks by _____(date).
   - Patient demonstrates effective use of compensatory memory strategies to increase patient's ability to carry out homemaking activities by _____(date).
   - Caregivers report improved communications related to homemaking needs by _____(date).
   - Other functional goals based on the patient's unique needs.

   OT:
   - Patient/caregiver will demonstrate adaptive techniques for safe homemaking tasks with (max/mod/min/no) assist by _____(date).
   - Patient/caregiver will demonstrate proper use of assistive devices for homemaking tasks by _____(date).
   - Patient will demonstrate safe functional mobility during homemaking tasks with (max/mod/min/no) assist by _____(date).
   - Patient/caregiver will demonstrate compliance with effective use of splinting or supportive techniques to protect UE during homemaking activities by _____(date).

◆ Patient/caregiver/therapist/social worker will obtain equipment/assistive devices or complete home modifications by _____(date).

◆ Patient/caregiver will demonstrate home program to increase UE strength/ROM/balance for homemaking tasks with (max/mod/min/no) assist by _____(date).

◆ Patient/caregiver will demonstrate home program for energy conservation/diaphragmatic breathing/relaxation techniques to 1reduce SOB with homemaking activities by _____(date).

◆ Other functional goals based on the patient's unique needs.

Performance Area: KITCHEN FUNCTIONING
Corresponding OASIS Components: (M0720, M0700)
(See also Equipment for Self-Care in Part Seven, and Kitchen Barriers and Adaptations -Box 3-12).

1. **Identified/Assessed Problems/Restricted Performance Areas**
   ◆ Access to kitchen/cupboards/cabinets/appliances/table/dishes/food/ utensils/sink
   ◆ Balance deficits
   ◆ Endurance limitations
   ◆ Impaired communication with caregiver related to assistance needs with meal preparation tasks
   ◆ Joint precautions
   ◆ Lower extremity weakness
   ◆ Pain
   ◆ Range of motion limitations
   ◆ Tonal abnormalities
   ◆ Upper extremity weakness
   ◆ Weight bearing limitations/precautions
   ◆ Other problems, based on the patient's unique medical history and environment

2. **Safety Checklist**
   ◆ Caregiver availability, capability and willingness to provide assistance
   ◆ Compliance with assistive device use during kitchen activities
   ◆ Compliance with joint precautions
   ◆ Compliance with weight bearing precautions/limitations
   ◆ History of falls
   ◆ Home safety assessment completed, including disaster evacuation plan
   ◆ Identified safety concerns documented and communicated to case manager
   ◆ Impaired judgement
   ◆ Kitchen layout, structure, and environment
   ◆ Lack of caregiver (specify, e.g., in daytime)
   ◆ Medication profile, history and side effects (e.g., bleeding precautions, orthostatic hypotension)
   ◆ Patient lives alone
   ◆ Sensory impairments (e.g., unawareness of dangerous temperatures)
   ◆ Other safety issues, based on the patient's unique medical history, environment, and support

3. Actions/Interventions/Activities

PT:

◆ Teach home exercise to increase endurance/strength/ROM/balance/ posture for mobility related to kitchen tasks.

◆ Increase independence and safety in kitchen tasks through use of assistive, protective, or supportive devices, or alternate mobility (e.g., wheelchair, walker with built in seat).

◆ Provide patient/caregiver fall prevention and kitchen safety measures.

◆ Teach home care aide in repetitive exercise program and techniques to support safety and function.

◆ Provide home program and teach caregivers and home care aide in strategies to support patient's PT goals.

◆ Other interventions/activities based on the patient's unique needs.

SLP:

◆ Address communication needs related to kitchen activities (e.g., amount and type of assistance needed, supplies needed).

◆ Teach patient and caregiver in alternative communication methods to facilitate kitchen tasks.

◆ Teach patient and caregivers in compensatory memory strategies to increase patient's ability to carry out multi-step kitchen tasks.

◆ Provide home program and teach caregivers and home care aide in strategies to support communication program and SLP goals.

◆ Other interventions/activities based on the patient's unique needs.

OT:

◆ Teach adaptive techniques and use of assistive devices for increased independence in meal preparation/cooking/clean-up and kitchen mobility tasks.

◆ Teach support or splinting interventions to protect impaired UE during kitchen activities.

◆ Teach safety measures regarding meal prep/cooking tasks, including home modification.

◆ Teach therapeutic exercises and provide home program to increase UE strength/ROM/balance for kitchen tasks.

◆ Teach energy conservation/diaphragmatic breathing/relaxation techniques to reduce SOB with homemaking tasks.

◆ Teach caregivers and home care aide in strategies to support patient's OT goals.

◆ Other interventions/activities based on the patient's unique needs.

4. **Specific Functional Goals**
   PT:
   ◆ Patient/caregiver will demonstrate home exercise program to increase endurance/strength/ROM/balance/posture for kitchen tasks with (max/mod/min/no) assist by _____(date).
   ◆ Patient/caregiver will demonstrate proper use of assistive, protective, or supportive devices during kitchen tasks by _____(date).
   ◆ Patient/caregiver/therapist/social worker will obtain equipment/complete home modifications to improve safe and effective function in kitchen tasks by _____(date).
   ◆ Patient/caregiver demonstrate compliance with fall prevention and home safety measures by _____(date).
   ◆ Other functional goals based on the patient's unique needs.
   SLP:
   ◆ Patient/caregiver will demonstrate effective communication needs related to kitchen activities by _____(date).
   ◆ Patient/caregiver will demonstrate effective use of alternative communications to facilitate kitchen tasks by _____(date).
   ◆ Patient/caregiver will demonstrate effective use of compensatory memory strategies to increase patient's ability to carry out homemaking activities by _____(date).
   ◆ Caregivers report improved communications related to homemaking needs by _____(date).
   ◆ Other functional goals based on the patient's unique needs.
   OT:
   ◆ Patient/caregiver will demonstrate adaptive kitchen techniques with (max/mod/min/no) assist by _____(date).
   ◆ Patient/caregiver will demonstrate proper use of assistive devices for kitchen skills by _____(date).
   ◆ Patient will demonstrate safe transport of food/dishes/other with (max/mod/min/no) assist by _____(date).
   ◆ Patient/caregiver will demonstrate safe mobility, access to and use of appliances/cabinets/other with (max/mod/min/no) assist by _____(date).
   ◆ Patient/caregiver/therapist/social worker will obtain assistive devices or equipment for kitchen tasks or complete kitchen modifications by _____(date).
   ◆ Patient/caregiver will demonstrate home program for energy conservation/diaphragmatic breathing/relaxation techniques to reduce SOB with kitchen tasks by _____(date).
   ◆ Other functional goals based on the patient's unique needs.

Performance Area: LAUNDRY
Corresponding OASIS Component: (M0740)
1. **Identified/Assessed Problems/Restricted Performance Areas**
   ◆ Ability to collect and transport dirty/clean clothing
   ◆ Access to washer/dryer/laundry supplies
   ◆ Balance deficits
   ◆ Endurance limitations
   ◆ Impaired communication with caregiver related to assistance needs
     for laundry activities
   ◆ Joint precautions
   ◆ Lower extremity weakness
   ◆ Pain
   ◆ Range of motion limitations
   ◆ Tonal abnormalities
   ◆ Upper extremity weakness
   ◆ Weight bearing limitations/precautions
   ◆ Other problems, based on the patient's unique medical history and
     environment

2. **Safety Checklist**
   ◆ Caregiver availability, capability and willingness to provide assistance
   ◆ Compliance with assistive device use during activities
   ◆ Compliance with joint precautions
   ◆ Compliance with weight bearing precautions/limitations
   ◆ History of falls
   ◆ Home layout, structure, and environment - location of laundry facilities
     within home
   ◆ Home safety assessment completed, including disaster evacuation plan
   ◆ Identified safety concerns documented and communicated to case
     manager
   ◆ Impaired judgment
   ◆ Medication profile, history and side effects (e.g., orthostatic
     hypotension)
   ◆ Patient lives alone
   ◆ Other safety issues, based on the patient's unique medical history,
     environment, and support

3. **Actions/Interventions/Activities**
   PT:
   ◆ Teach home exercise to increase endurance/strength/ROM/balance/
     posture for mobility related to laundry activities.

◆ Increase independence and safety in laundry tasks through use of assistive, protective, or supportive devices, or alternate mobility (e.g., wheelchair, walker with built in seat/basket, etc).

◆ Teach patient/caregiver fall prevention and home safety measures related to laundry tasks.

◆ Teach home care aide in repetitive exercise program and techniques to support safety and function.

◆ Provide home program and teach caregivers and home care aide in strategies to support patient's PT goals.

◆ Other interventions/activities based on the patient's unique needs.

SLP:

◆ Address communication needs related to laundry activities (e.g., amount and type of assistance needed, supplies needed).

◆ Teach patient/caregiver in alternative communication methods to laundry tasks.

◆ Teach patient/caregiver in compensatory memory strategies to increase patient's ability to carry out multi-step laundry tasks.

◆ Provide home program and teach caregivers and home care aide in strategies to support communication program and SLP goals

◆ Other interventions/activities based on the patient's unique needs

OT:

◆ Teach adaptive techniques and use of assistive devices for increased independence in management of laundry.

◆ Teach support or splinting interventions to protect impaired UE during laundry activities.

◆ Teach safety measures for laundry, including home modification.

◆ Teach use of assistive devices for management of laundry.

◆ Teach therapeutic exercises and provide home program to increase UE strength/ROM/balance for laundry tasks.

◆ Teach energy conservation/diaphragmatic breathing/relaxation techniques to reduce SOB with laundry tasks.

◆ Teach caregivers and home care aide in strategies to support patient's OT goals.

◆ Other interventions/activities based on the patient's unique needs.

4. **Specific Functional Goals**
   PT:
   ◆ Patient/caregiver will demonstrate home exercise program to increase endurance/strength/ROM/balance/posture for laundry tasks with (max/mod/min/no) assist by _____(date).

◆ Patient/caregiver will demonstrate proper use of assistive, protective, or supportive devices during laundry activities by _____(date).
◆ Patient/caregiver/therapist/social worker will obtain equipment/-complete home modifications to improve safe and effective function in laundry activities by _____(date).
◆ Provide patient and caregiver education related to fall prevention and home safety during laundry tasks.
◆ Teach home care aide in repetitive exercise program and techniques to support safety and function.
◆ Provide home program and teach caregivers and home care aide in strategies to support patient's PT goals.
◆ Other functional goals based on the patient's unique needs.

SLP:

◆ Patient demonstrates effective communication needs related to laundry activities by _____(date).
◆ Patient/caregiver demonstrate effective use of alternative communications to facilitate laundry activities by _____(date).
◆ Patient demonstrates effective use of compensatory memory strategies to increase patient's ability to carry out laundry tasks by _____(date).
◆ Caregivers report improved communications related to homemaking needs by _____(date).
◆ Other functional goals based on the patient's unique needs.

OT:

◆ Patient/caregiver will demonstrate adaptive techniques to do laundry safely with (max/mod/min/no) assist by _____(date).
◆ Patient/caregiver will demonstrate proper use of assistive devices for laundry tasks by _____(date).
◆ Patient will demonstrate safe transport of laundry to/from facilities with (max/mod/min/no) assist by _____(date).
◆ Patient/caregiver will demonstrate safe functional mobility during laundry tasks, access to and use of washer/dryer/supplies/other with (max/mod/min/no) assist by _____(date).
◆ Patient/caregiver/therapist/social worker will obtain assistive devices or equipment for laundry tasks or complete home modifications by _____(date).
◆ Patient/caregiver will demonstrate home program for energy conservation/diaphragmatic breathing/relaxation techniques to reduce SOB with laundry activities by _____(date).
◆ Other functional goals based on the patient's unique needs.

Performance Area: MEDICATION MANAGEMENT
Corresponding OASIS Components: (M0780, M0790, M0800)
1. **Identified/Assessed Problems/Restricted Performance Areas**
    ◆ Accessibility of medication bottles/vials/inhalers/supplies
    ◆ Balance deficits
    ◆ Impaired communication with caregiver related to assistance and
      needs related to medications
    ◆ Joint precautions
    ◆ Knowledge deficits related to medication administration
    ◆ Pain
    ◆ Range of motion limitations
    ◆ Tonal abnormalities
    ◆ Upper extremity weakness
    ◆ Other problems, based on the patient's unique medical history and
      environment

2. **Safety Checklist**
    ◆ Caregiver availability, capability and willingness to assist with
      medication administration
    ◆ Compliance with adaptive equipment use
    ◆ Compliance with joint precautions/ROM restrictions
    ◆ Identified safety concerns documented and communicated to case
      manager
    ◆ Impaired judgment
    ◆ Lack of caregiver (specify, e.g., at medication times)
    ◆ Medication profile, history and side effects (e.g., drug regimen review
      and identification of significant side effects, drug interactions, patient
      compliance with prescribed medications)
    ◆ Memory deficits affecting compliance/function
    ◆ Patient lives alone
    ◆ Patient high risk for aspiration/choking
    ◆ Visual deficits affecting performance in medication administration
    ◆ Other safety issues, based on the patient's unique medical history,
      environment, and support

3. **Actions/Interventions/Activities**
    PT:
    ◆ Teach home exercise to increase endurance/ROM/balance/posture
      to improve independence related to mobility activities required for
      medication management.

◆ Teach home care aide repetitive exercise program and techniques to support functional mobility, positioning and safety.
◆ Teach effects of medications prescribed as related to patient function and therapeutic activities/goals.
◆ Provide home program and teach caregivers and home care aide in strategies to support patient's PT goals.
◆ Other interventions/activities based on the patient's unique needs.

SLP:
◆ Address communication needs related to medication management activities (e.g., amount and type of assistance needed, when PRN medications needed?, etc.)
◆ Teach patient/caregiver alternative communication methods (e.g., communication board, bell, schedule, etc.)
◆ Teach safe swallowing techniques.
◆ Teach safety precautions related to aspiration.
◆ Teach patient/caregiver compensatory memory strategies to increase patient's ability to carry out multi-step medication administration activities.
◆ Teach caregiver and home care aide strategies to support communication program and SLP goals.
◆ Other interventions/activities based on the patient's unique needs.

OT:
◆ Teach adaptive techniques and use of assistive devices for opening bottles/self-injecting/organizing daily medication/other.
◆ Teach safety measures regarding medication.
◆ Teach environmental modification/seating to improve posture and promote independent/safe administration of medications.
◆ Assist in obtaining assistive devices for opening bottles/organizing doses.
◆ Provide written outline/instructions/visual cues to facilitate independent and safe medication administration.
◆ Teach therapeutic exercises and provide home program to increase UE fine motor skills/strength/ROM/coordination for self-administration of oral, injectable or inhalant/mist medications.
◆ Other interventions/activities based on the patient's unique needs.

4. Specific Functional Goals
PT:
◆ Patient/caregiver will demonstrate home program to improve endurance/ROM/balance/posture with medication management (max/mod/min/no) assist by _____(date).

◆ Patient/caregiver will demonstrate safe mobility necessary to allow compliant medication administration with (max/mod/min/no) assist by _____(date).
◆ Patient/caregiver will demonstrate compliance with prescribed medications to optimize therapeutic goals with (max/mod/min/no) assist by _____(date).
◆ Other functional goals based on the patient's unique needs.

SLP:
◆ Patient/caregiver uses adaptive communication techniques or compensatory memory strategies to achieve medication management goals by _____(date).
◆ Caregivers report improved communications related to medication needs by _____(date).
◆ Patient demonstrates safe swallowing techniques by _____(date).
◆ Patient/caregiver will demonstrate consistent preparation of medication (e.g., crushed in applesauce) for safe swallowing by _____(date).
◆ Other functional communication goals based on the patient's unique-needs.

OT:
◆ Patient/caregiver will demonstrate adaptive techniques to open medicine bottles/self-inject with (max/mod/min/no) assist by _____(date).
◆ Patient/caregiver will demonstrate safety precautions for swallowing with (min/no) coughing/choking by _____(date).
◆ Patient/caregiver will demonstrate safe and correct dose administration of medication, following written home program by _____(date).
◆ Patient will demonstrate proper effective and consistent use of assistive devices for opening bottles/self-injecting/taking pills by _____(date).
◆ Patient/caregiver will demonstrate proper positioning to prevent risk of aspiration by _____(date).
◆ Patient/Family/Therapist/Social Worker will obtain assistive devices for medication administration or positioning by _____(date).
◆ Patient will demonstrate home program for therapeutic exercises for increased strength/ROM/coordination needed for medication management with (max/mod/min/no) assist by _____(date).
◆ Other functional goals based on the patient's unique needs.

Performance Area: MONEY MANAGEMENT
Corresponding OASIS Components: (M0380)

1. Identified/Assessed Problems/Restricted Performance Areas
- ◆ Accessibility of money, money management supplies
- ◆ Cognitive impairment affecting money management
- ◆ Impaired communication with caregiver related to assistance and needs relative to money management
- ◆ Pain
- ◆ Range of motion limitations
- ◆ Tonal abnormalities
- ◆ Upper extremity weakness
- ◆ Other problems, based on the patient's unique medical history and environment

2. Safety Checklist
- ◆ Caregiver availability, capability and willingness to assist with money management activities
- ◆ Compliance with joint precautions/ROM restrictions
- ◆ Identified safety concerns documented and communicated to case manager
- ◆ Impaired judgment
- ◆ Lack of caregiver (specify, e.g., at specific times)
- ◆ Medication profile, history and side effects (e.g., alertness, concentration)
- ◆ Patient lives alone
- ◆ Visual deficits affecting performance in money management
- ◆ Other safety issues, based on the patient's unique medical history, environment, and support

3. Actions/Interventions/Activities
    PT:
- ◆ Teach home exercise to increase endurance/ROM/balance/posture to improve independence related to mobility activities required for money management.
- ◆ Teach home care aide repetitive exercise program and techniques to support functional mobility, positioning and safety.
- ◆ Provide home program and teach caregivers and home care aide in strategies to support patient's PT goals.
- ◆ Other interventions/activities based on the patient's unique needs.

SLP:
◆ Address communication needs related to money management activities (e.g., amount and type of assistance needed, etc.)
◆ Teach patient/caregiver alternative communication methods (e.g., communication board, bell, schedule, budget, etc.)
◆ Teach patient /caregiver compensatory memory strategies to increase patient's ability to carry out multi-step money management activities.
◆ Provide cognitive-communication treatment to improve cognitive deficits (attention/memory/problem solving) to improve money management skill.
◆ Teach caregivers and home care aide strategies to support communication program and SLP goals.
◆ Other interventions/activities based on the patient's unique needs.
OT:
◆ Teach adaptive techniques and use of assistive devices for handling/ organizing money/bills/other.
◆ Teach safety issues associated with money management, teach a system for double checking actions, if possible.
◆ Assist in obtaining assistive devices for handling money or organizing financial records.
◆ Provide written outline/instructions/visual cues to facilitate independent and accurate money management.
◆ Teach therapeutic exercises and provide home program to increase UE fine motor skills/strength/ROM/coordination for money management tasks.
◆ Provide cognitive retraining necessary for money management.
◆ Other interventions/activities based on the patient's unique needs.

4. **Specific Functional Goals**
   PT:
   ◆ Patient/caregiver will demonstrate home program to improve endurance/ROM/balance/posture to facilitate money management tasks with (max/mod/min/no) assist by _____(date).
   ◆ Patient/caregiver will demonstrate safe mobility necessary to allow money management activities with (max/mod/min/no) assist by _____(date).
   ◆ Other functional goals based on the patient's unique needs.
   SLP:
   ◆ Patient/caregiver uses adaptive communication techniques or compensatory memory strategies to achieve money management goals by _____(date).

◆ Caregivers report improved communications related to money management needs by _____(date).
◆ Patient demonstrates improved cognitive deficits (attention/memory/problem solving) resulting in improved money management by _____(date).
◆ Other functional communication goals based on the patient's unique needs.

OT:

◆ Patient/caregiver will demonstrate improved cognitive skills necessary for money management with (max/mod/min/no) assist by _____(date).
◆ Patient/caregiver will demonstrate safe and improved hand function necessary for money management with (max/mod/min/no) assist by _____(date).
◆ Patient/caregiver demonstrate adaptive techniques and use of assistive devices for handling/organizing money/bills/other by _____(date).
◆ Patient/caregiver demonstrates use of system for double checking financial actions by _____(date).
◆ Patient/caregiver/therapist/social worker will obtain assistive devices for handling money or organizing financial records by _____ (date).
◆ Patient demonstrates improved money management using written outline/instructions/visual cues by _____(date).
◆ Patient/caregiver demonstrates performance of home program to increase UE fine motor skills/strength/ROM/coordination for money management tasks with (max/mod/min/no) assist by _____(date).
◆ Other functional goals based on the patient's unique needs.

Performance Area: PAIN MANAGEMENT
Corresponding OASIS Components: (M0420, M0430)

1. Identified/Assessed Problems/Restricted Performance Areas
- ◆ Ineffective pain management affecting rehabilitation/function
- ◆ Impaired communication with caregiver related to assistance and related pain management needs
- ◆ Impaired coordination
- ◆ Injuries
- ◆ Limited functional mobility
- ◆ Weight bearing/ROM limitations/precautions
- ◆ Wounds
- ◆ Other problems, based on the patient's unique medical history and environment

2. Safety Checklist
- ◆ Caregiver availability, capability and willingness to provide care
- ◆ Compliance with adaptive equipment use
- ◆ Compliance with joint precautions/ROM restrictions
- ◆ Identified safety concerns documented and communicated to case manager
- ◆ Impaired judgment
- ◆ Lack of caregiver (specify, e.g., at times of pain)
- ◆ Medication profile, history and side effects (e.g., level of pain relief from medications)
- ◆ Patient lives alone
- ◆ Other safety issues, based on the patient's unique medical history, environment, and support

3. Actions/Interventions/Activities
PT:
- ◆ Teach home exercise to improve strength/ROM/balance/posture; where deficits are resulting in pain.
- ◆ Teach therapeutic use of physical agents or mechanical modalities (e.g., heat, cold, ultrasound, tens) for pain control, include safety precautions associated with use.
- ◆ Teach positioning techniques to reduce/minimize effects of pain.
- ◆ Teach adaptive techniques (e.g., biofeedback/relaxation) to reduce pain.
- ◆ Teach regarding use of assistive, adaptive, or supportive devices to reduce pain.
- ◆ Teach home care aide repetitive exercise program and techniques to support eating function, positioning and safety.

◆ Provide home program and teach caregivers and home care aide in strategies to support patient's PT goals.

◆ Other interventions/activities based on the patient's unique needs.

SLP:

◆ Address communication needs related to pain (e.g., location and severity of pain, pain relief measures desired, etc.)

◆ Teach patient/caregiver alternative communication methods (e.g., communication board, bell, schedule, etc.) to notify caregiver of pain.

◆ Teach patient/caregiver compensatory memory strategies to increase patient's ability to carry out multi-step pain management activities.

◆ Teach caregivers and home care aide strategies to support communication program and SLP goals.

◆ Other interventions/activities based on the patient's unique needs.

OT:

◆ Teach adaptive techniques and use of assistive devices for increased independence in communicating and minimizing pain.

◆ Teach use of ice/heat to reduce pain, including safety precautions associated with use.

◆ Teach functional position/edema control techniques to reduce pain.

◆ Assist in obtaining assistive devices and provide instructions for home modification to communicate pain needs and minimize aggravating factors.

◆ Teach energy conservation/diaphragmatic breathing/relaxation techniques to reduce SOB associated with pain.

◆ Other interventions/activities based on the patient's unique needs.

4. **Specific Functional Goals**
   PT:

   ◆ Patient/caregiver demonstrates home exercise to improve strength/ ROM/balance/posture; where deficits are resulting in pain, with (max/mod/min/no) assist by _____(date).

   ◆ Patient/caregiver demonstrate effective use of physical agents or mechanical modalities (e.g., heat, cold, ultrasound, tens) for pain control, include safety precautions associated with use, with (max/mod/min/no) assist by _____(date).

   ◆ Patient/caregiver demonstrate compliance with positioning techniques to reduce/minimize effects of pain with (max/mod/min/no) assist by _____(date).

◆ Patient/caregiver demonstrate performance of adaptive techniques (e.g., biofeedback/relaxation) to effectively reduce pain with (max/mod/min/no) assist by _____(date).

◆ Patient/caregiver demonstrate use of assistive, adaptive, or supportive devices to reduce pain with (max/mod/min/no) assist by _____(date).

◆ Teach home care aide repetitive exercise program and techniques to support eating function, positioning and safety.

◆ Provide home program and teach caregivers and home care aide in strategies to support patient's PT goals.

◆ Other functional goals based on the patient's unique needs.

SLP:

◆ Patient/caregiver will demonstrate effective communication in relating pain information and pain management needs to caregiver by _____(date).

◆ Patient/caregiver effectively utilize alternative communication methods for pain management by _____(date).

◆ Patient/caregiver will demonstrate use of compensatory memory strategies to effectively improve function in pain management activities by _____(date).

◆ Other cognitive/communication goals based on the patient's unique needs.

OT:

◆ Patient/caregiver will demonstrate effective communication of pain level and requests for pain control interventions by _____(date).

◆ Patient/caregiver will demonstrate use of proper functional positioning/edema reduction techniques to minimize pain with (max/mod/min/no) assist by _____(date).

◆ Patient/caregiver will demonstrate home program for use of ice/heat to reduce pain, including safety precautions associated with its use by _____(date).

◆ Patient/caregiver will demonstrate home program for energy conservation/diaphragmatic breathing/relaxation techniques to reduce SOB associated with pain by _____(date).

◆ Other functional goals based on the patient's unique needs.

Performance Area: TOILETING
Corresponding OASIS Components: (M0520, M0530, M0540,
M0680, M0690)
(See also Bathroom Equipment in Part Seven).
1. **Identified/Assessed Problems/Restricted Performance Areas**
    ◆ Access to toilet
    ◆ Balance deficits
    ◆ Clothing management (e.g., donning and doffing clothes)
    ◆ Impaired communication with caregiver related to continence
    ◆ Inability to self-manage incontinence products (e.g., protective
       undergarments)
    ◆ Inability to transfer
    ◆ Incontinence
    ◆ Lower extremity weakness
    ◆ Pain
    ◆ Range of motion limitations
    ◆ Upper extremity weakness
    ◆ Other problems, based on the patient's unique medical history and
       environment

2. **Safety Checklist**
    ◆ Caregiver availability, capability and willingness to provide care
    ◆ History of falls
    ◆ Home layout, structure, and environment
    ◆ Home safety assessment completed, including disaster evacuation plan
    ◆ Identified safety concerns documented and communicated to case
       manager
    ◆ Lack of caregiver (specify, e.g., in daytime, at nighttime)
    ◆ Medication profile, history and side effects (e.g., related to bowel/
       bladder function [diarrhea, urinary frequency, etc.], orthostatic
       hypotension)
    ◆ Patient lives alone
    ◆ Other safety issues, based on the patient's unique medical history,
       environment, and support

3. **Actions/Interventions/Activities**
    PT:
    ◆ Instruct in therapeutic exercise to increase endurance/strength/ROM/
       balance/posture related to toileting activities.
    ◆ Increase independence and safety in toileting through use of adaptive
       techniques, assistive devices, equipment or environment modification.

◆ Teach patient/caregiver fall prevention and bathroom safety measures.
◆ Provide home program and instruct home care aide in repetitive exercise program to improve toileting function (e.g., Kegel's exercises).
◆ Instruct caregivers and home care aide in strategies to support patient's PT goals.
◆ Other interventions/activities based on the patient's unique needs.

SLP:
◆ Address communication needs related to toileting activities.
◆ Instruct patient/caregiver in alternative communications (e.g., bell, bed moisture alarm).
◆ Instruct caregivers and home care aide in strategies to support communication program and SLP goals.
◆ Other interventions/activities based on the patient's unique needs.

OT:
◆ Teach adaptive techniques and use of assistive devices to increase independence in toileting and clothing management.
◆ Teach safety measures and fall prevention for toileting, including functional mobility in bathroom.
◆ Instruct in bathroom modifications, including proper installation of grab bars, toilet safety frames, doorway widening, etc.
◆ Assist in obtaining assistive toileting devices.
◆ Teach therapeutic exercises and provide home program to increase UE strength/ROM/balance/coordination for toileting/clothing management/related transfers.
◆ Teach ROM precautions/restrictions (e.g., total hip precautions) related to toileting activities.
◆ Teach energy conservation/diaphragmatic breathing/relaxation techniques to reduce SOB with toileting activities.
◆ Other interventions/activities based on the patient's unique needs.

4. **Specific Functional Goals**
   PT:
   ◆ Patient/caregiver will demonstrate safe effective toileting with (max/mod/min/no) assist by _____(date).
   ◆ Patient/caregiver will demonstrate home exercise program to increase endurance/strength/ROM/balance/posture related to toileting activities with (max/mod/min/no) assist by _____(date).
   ◆ Patient/caregiver will demonstrate use of adaptive techniques, assistive devices, equipment or environment modification for safe and effective toileting with (max/mod/min/no) assist by _____(date).

◆ Patient/caregiver demonstrate compliance with fall prevention instruction by _____(date).

◆ Patient/ Family/Therapist/Social Worker will arrange obtain equipment/ complete home modification needs by _____(date).

◆ Other functional goals based on the patient's unique needs.

SLP:

◆ Patient/caregiver will demonstrate use of adaptive communication techniques to achieve toileting goals by _____(date).

◆ Caregivers report improved communications related to toileting needs by _____(date).

◆ Other functional communication goals based on the patient's unique needs.

OT:

◆ Patient/caregiver will demonstrate adaptive techniques for safe toilet transfers with (max/mod/min/no) assist by _____(date).

◆ Patient/caregiver will demonstrate safe clothing management before and after toileting with (max/mod/min/no) assist by _____(date).

◆ Patient/caregiver will verbalize/demonstrate self-care/hygiene needs and activities with (max/mod/min/no) assist by _____(date.)

◆ Patient/caregiver will demonstrate proper use of assistive devices/ protective undergarments for toileting by _____(date).

◆ Patient/caregiver/therapist/social worker will obtain assistive devices or equipment/ complete bathroom modifications by _____(date).

◆ Patient/caregiver will demonstrate home program for energy conservation/diaphragmatic breathing/relaxation techniques to reduce SOB by _____(date).

◆ Other functional goals based on the patient's unique needs.

Performance Area: TRANSFERS
Corresponding OASIS Component: (M0690)
1. **Identified/Assessed Problems/Restricted Performance Areas**
   - ◆ Balance deficits
   - ◆ Endurance limitations
   - ◆ Impaired communication with caregiver related to transfer assistance needs
   - ◆ Joint precautions
   - ◆ Lower extremity weakness
   - ◈ Pain
   - ◆ Range of motion limitations
   - ◆ Tonal abnormalities
   - ◆ Upper extremity weakness
   - ◆ Weight bearing limitations/precautions
   - ◆ Other problems, based on the patient's unique medical history and environment

2. **Safety Checklist**
   - ◆ Caregiver availability, capability and willingness to provide care
   - ◆ Compliance with assistive/adaptive device use
   - ◆ Compliance with joint precautions
   - ◆ Compliance with weight bearing precautions/limitations
   - ◆ History of falls
   - ◆ Home layout, structure, and environment
   - ◆ Home safety assessment completed, including disaster evacuation plan
   - ◆ Identified safety concerns documented and communicated to case manager
   - ◆ Impaired judgment
   - ◆ Lack of caregiver (specify, e.g., in daytime, at nighttime)
   - ◆ Medication profile, history and side effects (e.g., orthostatic hypotension)
   - ◆ Patient lives alone
   - ◆ Other safety issues, based on the patient's unique medical history, environment, and support

3. **Actions/Interventions/Activities**
   PT:
   - ◆ Teach home exercise to increase endurance/strength/ROM/balance/ posture to improve transfer function.

◆ Increase independence and safety in transfers through use of adaptive techniques or assistive/orthotic/ protective/supportive or prosthetic devices.

◆ Teach environment modification to increase transfer independence and safety.

◆ Teach patient/caregiver fall prevention and home safety measures related to transfer activities.

◆ Teach home care aide in repetitive exercise program and techniques to support transfer safety and function.

◆ Provide home program and teach caregivers and home care aide in strategies to support patient's PT goals.

◆ Other interventions/activities based on the patient's unique needs.

SLP:

◆ Address communication needs related to transfer activities (e.g., amount and type of assistance needed, when transfer is desired).

◆ Teach patient/caregiver in alternative communications (e.g., communication board, bell).

◆ Teach patient/caregiver in compensatory memory strategies to increase patient's ability to carry out PT and/or OT instructions related to transfer activities (e.g., weight bearing precautions, use of assistive device, multi-step activities).

◆ Provide home program and teach caregivers and home care aide in strategies to support communication program and SLP goals.

◆ Other interventions/activities based on the patient's unique needs.

OT:

◆ Teach adaptive techniques and use of assistive/supportive devices for increased independence in transfers.

◆ Teach safety and fall prevention measures for transfers.

◆ Assist in obtaining assistive transfer devices.

◆ Teach therapeutic exercises and provide home program to increase UE strength/ROM/balance/coordination for transfers.

◆ Teach energy conservation/diaphragmatic breathing/relaxation techniques to reduce SOB with transfers.

◆ Teach in-home modification measures to increase safety and function for transfers.

◆ Teach caregivers and home care aide in strategies to support patient's OT goals.

◆ Other interventions/activities based on the patient's unique needs.

4. Specific Functional Goals
PT:

◆ Patient/caregiver will demonstrate home program to increase endurance/strength/ROM/balance/posture to improve transfer function with (max/mod/min/no) assist by _____(date).

◆ Patient/caregiver will demonstrate proper use of adaptive techniques or assistive/orthotic/ protective/supportive or prosthetic devices for effective/safe transfers with (max/mod/min/no) assist by ____(date).

◆ Patient/caregiver/therapist/social worker will obtain assistive devices/ equipment or complete home modification by _____(date).

◆ Patient/caregiver will demonstrate compliance with fall prevention and home safety measures with (max/mod/min/no) assist by _____(date).

◆ Patient/caregiver will demonstrate safe transfers in home with (max/mod/min/no) assist for by _____(date).

◆ Patient/caregiver will demonstrate appropriate use of (assistive, adaptive, orthotic, protective, supporting, prosthetic devices) for gait by _____(date).

◆ Patient/caregiver will demonstrate compliance with (prescribed device use, weight bearing status) by _____(date).

◆ Other functional goals based on the patient's unique needs.

SLP:

◆ Patient/caregiver demonstrates effective use of adaptive/alternative communication techniques to achieve transfer goals by _____(date).

◆ Caregivers report improved communications related to transfer needs by _____(date).

◆ Patient/caregiver demonstrate effective use of compensatory memory strategies to increase patient's ability to carry out PT and/or OT instructions related to transfer activities (e.g., weight bearing precautions, use of assistive device, multi-step activities).

◆ Other functional communication goals based on the patient's unique needs.

OT:

◆ Patient/caregiver will demonstrate adaptive techniques for safe transfers, with (max/mod/min/no) assist by _____(date).

◆ Patient/caregiver will demonstrate proper use of assistive devices for transfers by ____(date).

◆ Patient/caregiver/therapist/social worker will obtain assistive transfer devices/complete home modifications by ____(date).

◆ Patient/caregiver will demonstrate home program for therapeutic exercises for increased strength/ROM/balance/coordination required for transfers with (max/mod/min/no) assist by ____(date).

◆ Patient/caregiver will demonstrate home program for energy conservation/diaphragmatic breathing/relaxation techniques to reduce SOB for transfers by ____(date).

◆ Other functional goals based on the patient's unique needs.

Performance Area: WHEELCHAIR FUNCTION
Corresponding OASIS Component: (M0700)
(See also Home Access Barriers and Adaptations - Box 3-13,
and Wheelchair Assessment - Box 7-1.)

1. **Identified/Assessed Problems/Restricted Performance Areas**
   - Ability to enter/exit home in wheelchair
   - Accessibility to necessary rooms/areas in home with wheelchair
   - Balance deficits
   - Coordination
   - Endurance limitations
   - Impaired communication with caregiver related to assistance needs for wheelchair activities
   - Impaired judgement
   - Impaired sensory status (e.g., wound presence or risk, visual deficits)
   - Joint precautions
   - Lower extremity weakness
   - Pain
   - Range of motion limitations
   - Tonal abnormalities
   - Upper extremity weakness
   - Weight bearing limitations/pressure precautions
   - Other problems, based on the patient's unique medical history and environment

2. **Safety Checklist**
   - Caregiver availability, capability and willingness to provide assistance
   - Compliance with assistive/adaptive/supportive devices use during wheelchair function
   - Compliance with joint precautions
   - Compliance with weight bearing precautions/limitations
   - History of falls from chair
   - Home layout, structure, and environment
   - Home safety assessment completed, including disaster evacuation plan
   - Identified safety concerns documented and communicated to case manager
   - Impaired judgment
   - Lack of caregiver
   - Medication profile, history and side effects
   - Patient lives alone
   - Other safety issues, based on the patient's unique medical history, environment, and support

3. Actions/Interventions/Activities

PT:

◆ Teach home exercise to increase endurance/strength/ROM/balance/ posture for mobility related to wheelchair positioning/function.

◆ Instruct in wheelchair features and proper use (e.g., locks, elevating/ swing-a-way leg rests, reclining back).

◆ Increase independence and safety in wheelchair tasks through use of assistive, protective, or supportive devices, or wheelchair modification (e.g., lightweight, one-handed drive, hemi-chair).

◆ Teach patient/caregiver fall prevention and home safety measures related to wheelchair function (e.g., use of locks, lap belts).

◆ Teach skin care/pressure relief techniques, including use of pressure relief cushion.

◆ Teach home modification related to wheelchair mobility (e.g., widening doorways, floor surfaces, furniture placement).

◆ Teach home care aide in repetitive exercise program and techniques to support safety and function.

◆ Provide home program and teach caregivers and home care aide in strategies to support patient's PT goals.

◆ Other interventions/activities based on the patient's unique needs.

SLP:

◆ Address communication needs related to wheelchair function (e.g., amount and type of assistance needed, comfort of chair).

◆ Teach patient/caregiver in alternative communication methods to facilitate wheelchair function.

◆ Teach patient/caregiver in compensatory memory strategies to increase patient's ability to carryout multi-step tasks (e.g., locking/unlocking chair, removing leg rests).

◆ Provide home program and teach caregivers and home care aide in strategies to support communication program and SLP goals.

◆ Other interventions/activities based on the patient's unique needs.

OT:

◆ Teach adaptive techniques and use of assistive/supportive/positioning devices/techniques for increased independence in mobility/management of wheelchair.

◆ Teach safety measures regarding wheelchair function, including home modification.

◆ Coordinate arrangements to obtain new wheelchair/equipment and/or make home modifications (e.g., extended locking lever, removable arm rests, portable or permanent ramp).

◆ Teach therapeutic exercises and provide home program to increase UE coordination/strength/ROM/balance necessary for wheelchair function.

◆ Teach adaptive techniques for wheelchair function, in presence of ROM limitations/precautions (e.g., total hip precautions).

◆ Instruct in wheelchair features and proper use for patient needs (e.g., use of desk arm rests to improve position at table).

◆ Teach energy conservation/diaphragmatic breathing/relaxation techniques to reduce SOB related to wheelchair functioning.

◆ Teach support or splinting interventions to protect impaired UE during wheelchair activities (e.g., splint, sling, tray table).

◆ Teach patient methods to allow safe transportation of food/drink/phone/ other by patient in wheelchair.

◆ Teach therapeutic exercises and provide home program to increase UE strength/ROM/balance for laundry tasks.

◆ Teach energy conservation/diaphragmatic breathing/relaxation techniques to reduce SOB with laundry tasks.

◆ Teach caregivers and home care aide in strategies to support patient's OT goals.

◆ Other interventions/activities based on the patient's unique needs.

4. Specific Functional Goals
   PT:

◆ Patient/caregiver will demonstrate home exercise to increase endurance/strength/ROM/balance/posture for mobility related to wheelchair positioning/function with (max/mod/min/no) assist by ____(date).

◆ Patient/caregiver will demonstrate safe and effective use of assistive, protective, or supportive devices, for wheelchair functioning with (max/mod/min/no) assist by ____(date).

◆ Patient/caregiver demonstrates proper use of wheelchair features (e.g. elevating leg rests/lap tray) to promote therapeutic goals with (max/mod/min/no) assist by ____(date).

◆ Patient/caregiver will demonstrate compliance with fall prevention and home safety measures related to wheelchair function (e.g. use of locks, lap belts) with (max/mod/min/no) assist by ____(date).

◆ Patient/caregiver will demonstrate effective performance of skin care/pressure relief techniques/use of pressure relief cushion with (max/mod/min/no) assist by ____(date).

◆ Patient/caregiver/therapist/social worker will obtain assistive/adaptive/ supportive devices or complete home modifications by _____(date).
◆ Other functional goals based on the patient's unique needs.

SLP:
◆ Patient/caregiver will demonstrate effective communication of needs related to wheelchair function activities by _____(date).
◆ Patient demonstrates effective use of compensatory memory strategies to increase patient's ability to carry out complex wheelchair function tasks by _____(date).
◆ Caregivers report improved communications related to homemaking needs by _____(date).
◆ Other functional goals based on the patient's unique needs.

OT:
◆ Patient/caregiver will demonstrate safe functional mobility throughout necessary areas of home using wheelchair with (max/mod/min/no) assist by _____(date).
◆ Patient/caregiver will demonstrate safe wheelchair mobility in/out of home with (max/mod/min/no) assist by ____(date).
◆ Patient/caregiver will demonstrate proper positioning in wheelchair to promote function and limit pressure/deformity with (max/mod/min/no) assist by ____(date).
◆ Patient/caregiver will demonstrate proper use of wheelchair features (locks/lap belt/footrests/arm rests) with (max/mod/min/no) assist by ____(date).
◆ Patient/caregiver/therapist/social worker will obtain wheelchair/ cushion/assistive devices or complete wheelchair or home modifications by ____(date).
◆ Patient/caregiver will demonstrate home program for therapeutic exercises for increased strength/ROM/coordination/balance needed for wheelchair function with (max/mod/min/no) assist by ____(date).
◆ Patient/caregiver will demonstrate home program for energy conservation/diaphragmatic breathing/relaxation techniques to reduce SOB related to wheelchair function by ____(date).
◆ Patient will demonstrate safe transport of items while in wheelchair (max/mod/min/no) assist by _____(date).
◆ Other functional goals based on the patient's unique needs.

PART SEVEN
Optimizing Home Safety
Equipment Considerations: Assistive and Adaptive Devices

Assistive and Adaptive Devices: Gait Considerations

Canes	**Styles:** • Straight cane • Narrow-based quad cane • Wide-based quad cane • Hemi-cane/hemi-walker	• Assistive devices which provide support for patients with lower extremity weakness, balance deficits, or weight bearing limitations. Cane styles vary by the number of "feet" (one on a straight cane, to four on a quad cane) and by the base of support offered by the position of the cane feet (narrow vs. wide). The hemi-cane (hemi-walker) provides the greatest amount of support available in an ambulation assistive device, which requires only one upper extremity for use. • With the increased support from additional cane feet and base of support, comes additional weight and bulkiness. *As a general rule, the least restrictive assistive device which meets the patient's safety and support needs should be utilized.*

Crutches	**Styles:** • Axillary crutches • Lofstrand/ Canadian crutches	• Assistive devices which provide support for patients with lower extremity weakness or weight bearing limitations. Crutch styles include axillary (underarm styles), or Lofstrand/Canadian (forearm/ cuff styles). • A single crutch or a pair of crutches may be used, based on the need for unilateral or bilateral support. Bilateral use can be transitioned to unilateral use as strength and/or balance improves. • Caution should be taken with axillary crutches to ensure proper axillary fit and use to avoid nerve injury due to pressure.
Walkers	**Styles:** • Standard, non-folding • Standard, folding • Wheeled- walkers **Accessories:** • Glide brakes • Swivel wheels • Platform attachments • Baskets/trays	• Assistive devices which provide support for patients with lower extremity weakness, balance deficits, weight bearing limitations or endurance deficits. • Walker features vary and as a general rule, the least restrictive style which meets the patient's safety and support needs should be utilized. *A standard walker is appropriate for patients whose support needs are not met using a cane.* Folding features will increase ease of walker transport in a car, but add additional weight to the walker. • Wheels eliminate the need for the patient to lift the walker for gait which is helpful for patients with back pain or upper extremity weakness, and allow a continuous gait pattern. Smaller wheels are appropriate for indoor use and on smooth surfaces. Larger wheels

		are appropriate for outdoor use or for use on uneven surfaces. • Glide brakes allow a means of stabilizing a wheeled-walker through direct downward pressure into the walker handgrips. • Platform attachments allow walker use in the presence of limited upper extremity function. • Baskets and trays improve function and safety, allowing patients to carry items safely while walking.

Assistive and Adaptive Devices: Bathroom Equipment

Free-Standing Commodes	**Styles:** • Bed-side commode • 3-in-1 commode ("backless commode") • Rolling commode	• Assistive and safety devices appropriate when mobility limitations prevent safe and timely transfer to the bathroom commode. • Features including adjustable height, presence of armrests and back support, swing-away, or drop arm rests, and weight and base of support of commode seat should be considered in light of the patient's individual mobility status, support needs, and environment. • The 3-in-1 style is useful in cases of anticipated patient progression or deterioration, as its use can change as patient function changes. It can be used as a bedside commode or as an elevated toiled seat over the bathroom commode, and as a bathtub seat. • Rolling commodes are helpful in home environments where frequent mobility of the commode is necessary.
Elevated Toilet Seats	**Styles:**	• Assistive and safety devices appropriate when toilet transfers are limited by strength, range of

	• Portable elevated seats • Clamp-On seats • Arm rests	motion or balance deficits, or by weight bearing limitations or positional restrictions, such as those for post-surgical hip precautions. • Portable styles are lightweight and easily removable. There is a potential to dislodge or move during transfer. • Clamp-on styles are sturdier that portable, and require clamping to the commode. May pose inconvenience for other family members sharing bathroom. • Arm rests assist in transfer safety, and assist the patient in stabilization during hygiene or clothing management activities.
Tub/Shower Chairs/Benches	**Styles:** • Stool • Chair • Bench **Features:** • Padded • Arm rests • Adjustable height	• Assistive and safety devices appropriate for patients unable to stand to shower due to strength, balance, and endurance deficits. • Chair features vary to include degrees of support from arm and back rests to comfort features, such as padding. • The stool style is the most light weight and inexpensive, but provides no arm or back support. The stool, or chair style require the patient be able to transfer into the tub or shower. • The transfer tub bench provides an option for the patient who is unable to step over the tub wall/edge. A portion of the bench extends out of the tub and may not be feasible in some bathrooms due to space constraints.
Grab Bars	**Styles:**	• Assistive and safety devices appropriate for patients requiring support or assistance during transfers or activities.

	• Permanently attached to wall • Removable bar attached to tub edge • Floor to ceiling pole	• Permanent grab bars may be attached into tub or shower wall, at entrance/exit to tub or shower, or on wall or cabinet near commode to provide support during transfers. Placement may be vertical, horizontal, or diagonal based on patient need. Simulation of the patient's transfer will assist in identifying appropriate bar orientation and height. For placement in the tub, consider diagonal placement, to allow multi-height use of the bar for support if patient is standing, or sitting on a tub chair. Diagonal placement may be necessary to allow bar fixation into support studs. • Floor to ceiling poles may be necessary in situations where permanent wall bar placement is not possible or desired. Spring tension poles can give support for transfers without permanent placement requirements.

Assistive and Adaptive Devices: Equipment for Self-Care

Bathing	**Equipment:** • Hand-held shower head • Reacher • Long-handled sponge/brush • Soap-on-a-rope • Soap mitt • Rubber tub/shower mat	• Assistive and adaptive devices appropriate when independence is limited by strength, endurance, shortness of breath, balance, sensory or range of motion deficits. • Hand-held showerhead which allows water and temperature control can minimize forward reaching for patients with hip precautions or poor sitting balance. • Reacher may assist in retrieving towels or manipulating shower curtain. • Soap-on-a-rope- tied to tub chair

		or grab bar, will prevent soap from dropping, and will free-up patient's hands for stabilizing self, holding shower head, or washing self.
Grooming	**Equipment:** • Suction toothbrushes • Adaptive combs and brushes • Toothpaste tube squeezers	• Assistive and adaptive devices appropriate when independence is limited by strength, endurance, shortness of breath, balance, sensory or range of motion deficits. • Grooming devices with built-up handles to improve patient's functional grip, or modifications allowing one-handed use reduce functional limitations.
Dressing	**Equipment:** • Dressing stick • Reacher • Long shoe horn • Sock aid • Elastic laces • Button aide • Zipper pull	• Assistive and adaptive devices appropriate when independence is limited by strength, endurance, shortness of breath, balance, sensory or range of motion deficits. • Long-handled devices, sock aids, and elastic laces minimize the need for forward reaching for patients with hip precautions or poor balance. • Button aides compensate for functional limitations due to fine motor and bilateral hand use deficits. • Slip-on shoes and pull-on clothes increases independence and safety in dressing and toileting.
Eating	**Equipment:** • Adapted eating utensils/ Built-up handles • Handled cups, travel mug • Rocker knives/ Pizza cutters • Divided plates/ Scoop bowl	• Assistive and adaptive devices appropriate when independence is limited by strength, endurance, sensory, or range of motion deficits. • Eating utensils with built-up handles improve patient's functional grip. • Rocker knives, pizza cutters, and adapted/stabilized bowls or plates allowing one-handed function. • Rubber mat or Dycem under dishes

	• Plate guards • Dycem, rubber pad • Long straw	keeps them stabilized on table. • Travel-type mug reduces spillage.
Meal Preparation	**Equipment:** • Knob turners • Reacher • Long-handled utensils • Pull-out storage units or turntables for cupboard contents • Utility cart on wheels • Rubber pads/ Jar openers • Unilateral can opener • Adaptive cutting board	• Assistive and adaptive devices appropriate when independence is limited by strength, endurance, shortness of breath, balance, sensory or range of motion deficits. • Pull-out storage units, turntables, long-handled utensils and reachers compensate for range of motion, balance, or visual deficits, and/or increase function for wheelchair-bound patients. • Rolling utility cart can assist in transporting food or supplies. • Knob turners, rubber pads, and jar openers improve functional grip. • Adaptive can openers and cutting boards allow unilateral use. • Jar openers mounted under cabinets or on walls enable unilateral function. • Rubber pads both under a jar and on lid enable pressure and stability to open jars unilaterally.
Housekeeping	**Equipment:** • Long-handle dusters, mops, brooms and dust pans • Reacher • Utility cart on wheels	• Assistive and adaptive devices appropriate when independence is limited by strength, endurance, shortness of breath, balance, sensory or range of motion deficits. • Long-handled equipment compensates for range of motion or balance deficits, minimizes forward reaching for compliance with hip precautions, and increases function for wheelchair-bound patients. • Rolling utility cart can assist in transporting laundry, cleaning equipment or supplies.

Box 7-1   Wheelchair Assessment

Patient Name: _____ **Record #:**_____ **Date:** _____

Date of Birth: _____ **Sex:** ___ **Height:** _____ **Weight:** _____

Primary Diagnosis:	
Secondary Diagnosis:	
Medical & Surgery History:	
Caregiver Support:	(Ability, availability, willingness, competence, etc.)
Current Equipment:	(DME, Orthotics, Prosthetics, Adaptive Equipment, Oxygen, Ventilator, Suction machine, Infusion, Enteral/Parenteral nutrition, etc.)
Cognitive Level:	(Alertness, orientation, memory, judgment, carryover from learning, etc.)
Vision:	(Acuity, depth perception, etc.)
Hearing:	(Deficits, aids, etc.)
Communication:	(Verbal & nonverbal expressive and receptive language, augmentative devices, aids, etc.)
Respiration:	(Breathing patterns, adequacy for breath support & speech production, ventilatory support, oxygen, etc.)
Sensation:	(Light touch, pressure, joint position, etc.)
Skin Integrity:	(Color, temperature, turgor, lesions, etc.)
Pressure relief:	(Level of assistance, effectiveness, etc.)
Skin inspection:	(Level of assistance, effectiveness, etc.)

Box 7-1   Wheelchair Assessment (cont'd)

Bowel:	(Continent, incontinent, training, continent w/occasional accidents, etc.)
Bladder:	(Continent, incontinent, traiing, catheterized, intermittent catheterization, etc.)
Posture:	(Scoliosis, kyphosis, pelvic obliquity, etc.)
Strength:	(Note any strength limitations having functional limitations for transfers or sitting)
Tone:	(Note any tonal abnormalities having functional limitations for transfers or sitting)
ROM:	(Note any strength limitations having functional limitations for transfers or sitting)
Sitting Balance:	(Supported, unsupported, righting / equilibrium / protective responses, etc.)
Transfers:	(Level of assist & equipment needed)
Ambulation:	(Assist, equipment, surface, distance, limiting factors, etc.)
Environment:	(Steps, ramps, door widths, etc.)
Transportation:	(Personal vehicle, vehicle type, storage area, door dimensions, ramp/lift, etc.)
Current Seating:	Manual / companion / power chair: Manufacture / Model: Purchased from / Date: Funded by: Dimensions- seat / back: Accessories: headrest, anterior chest support, lap belt, chest strap, lateral trunk support, lateral hip support, medial / anterior / lateral knee support, foot controllers, etc.) Problems: (outgrown, disrepair, insufficient support, doesn't accommodate limited ROM, insufficient pressure relief, does not tilt/recline, user cannot push functionally, etc.)

Box 7-1   Wheelchair Assessment (cont'd)

All measurements taken in sitting

Enter measurements in inches with accomodation of all range of motion limitations.

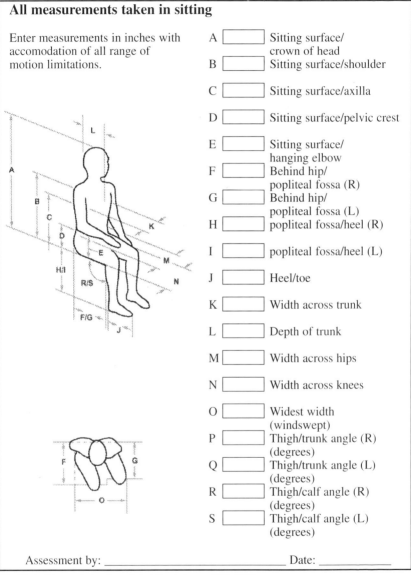

A [ ] Sitting surface/crown of head

B [ ] Sitting surface/shoulder

C [ ] Sitting surface/axilla

D [ ] Sitting surface/pelvic crest

E [ ] Sitting surface/hanging elbow

F [ ] Behind hip/popliteal fossa (R)

G [ ] Behind hip/popliteal fossa (L)

H [ ] popliteal fossa/heel (R)

I [ ] popliteal fossa/heel (L)

J [ ] Heel/toe

K [ ] Width across trunk

L [ ] Depth of trunk

M [ ] Width across hips

N [ ] Width across knees

O [ ] Widest width (windswept)

P [ ] Thigh/trunk angle (R) (degrees)

Q [ ] Thigh/trunk angle (L) (degrees)

R [ ] Thigh/calf angle (R) (degrees)

S [ ] Thigh/calf angle (L) (degrees)

Assessment by: _____ Date: _____

Modified with permission from RehabCentral.com, LLC, 1999.

A Home Safety Program: Guidelines and Assessment

(For physicians and other health care professionals making referrals.)

The S.A.F.E. Home Safety Program
Safety Assessment for Functional Effectiveness

Safety in the home is good preventative medicine!

_____, Therapist   Referring Physician_____

Home Safety Program Goals

The S.A.F.E. Home Safety Program provides assessment and individualized instructions on safe functioning for patients with physical impairment or disability. Through training in adaptive techniques and use of assistive devices, patients learn to safely perform Activities of Daily Living (ADL) and functional mobility with improved independence. This helps achieve improved quality of life and lower medical costs by preventing accidents, and it gives families more peace of mind.

Providing Individualized Services

The physician refers the patient for an occupational therapy or physical therapy evaluation and a home safety assessment. Using the treatment team approach, the therapist performs the initial evaluation and provides most of the training pertaining to safe functioning within the home. The therapist develops the plan of care, coordinates with the physician and other home health personnel, helps the patient obtain necessary adaptive equipment, and coordinates with home design specialists or contractors for home modifications when needed. The occupational therapist teaches adaptive techniques and use of assistive devices to improve independence in self-care, and also provides therapeutic exercises for improving use of arm and hand use. The physical therapist provides assessment and training when functional mobility problems need addressing.

Training sessions include the patient's family or caregiver and provide outlined instructions to help promote consistency with carry over. The therapist usually makes 3 or more visits, and will provide a written list of recommendations to make the patient safer in the home. Changes to the home environment may be as simple as rearranging the furniture or improving access in the kitchen, or more involved such as structural changes for the home. The therapist also insures the patient has a thorough plan for any emergency that may occur.

Medicare and many insurance companies cover most of the cost of this program and some of the adaptive equipment. For other assistive devices not covered, patients are given information on ordering directly from companies who specialize in selling these devices directly to the patient. If modifications to the home are recommended, the therapist will help coordinate arrangements between the patient and the handyman or contractor.

Patient Training and Education

Problem areas that the therapists address for improving the patient's ability to manage safely at home with optimum independence:

- Activities of Daily Living (ADL): bathing, dressing, toileting, grooming, feeding/eating/drinking
- Transfer training: in/out of bed, in/out of tub or shower, in/out of the house or car
- Mobility training: walking, climbing stairs, propelling a wheelchair
- Homemaking skills: simple kitchen skills, simple cleaning, laundry
- Adaptive equipment: grab bar, raised toilet, tub/shower seat, cordless phone
- Minor home alterations: arrangement of furniture, easier access to items for ADL and kitchen skills
- Major home modification: ramp, stair rail, widening doorways, kitchen and bath renovations

Reprinted with permission of Carroll Tollner Fernstrom, OTR/L, 1999.

S.A.F.E. HOME SAFETY ASSESSMENT
Safety Assessment for Functional Effectiveness

Circle: e.g. yes / no OR problem areas.   I=independence min= min assistance mod=mod assistance max=max assistance   √ = Within Functional Limits

pt:	**MD:**
	therapist:
age/mar. stat/sex:	**tx dx:**
loc/home:	**onset:**
	med. hx:
phone:	
	precautions/falls:
date of assessment:	

Patient/Caregiver/Family Feedback	**Caregiver Availability**	
Patient's concerns-	caregiver(s) name, relation-	
	day- night-	
fam / cg concerns-		
	alone: day / night-	
alcohol use- no / yes	c.giver experience-	
pain-		

Structural layout of Home/Apt/Room	**DME /Equip & Ability to Use**	**Ass't Devices & Splints**
1/2/3 story, exterior access_____ steps / rail / ramp	hosp bed-	ADL-
interior #____ steps/NA ____R/L rail landing- yes / no		
furniture hindrance-	w/chair-	
floor: rugs / clutter-		
lights: adequate / access-	walker (type)-	
doors' width-		UE / LE splint-
smoke detect: yes/no	cane(type)-	
night light: yes/no		sling-
hot water temperature(unsafe)-	crutches-	
pets- no / yes type/restrained?-		

Functional impairments	**Functional Mobility**
visual or hearing-	mobility: equip-
communication: rec / exp- read / write-	I / min / mod / max ass't
R / L UE weakness -	get up from fall-
sensory-	open / close / lock / un / exterior door-
R / L LE weakness -	chair transfer-
sensory-	bed transfer-
endur / SOB-	pick object off floor-
other-	
	balance-

UE Impairment	**Cognitive Skills**
hand dom: R L	RO: person place time
effected: R L	Memory: ST- LT-
grip strength: R L	
sensory: touch proprioc- stereog-	attention span / concentration-
coordination: right hand: P F G N	judgment-
left hand: P F G N	follow direct-
ROM-	sequencing-
	problem solving-
strength-	decision making-
	frust. Tolerance-

Reprinted with permission of Carroll Tollner Fernstrom, OTR/L, 1999.

S.A.F.E. Home Safety Assessment

Dressing/ADL Skills

ass't devices-

clothes from closet / dresser-
UE dressing-

LE dressing-

grooming-

splint / sling / brace-

Bathroom Skills

Ass't devices-

toilet transfer-
hygiene / flush-
toilet @ night-
continence: day-   night-
tub or shower transfer-

wash hands-
reach towels-
oral care-   shave-

Kitchen Skills

feed/eat-
    drink-
cup / plate / fork access & transport-
food /drink from frig-
cabinet access: food /dishes/equip-
hot water-
open pkg-
use of stove/oven/toaster oven-
transport food / drink-

Daily Activities & Emergency Skills/Plans

phone use / access-
    ph. no. & contacts for emerg.-
meds / insulin / ostomy care-

emergency call plan
    contact person-   Life Line: yes / no

loss of power or phone-
fire plan / exist-

Lives Alone

In home: pay bills/budget-
        open/close curtains-
        laundry-

Outside home:
    cash transaction-
    transportation transfers-
    shopping-

Other Significant Findings/Factors Effecting Safety

Problem Areas	Skilled Intervention	Treatment Goals	Recommend. to Pt/Fam/CG

Referrals to other Home Health Services:

Reprinted with permission of Carroll Tollner Fernstrom, OTR/L, 1999.

PART EIGHT
Human Resource Management

COMPETENCE ASSESSMENT

Purpose: To outline the ongoing processes for assuring competence of all staff members.

Policy:
1. The competency of all agency staff (employed and contract) will be assessed during orientation, during the introductory period, periodically throughout the course of a year and during the annual performance evaluation.

2. Educational activities will be based, in part, on the outcomes of the competency evaluations.

3. Competency validation will include the following components:
   a. Licensure/Certification
   b. Orientation Program (including competency testing)
   c. Core competencies Validation Annually
   d. Education/Contingency Education
   e. Performance Appraisals
   f. Ongoing Competencies
   g. Performance Improvement Activities
   h. Incident Reporting
   i. Infection Reporting
   j. Satisfaction Surveys

4. Competency is defined as the demonstration of knowledge, interpersonal relationships, technical and critical thinking skills in the delivery of patient care/services.

5. Guidelines for correcting deficiencies in employee performance and behavior changes are maintained in the Baptist Health Systems Human Resource Manual entitled: Corrective Action.

Procedure:

Orientation and Probationary Period

1. As part of the orientation process, a preceptor will be assigned to each new employee.

2. Using the skills/orientation checklist, the Director and/or designee will observe the new employee performing the required skills and activities.

3. Upon completion of the checklists, the new employee will end their orientation period.

4. A performance review for probationary employees will then be done at the end of the first 90 days.

Ongoing Assessments

1. At least once during the year (prior to the annual performance evaluation), every employee will make at least one (1) joint visit with a clinical supervisor.

2. Using the skills checklist, competency test and competency/review evaluation form, the Director of Professional Services and/or designee will evaluate the staff's competence in performing and rendering care/service according to agency policies and standards of practice.

3. Based on the ongoing reviews, the inservice education plan will incorporate any areas where there are trends and patterns across all staff within the agency.

4. Isolated episodes, relating to one or two individual's performance, will be dealt with on an individual basis. Actions may include, but are not limited to, one on one counseling, reviewing resource information, etc.

5. Random visits to a patient's home will be made by a clinical supervisor to assess patient satisfaction and field staff compliance to agency standard. Based on the visit findings, each field staff member will be dealt with on an individual basis.

6. A supervisory visit is made on new IV cases one week after start of care.

7. As part of the ongoing review of staff competence, there will be a tracking and trending of measures, including but not limited to:

   a. Employee Injuries
   b. Incidents relating to both patients and staff
   c. Infections among patients and staff
   d. Patient complaints
   e. Employee opinion surveys
   f. Patient satisfaction surveys
   g. Physician satisfaction surveys

8. The above will be used to improve the staff competence, as well as, plan for educational activities. Any identified trends will be considered as part of the agency performance improvement plan.

Annual Performance Evaluation

1. During the annual performance evaluation, each staff member's competence in performing the activities specified in their job description will be evaluated.

2. Each staff member will be asked to re-demonstrate their core competencies in specific areas relating to their job description and functions (i.e., home health aides demonstrate skills ADL assistance bathing, toileting, etc., RN's performing IV therapy demonstrate skills for venipuncture, accessing ports, etc.) as identified on the evaluation forms.

3. Competency improvement will be the focus of the annual performance evaluation and performance plans for the next year.

Reprinted with permission from South Miami Hospital Home Health, 1999.

SCOPE OF COMPETENCY PROGRAM

Purpose: To outline policies, procedures and processes designed to ensure that the competence of agency personnel is assessed, maintained and improved on a continuing basis.

Policy:

1. The Agency defines and implements an objective measurable assessment system to evaluate the competency of its personnel, which includes contracted personnel.

2. Agency personnel demonstrate knowledge and proficiency of skills appropriate to their assigned responsibilities, including an ability to perform specified duties determined by the agency.

3. On-going skills are maintained and improved through continuing education programs, based in part by the analysis of data trends and outcomes of the Clinical Competency Program, on-site supervision and on-going reviews.

4. All direct care agency personnel and their immediate Field Supervisor are included in the Clinical Competency Program. Administration, clerical and support personnel are not included.

   Care related agency personnel (i.e., Field Supervisor, PI Coordinator) may require competency evaluation. This will be performed by the Director of Professional Services/or designee based upon the existence and function/duties of these personnel.

5. The proficiency demonstration component of the Clinical Competency Program will be conducted by qualified evaluators.

   Proficiency demonstration will occur when the following conditions exist:

   a. At least annually as part of the agency personnel evaluation process using the agency Competency review forms.

   b. Agency personnel are performing a new procedure, or using a piece of equipment for the first time.

   c. The skill checklist indicated retraining is needed or in which little or no knowledge/experience exist.

   d. Care is provided in a specialized area for the first time.

   e. Reporting systems indicated that agency personnel require additional training or supervision.

   f. Whenever agency personnel request it.

6. Skill proficiency can be determined by verbal or written examination; skill demonstration in a lab setting or a patient's/client's home; or by completing a specialized training course specific to a clinical procedure (i.e., PICC certification)

Procedure:

1. The agency established and periodically re-evaluates job specific "Skills Checklists" that reflect duties commonly required in the routine performance of the position.

2. The agency also establishes and periodically re-evaluates a group of mandatory skills found on the skills checklist/competency review forms that are related to the patient/client care responsibilities and complexity of care of direct care staff. The competencies must be successfully demonstrated before agency personnel completes orientation and must be documented on the skills checklists/competency review forms.

3. The agency further defines the core competencies in terms of objective measurable behavior sites, personnel must demonstrate which are called "Performance Criteria". Agency personnel are deemed proficient when each core competency is met. Performance criteria are found in the policies/ procedures.

4. High risk, problem prone, specialty services or area of care are defined. These services require specialty training and experience and mandatory demonstration of proficiency before personnel provide these services independently.

5. A preceptor will be assigned to each new staff member as part of the orientation process. The preceptor/supervisor will observe/deem proficient the indicated skills and core competencies. If necessary, additional training, inservice education, will be provided to the staff member. Agency personnel will not provide the care or service independently until competency is attained.

6. Clinical competency of evaluating agency personnel (preceptors, supervisors, peers, clinical specialists) is performed by the Director of Professional Services and/or designee and regularly evaluated.

7. Agency personnel will re-demonstrate required competency review areas annually as part of the evaluation process.

Reprinted with permission from South Miami Hospital Home Health, 1999.

SOUTH MIAMI HOSPITAL HOME HEALTH
PHYSICAL THERAPIST COMPETENCE
REVIEW/EVALUATION FORM

	RATING SCALE
D/C	DEMONSTRATING COMPETENCE
V/C	VERBALIZE COMPETENCE
N/P	NOT PROFICIENT
N/A	NOT APPLICABLE

DATE: _____

PHYSICAL THERAPIST: _____

EVALUATING PHYSICAL THERAPIST: _____

SPECIFIC UNIT: HOME CARE
Care of the Patient in the Home Environment - All Ages
PROCESSES

___ a. Assess Patient
___ b. Develop Problem List
___ c. Select, Develop and Individualize Plan of Care
___ d. Implement Plan of Care
___ e. Evaluate Plan of Care
___ f. Communication/Documentation
___ g. Supervise Delegated Functions
___ h. Age Appropriate Care
___ i. Knowledge of Growth and Development
___ j. Discharge Planning

PROCEDURES

___ a. Application of TENS Unit   ___ d. Fit/Adjust Assist Devices
___ b. Ultrasound   ___ e. Application CPM
___ c. Stump Condition

EQUIPMENT

___ a. TENS Unit   ___ d. Prosthesis
___ b. Ultrasound   ___ e. CPM
___ c. Assistive Devices   ___ f. PPE

QUALITY

____ a. Performance Improvement
  ❏ Philosophy
  ❏ Systems of Focus
  ❏ Methodology
  ❏ Quality Improvement Tools
  ❏ Meeting Skills
  ❏ Demonstrates Initiative for Continuous Education/ Training

Performance Improvement (continued)
  ❏ Group Decision Making
  ❏ Assessment
  ❏ Data Collection
____ b. Patient Complaints/ Compliments
____ c. Incidents

MANDATORY EDUCATION/TRAINING

____ a. CPR Certification _____ (Expiration Date)
____ b. Safety Inservice _____ (Expiration Date)
  ❏ Fire
  ❏ Electrical
  ❏ Infection Control
  ❏ Haz/Mat
  ❏ Lifting (Proper Body Mechanics)
____ c. Bloodborne Pathogens _____ (Expiration Date)
____ d. Department Safety, Education Training
____ e. Advance Directives
____ f. Abuse/Neglect

Reprinted with permission from South Miami Hospital Home Health, 1999.

SOUTH MIAMI HOSPITAL HOME HEALTH
SPEECH LANGUAGE PATHOLOGIST COMPETENCE
REVIEW/EVALUATION FORM

RATING SCALE
D/C   DEMONSTRATING COMPETENCE
V/C   VERBALIZE COMPETENCE
N/P   NOT PROFICIENT
N/A   NOT APPLICABLE

DATE: _____ _____

SPEECH LANGUAGE PATHOLOGIST: _____

EVALUATING SPEECH LANGUAGE PATHOLOGIST: _____

SPECIFIC UNIT: HOME CARE
Care of the Patient in the Home Environment - All Ages
PROCESSES

____ a. Assess Patient
____ b. Develop Problem List
____ c. Select, Develop and Individualize Plan of Care
____ d. Implement Plan of Care
____ e. Evaluate Plan of Care
____ f. Communication/Documentation
____ g. Supervise Delegated Functions
____ h. Age Appropriate Care
____ i. Knowledge of Growth and Development
____ j. Discharge Planning

PROCEDURES

____ a. Dysarthria Treatment   ____ d. Aphasia Treatment
____ b. Apraxia Treatment   ____ e. Dysphagia Treatment
____ c. Prosthesis

EQUIPMENT

____ a. Picture/Word Book   ____ c. Mirror
____ b. Prosthesis   ____ d. PPE

QUALITY

___ a. Performance Improvement
  ❏ Philosophy
  ❏ Systems of Focus
  ❏ Methodology
  ❏ Quality Improvement Tools
  ❏ Meeting Skills
  ❏ Demonstrates Initiative for Continuous Education/ Training

Performance Improvement (continued)
  ❏ Group Decision Making
  ❏ Assessment
  ❏ Data Collection
  ___ b. Patient Complaints/ Compliments
  ___ c. Incidents

MANDATORY EDUCATION/TRAINING

___ a. CPR Certification _____ (Expiration Date)
___ b. Safety Inservice _____ (Expiration Date)
  ❏ Fire
  ❏ Electrical
  ❏ Infection Control
  ❏ Haz/Mat
  ❏ Lifting (Proper Body Mechanics)
___ c. Bloodborne Pathogens _____ (Expiration Date)
___ d. Department Safety, Education Training
___ e. Advance Directives
___ f. Abuse/Neglect

Reprinted with permission from South Miami Hospital Home Health, 1999.

SOUTH MIAMI HOSPITAL HOME HEALTH
OCCUPATIONAL THERAPIST COMPETENCE
REVIEW/EVALUATION FORM

	RATING SCALE
D/C	DEMONSTRATING COMPETENCE
V/C	VERBALIZE COMPETENCE
N/P	NOT PROFICIENT
N/A	NOT APPLICABLE

DATE: _____ ___

OCCUPATIONAL THERAPIST: _____

EVALUATING PHYSICAL/OCCUPATIONAL THERAPIST: _____

SPECIFIC UNIT: HOME CARE
Care of the Patient in the Home Environment - All Ages
PROCESSES

___ a. Assess Patient
___ b. Develop Problem List
___ c. Select, Develop and Individualize Plan of Care
___ d. Implement Plan of Care
___ e. Evaluate Plan of Care
___ f. Communication/Documentation
___ g. Supervise Delegated Functions
___ h. Age Appropriate Care
___ i. Knowledge of Growth and Development
___ j. Discharge Planning

PROCEDURES

___ a. Develop ADL Program   ___ d. Environment Adaptation
___ b. Muscle Reeducation Program ___ e. Work Capacity Evaluation
___ c. Neuro-Development and Training

EQUIPMENT

___ a. Orthotics   ___ c. Adaptive Equipment
___ b. Splints   ___ d. PPE

QUALITY

___ a. Performance Improvement
- ❏ Philosophy
- ❏ Systems of Focus
- ❏ Methodology
- ❏ Quality Improvement Tools
- ❏ Meeting Skills
- ❏ Demonstrates Initiative for Continuous Education/ Training

Performance Improvement (continued)
- ❏ Group Decision Making
- ❏ Assessment
- ❏ Data Collection
- ___ b. Patient Complaints/ Compliments
- ___ c. Incidents

MANDATORY EDUCATION/TRAINING

___ a. CPR Certification _____ (Expiration Date)
___ b. Safety Inservice _____ (Expiration Date)
- ❏ Fire
- ❏ Electrical
- ❏ Infection Control
- ❏ Haz/Mat
- ❏ Lifting (Proper Body Mechanics)
___ c. Bloodborne Pathogens _____ (Expiration Date)
___ d. Department Safety, Education Training
___ e. Advance Directives
___ f. Abuse/Neglect

Reprinted with permission from South Miami Hospital Home Health, 1999.

Job Descriptions for:
Physical Therapist
Speech-Language Pathologist
Occupational Therapist
in Home Care

JOB DESCRIPTION: PHYSICAL THERAPIST

ESSENTIAL JOB FUNCTIONS

1. Performs physical therapist treatment and evaluation as prescribed by the physician, evaluating and treating clients by applying diagnostic and prognostic muscle, nerve joint and functional abilities tests.

2. Guides the client in use of therapeutic and self care activities for the purpose of improving function and increasing independence.

3. Instructs the client, family members and other health team members to incorporate therapeutic and self care activities into the treatment program, encouraging them to follow those procedures so they can safely perform or supervise the activities.

4. Plans and exchanges information with staff members and community agencies that service the client to promote continuity of client care.

5. Maintains current agency documentation standards assisting in the formulation and review of the patient's plan of treatment and care.

6. Initiates contact with physician for orders and treatment plan formulation and/or revision as the patient's condition requires.

MARGINAL JOB FUNCTIONS

1. Provides continuing education programs and educational experiences to nursing and home health aide staff as requested by the Director of Professional Services to promote the agency quality care standards.

2. Follows proper safety procedures and lifting techniques, reporting all injuries and unsafe practices to immediate supervisor, following agency safety policies and procedures.

3. Performs other assigned duties as required to ensure the agency systems and quality standard policies are met.

Reprinted with permission from South Miami Hospital Home Health, 1999.

EXCEEDS EXPECTATIONS	FULLY MEETS EXPECTATIONS	MINIMALLY MEETS EXPECTATIONS	DOES NOT MEET EXPECTATIONS

EXCEEDS EXPECTATIONS	FULLY MEETS EXPECTATIONS	MINIMALLY MEETS EXPECTATIONS	DOES NOT MEET EXPECTATIONS

JOB DESCRIPTION: SPEECH-LANGUAGE PATHOLOGIST

ESSENTIAL JOB FUNCTIONS

1. Performs speech pathology treatment and evaluation as prescribed by the physician, evaluating and treating clients by applying diagnostic and prognostic speech functional abilities tests.

2. Guides the client in use of therapeutic and self care activities for the purpose of improving function and increasing independence.

3. Instructs the client, family members and other health team members to incorporate therapeutic and self care activities into the treatment program, encouraging them to follow those procedures so they can safely perform or supervise the activities.

4. Plans and exchanges information with staff members and community agencies that service the client to promote continuity of client care.

5. Maintains current agency documentation standards assisting in the formulation and review of the patient's plan of treatment and care.

6. Initiates contact with physician for orders and treatment plan formulation and/or revision as the patient's condition requires.

7. Supervises field competency of speech pathologists to ensure agency quality care standards are met as requested by the Director of Professional Services.

MARGINAL JOB FUNCTIONS

1. Provides continuing education programs and educational experiences to nursing and home health aide staff as requested by the Director of Professional Services to promote the agency quality care standards.

2. Follows proper safety procedures and lifting techniques, reporting all injuries and unsafe practices to immediate supervisor, following agency safety policies and procedures.

3. Performs other assigned duties as required to ensure the agency systems and quality standard policies are met.

Reprinted with permission from South Miami Hospital Home Health, 1999.

EXCEEDS EXPECTATIONS	FULLY MEETS EXPECTATIONS	MINIMALLY MEETS EXPECTATIONS	DOES NOT MEET EXPECTATIONS

EXCEEDS EXPECTATIONS	FULLY MEETS EXPECTATIONS	MINIMALLY MEETS EXPECTATIONS	DOES NOT MEET EXPECTATIONS

JOB DESCRIPTION: OCCUPATIONAL THERAPIST

ESSENTIAL JOB FUNCTIONS

1. Performs occupational therapist treatment and evaluation as prescribed by the physician, evaluating and treating clients by applying diagnostic and prognostic muscle, nerve joint and functional abilities tests.

2. Guides the client in use of therapeutic and self care activities for the purpose of improving function and increasing independence.

3. Instructs the client, family members and other health team members to incorporate therapeutic and self care activities into the treatment program, encouraging them to follow those procedures so they can safely perform or supervise the activities.

4. Plans and exchanges information with staff members and community agencies that service the client to promote continuity of client care.

5. Maintains current agency documentation standards assisting in the formulation and review of the patient's plan of treatment and care.

6. Initiates contact with physician for orders and treatment plan formulation and/or revision as the patient's condition requires.

7. Supervises field competency of Occupational Therapist to ensure agency quality care standards are met as requested by the Director of Professional Services.

MARGINAL JOB FUNCTIONS

1. Provides continuing education programs and educational experiences to nursing and home health aide staff as requested by the Director of Professional Services to promote the agency quality care standards.

2. Follows proper safety procedures and lifting techniques, reporting all injuries and unsafe practices to immediate supervisor, following agency safety policies and procedures.

3. Performs other assigned duties as required to ensure the agency systems and quality standard policies are met.

Reprinted with permission from South Miami Hospital Home Health, 1999.

EXCEEDS EXPECTATIONS	FULLY MEETS EXPECTATIONS	MINIMALLY MEETS EXPECTATIONS	DOES NOT MEET EXPECTATIONS

EXCEEDS EXPECTATIONS	FULLY MEETS EXPECTATIONS	MINIMALLY MEETS EXPECTATIONS	DOES NOT MEET EXPECTATIONS

312

PART NINE
Excerpts from The
Medicare Home Health Agency Manual
(HCFA Pub-11)

Coverage of Services for Skilled Therapy

205.2　　Skilled Therapy Services.—

　　A.　General Principles Governing Reasonable and Necessary Physical Therapy, Speech-Language Pathology Services, and Occupational Therapy.—

　　1.　The service of a physical, speech-language pathologist or occupational therapist is a skilled therapy service if the inherent complexity of the service is such that it can be performed safely and/or effectively only by or under the general supervision of a skilled therapist. To be covered, the skilled services must also be reasonable and necessary to the treatment of the patient's illness or injury or to the restoration of maintenance of function affected by the patient's illness or injury. It is necessary to determine whether individual therapy services are skilled and whether, in view of the patient's overall condition, skilled management of the services provided is needed although many or all of the specific services needed to treat the illness or injury do not require the skills of a therapist.

　　2.　The development, implementation management and evaluation of a patient care plan based on the physician's orders constitute skilled therapy services when, because of the patient's condition, those activities require the involvement of a skilled therapist to meet the patient's needs, promote recovery and ensure medical safety. Where the skills of a therapist are needed to manage and periodically reevaluate the appropriateness of a maintenance program because of an identified danger to the patient, such services would be covered even if the skills of a therapist are not needed to carry out the activities performed as part of the maintenance program.

　　3.　While a patient's particular medical condition is a valid factor in deciding if skilled therapy services are needed, the diagnosis or prognosis should never be the sole factor in deciding that a service is or is not skilled. The key issue is whether the skills of a therapist are needed to treat the illness or injury, or whether the services can be carried out by nonskilled personnel.

　　4.　A service that is ordinarily considered nonskilled could be considered a skilled therapy service in cases in which there is clear documentation that, because of special medical complications, skilled rehabilitation personnel are required to perform or supervise the service or to observe the patient. However, the importance of a particular service to a patient or the frequency with which it must be performed does not, by itself, make a nonskilled service into a skilled service.

Part Nine: Excerpts from Medicare *Home Health Agency Manual* **313**

205.2 (Cont.)   COVERAGE OF SERVICES   04-96

5.   The skilled therapy services must be reasonable and necessary to the treatment of the patient's illness or injury within the context of the patient's unique medical condition. To be considered reasonable and necessary for the treatment of the illness or injury:

     a.   The services must be consistent with the nature and severity of the illness or injury, the patient's particular medical needs, including the requirement that the amount, frequency and duration of the services must be reasonable;

     b.   The services must be considered, under accepted standards of medical practice, to be specific, safe, and effective treatment for the patient's condition; and

     c.   The services must be provided with the expectation, based on the assessment made by the physician of the patient's rehabilitation potential, that:

     +   The condition of the patient will improve materially in a reasonable and generally predictable period of time; or

     +   The services are necessary to the establishment of a safe and effective maintenance program.

Services involving activities for the general welfare of any patient, e.g., general exercises to promote overall fitness or flexibility and activities to provide diversion or general motivation, do not constitute skilled therapy. Those services can be performed by nonskilled individuals without the supervision of a therapist.

     d.   Services of skilled therapists for the purpose of teaching the patient, family or caregivers necessary techniques, exercises or precautions are covered to the extent that they are reasonable and necessary to treat illness or injury. However, visits made by skilled therapists to a patient's home solely to train other HHA staff (e.g., home health aides) are not billable as visits since the HHA is responsible for ensuring that its staff is properly trained to perform any service it furnishes. The cost of a skilled therapist's visit for the purpose of training HHA staff is an administrative cost to the agency.

EXAMPLE: A patient with a diagnosis of multiple sclerosis has recently been discharged from the hospital following an exacerbation of her condition that has left her wheelchair bound and, for the first time, without any expectation of achieving ambulation again. The physician has ordered physical therapy to select the proper wheelchair for her long term use, to teach safe use of the wheelchair and safe transfer techniques to the patient and family. Physical therapy would be reasonable and necessary to evaluate the patient's overall needs, to make the selection of the proper wheelchair and to teach the patient and family safe use of the wheelchair and proper transfer techniques.

     e.   The amount, frequency, and duration of the services must be reasonable.

     B.   Application of the Principles to Physical Therapy Services.—The following discussion of skilled physical therapy services applies the principles in §205.2A to specific physical therapy services about which questions are most frequently raised.

1. <u>Assessment</u>.—The skills of a physical therapist to assess a patient's rehabilitation needs and potential or to develop and/or implement a physical therapy program are covered when they are reasonable and necessary because of the patient's condition. Skilled rehabilitation services concurrent with the management of a patient's care plan include objective tests and measurements such as, but not limited to, range of motion, strength, balance coordination endurance or functional ability.

2. <u>Therapeutic Exercises</u>.—Therapeutic exercises which must be performed by or under the supervision of the qualified physical therapist to ensure the safety of the patient and effectiveness of the treatment, due either to the type of exercise employed or to the condition of the patient, constitute skilled physical therapy.

3. <u>Gait Training</u>.—Gait evaluation and training furnished to a patient whose ability to walk has been impaired by neurological, muscular or skeletal abnormality require the skills of a qualified physical therapist and constitute skilled physical therapy and are considered reasonable and necessary if training can be expected to improve materially the patient's ability to walk.

Gait evaluation and training that is furnished to a patient whose ability to walk has been impaired by a condition other than a neurological, muscular or skeletal abnormality would nevertheless be covered where physical therapy is reasonable and necessary to restore the lost function.

EXAMPLE 1:   A physician has ordered gait evaluation and training for a patient whose gait has been materially impaired by scar tissue resulting from burns. Physical therapy services to evaluate the patient's gait, establish a gait training program, and provide the skilled services necessary to implement the program would be covered.

EXAMPLE 2:   A patient who has had a total hip replacement is ambulatory but demonstrates weakness and is unable to climb stairs safely. Physical therapy would be reasonable and necessary to teach the patient to safely climb and descend stairs.

Repetitive exercises to improve gait, or to maintain strength and endurance and assistive walking are appropriately provided by nonskilled persons and ordinarily do not require the skills of a physical therapist. Where such services are performed by a physical therapist as part of the initial design and establishment of a safe and effective maintenance program, the services would, to the extent that they are reasonable and necessary, be covered.

EXAMPLE: A patient who has received gait training has reached his maximum restoration potential and the physical therapist is teaching the patient and family how to perform safely the activities that are a part of a maintenance program. The visits by the physical therapist to demonstrate and teach the activities (which by themselves do not require the skills of a therapist) would be covered since they are needed to establish the program.

4. <u>Range of Motion</u>.—Only a qualified physical therapist may perform range of motion tests and, therefore, such tests are skilled physical therapy.

Range of motion exercises constitute skilled physical therapy only if they are part of an active treatment for a specific disease state, illness, or injury, that has resulted in a loss or restriction of mobility (as evidenced by physical therapy notes showing the degree of motion lost and the degree to be restored). Range of motion exercises unrelated to the restoration of a specific loss of function often may be provided safely and effectively by nonskilled individuals. Passive exercises to maintain range of motion in paralyzed extremities that can be carried out by nonskilled persons do not constitute skilled physical therapy.

However, as indicated in §205.2A4, where there is clear documentation that, because of special medical complications (e.g., susceptible to pathological bone fractures), the skills of a therapist are needed to provide services that ordinarily do not need the skills of a therapist, then the services would be covered.

   5.   Maintenance Therapy.—Where repetitive services that are required to maintain function involve the use of complex and sophisticated procedures, the judgment and skill of a physical therapist might be required for the safe and effective rendition of such services. If the judgment and skill of a physical therapist is required to treat the illness or injury safely and effectively, the services would be covered as physical therapy services.

EXAMPLE: Where there is an unhealed, unstable fracture that requires regular exercise to maintain function until the fracture heals, the skills of a physical therapist would be needed to ensure that the fractured extremity is maintained in proper position and alignment during maintenance range of motion exercises.

Establishment of a maintenance program is a skilled physical therapy service where the specialized knowledge and judgment of a qualified physical therapist is required for the program to be safely carried out and the treatment aims of the physician achieved.

EXAMPLE: A Parkinson's patient or a patient with rheumatoid arthritis who has not been under a restorative physical therapy program may require the services of a physical therapist to determine what type of exercises are required to maintain his/her present level of function. The initial evaluation of the patient's needs, the designing of a maintenance program appropriate to the capacity and tolerance of the patient and the treatment objectives of the physician, the instruction of the patient, family or caregivers to carry out the program safely and effectively and such reevaluations as may be required by the patient's condition, would constitute skilled physical therapy.

While a patient is under a restorative physical therapy program, the physical therapist should regularly reevaluate his condition and adjust any exercise program the patient is expected to carry out himself or with the aid of supportive personnel to maintain the function being restored. Consequently, by the time it is determined that no further restoration is possible (i.e., by the end of the last restorative session) the physical therapist will already have designed the maintenance program required and instructed the patient or caregivers in carrying out the program.

   6.   Ultrasound, Shortwave, and Microwave Diathermy Treatments.—These treatments must always be performed by or under the supervision of a qualified physical therapist and are a skilled therapy.

7.   Hot Packs, Infra-Red Treatments, Paraffin Baths and Whirlpool Baths.—Heat treatments and baths of this type ordinarily do not require the skills of a qualified physical therapist. However, the skills, knowledge and judgment of a qualified physical therapist might be required in the giving of such treatments or baths in a particular case, e.g., where the patient's condition is complicated by circulatory deficiency, areas of desensitization, open wounds, fractures or other complications.

C.   Application of the General Principles to Speech-Language Pathology Services.—Speech-language pathology services are those services necessary for the diagnosis and treatment of speech and language disorders that result in communication disabilities and for the diagnosis and treatment of swallowing disorders (dysphagia), regardless of the presence of a communication disability. The following discussion of skilled speech-language pathology services applies the principles to specific speech-language pathology services about which questions are most frequently raised.

1.   The skills of a speech-language pathologist are required for the assessment of a patient's rehabilitation needs (including the causal factors and the severity of the speech and language disorders), and rehabilitation potential. Reevaluation would only be considered reasonable and necessary if the patient exhibited a change in functional speech or motivation, clearing of confusion or the remission of some other medical condition that previously contraindicated speech-language pathology services. Where a patient is undergoing restorative speech-language pathology services, routine reevaluations are considered to be a part of the therapy and could not be billed as a separate visit.

2.   The services of a speech-language pathologist would be covered if they are needed as a result of an illness or injury and are directed towards specific speech/voice production.

3.   Speech-language pathology would be covered where the service can only be provided by a speech-language pathologist and where it is reasonably expected that the service will materially improve the patient's ability to independently carry out any one or combination of communicative activities of daily living in a manner that is measurably at a higher level of attainment than that prior to the initiation of the services.

4.   The services of a speech-language pathologist to establish a hierarchy of speech-voice-language communication tasks and cueing that directs a patient toward speech-language communication goals in the plan of care would be covered speech-language pathology services.

5.   The services of a speech-language pathologist to train the patient, family, or other caregivers to augment the speech-language communication, treatment or to establish an effective maintenance program would be covered speech-language pathology services.

6.   The services of a speech-language pathologist to assist patients with aphasia in rehabilitation of speech and language skills are covered when needed by a patient.

7.   The services of a speech-language pathologist to assist patients with voice disorders to develop proper control of the vocal and respiratory systems for correct voice production are covered when needed by a patient.

D.   Application of the General Principles to Occupational Therapy.—The following discussion of skilled occupational therapy services applies the principles to specific occupational therapy services about which questions are most frequently raised.

1.   Assessment.—The skills of an occupational therapist to assess and reassess a patient's rehabilitation needs and potential or to develop and/or implement an occupational therapy program are covered when they are reasonable and necessary because of the patient's condition.

2.   Planning, Implementing and Supervision of Therapeutic Programs.—The planning, implementing and supervision of therapeutic programs including, but not limited to those listed below are skilled occupational therapy services, and if reasonable and necessary to the treatment of the patient's illness or injury would be covered.

a.   Selecting and teaching task oriented therapeutic activities designed to restore physical function.

EXAMPLE: Use of woodworking activities on an inclined table to restore shoulder, elbow and wrist range of motion lost as a result of burns.

b.   Planning, implementing and supervising therapeutic tasks and activities designed to restore sensory-integrative function.

EXAMPLE: Providing motor and tactile activities to increase sensory output and improve response for a stroke patient with functional loss resulting in a distorted body image.

c.   Planning, implementing and supervising of individualized therapeutic activity programs as part of an overall "active treatment" program for a patient with a diagnosed psychiatric illness.

EXAMPLE: Use of sewing activities which require following a pattern to reduce confusion and restore reality orientation in a schizophrenic patient.

d.   Teaching compensatory techniques to improve the level of independence in the activities of daily living.

EXAMPLE 1:   Teaching a patient who has lost use of an arm how to pare potatoes and chop vegetables with one hand.

EXAMPLE 2:   Teaching a stroke patient new techniques to enable him to perform feeding, dressing, and other activities of daily living as independently as possible.

e.   The designing, fabricating, and fitting of orthotic and self-help devices.

EXAMPLE 1:   Construction of a device that would enable a patient to hold a utensil and feed himself independently.

EXAMPLE 2:   Construction of a hand splint for a patient with rheumatoid arthritis to maintain the hand in a functional position.

318 **Part Nine: Excerpts from Medicare** *Home Health Agency Manual*

205.2 (Cont.)   COVERAGE OF SERVICES   04-96

       f.   Vocational and prevocational assessment and training that is directed toward the restoration of function in the activities of daily living lost due to illness or injury would be covered. Where vocational or prevocational assessment and training is related solely to specific employment opportunities, work skills or work settings, such services would not be covered because they would not be directed toward the treatment of an illness or injury.

       3.   Illustration of Covered Services.—

EXAMPLE 1:   A physician orders occupational therapy for a patient who is recovering from a fractured hip and who needs to be taught compensatory and safety techniques with regard to lower extremity dressing, hygiene, toileting and bathing. The occupational therapist will establish goals for the patient's rehabilitation (to be approved by the physician), and will undertake the teaching of the techniques necessary for the patient to reach the goals. Occupational therapy services would be covered at a duration and intensity appropriate to the severity of the impairment and the patient's response to treatment.

EXAMPLE 2:   A physician has ordered occupational therapy for a patient who is recovering from a CVA. The patient has decreased range of motion, strength and sensation in both the upper and lower extremities on the right side and has perceptual and cognitive deficits resulting from the CVA. The patient's condition has resulted in decreased function in activities of daily living (specifically bathing, dressing, grooming, hygiene and toileting). The loss of function requires assistive devices to enable the patient to compensate for the loss of function and to maximize safety and independence. The patient also needs equipment such as himislings to prevent shoulder subluxation and a hand splint to prevent joint contracture and deformity in the right hand. The services of an occupational therapist would be necessary to assess the patient's needs, develop goals (to be approved by the physician), manufacture or adapt the needed equipment to the patient's use, teach compensatory techniques, strengthen the patient as necessary to permit use of compensatory techniques, and provide activities that are directed towards meeting the goals governing increased perceptual and cognitive function. Occupational therapy services would be covered at a duration and intensity appropriate to the severity of the impairment and the patient's response to treatment.

Medicare
Home Health Agency Manual

Department of Health
and Human Services

Health Care Financing
Administration

Completion of the Plan of Care (HCFA Form 485)

234.6   Form HCFA-485, Home Health Certification and Plan of Care.—Form HCFA-485 contains the data necessary to meet regulatory and national survey requirements for the physician's plan of care and certification.

Form HCFA-485 is also used by the RHHI alone or with other medical information to make decisions on home health coverage.

HCFA requires you to obtain a signed certification as soon as practicable after the start of care and prior to submitting a claim to the intermediary. You may provide services prior to obtaining the physician's written plan of care based on documented verbal orders. If care continues beyond the certification period, you must obtain a recertification from the physician. The signed HCFA-485 must be retained in your files and available upon request by the intermediary. Complete the form in it's entirety. Do not leave any items blank. However, there are items where "not applicable" (N/A) is acceptable. These items are specified.

You may submit Form HCFA-485 via electronic media, if acceptable to your intermediary. Specifications for electronic transmissions are in Addenda A and D. If you choose to use the abbreviated format for electronic submission, complete those items identified in the Addenda with an asterisk.

When the intermediary needs additional information to determine if the services furnished by you are Medicare covered services, a copy of Form HCFA-485, additional medical documentation, and/or copies of your medical record will be requested.

The intermediary may also pay or deny visits/services based only upon information provided on Form HCFA-485. However, additional information must be requested when objective clinical evidence needed to support a decision is not clearly present. (See S203.1.) Claims are not denied because a necessary field on Form HCFA-485 has not been completed. If the missing information is needed to make a coverage determination, request the necessary information. The claim is denied if the missing information is not submitted within 35 days of the date of the request for documentation or if you indicate that the information is not available. Intermediaries follow the procedures below for the items noted.

   o   Missing or Incomplete Physician's Orders - (HCFA-485, Item 21).

        1.   Visits for a discipline are billed but there is no physician order or the physician's order is present but it is not specific or there is no frequency.

        —   The physician's order for the services is requested. A documented verbal order or signed written order is accepted. (See below for acceptable verbal orders). Orders signed after the service(s) is rendered are not acceptable unless there is evidence of a pre-existing verbal order. If you furnish services without a physician's order, the services are denied. Such findings may be reported to the State survey office.

Part Nine: Excerpts from Medicare *Home Health Agency Manual* 321

234.6 (Cont.)   COVERAGE OF SERVICES   02-98

2.   Physician order for discipline and frequency is present but there is no duration of visits.

—   Make medical necessity determination on the duration billed.

o   You provide fewer visits than the physician orders.

—   Visits are not denied because you provide fewer visits. However, report the decrease to the physician. Where you consistently decrease visits without reporting to the physician, the State survey office may be notified.

o   Documentation of physician's verbal orders. Any of the following is acceptable:

—   Receipt of verbal orders is identified by the signature of a registered nurse, qualified therapist, social worker or any other health professional responsible for furnishing or supervising the patient's care and the date in Item 23 of Form HCFA-485 and the form is signed by the physician;

—   The HCFA-485 is signed by the physician and contains the verbal order(s) that has been written, signed and dated in the clinical record;

—   The form on which the verbal order is written, signed, or dated by agency staff is countersigned by the physician; or

—   A document signed by the physician contains the written signed and dated verbal order in the clinical record.

There is no required form or format for documentation or confirmation of verbal orders. In the absence of documentation of verbal orders, the FI will accept a notarized statement from the physician that he/she gave verbal orders before the services were rendered.

o   Physician Certification/Recertification:

—   The intermediary is required to investigate whether the physician certifying or recertifying the need for home health services has a financial interest or ownership in your agency.

—   Submit a listing of physicians associated with your agency who have such an interest or relationship. For each physician, identify their UPIN. (See §475.)

—   Once a year, the intermediary asks you to verify and update the listing. Notify the intermediary of any changes in ownership in the interim.

—   The intermediary automates the list and establishes edits to match the list against the UPIN. The intermediary denies claims that show a matching UPIN.

234.7   Completion of Form HCFA-485, Home Health Certification and Plan of Care.—
Form HCFA-485 meets the regulatory requirements (State and Federal) for both the physician's home health plan of care and home health certification and recertification requirements. HCFA requires you to obtain a signed certification as soon as practicable after the start of care and prior to submitting a claim to the intermediary. You may provide services prior to obtaining the physician's written plan of care based on documented verbal orders. If care continues beyond the certification period, you must obtain a recertification from the physician. The signed HCFA-485 must be retained in your files and a copy of the signed form made available upon request by the intermediary.

Complete the following:

1.   Patient's HICN.--Enter the HICN (numeric plus alpha indicator(s)) as shown on the patient's health insurance card, certificate award, utilization notice, temporary eligibility notice, or as reported by the SSO.

2.   Start of Care Date.--Enter the 6 digit month, day, year on which covered home health services began, i.e., MMDDYY (e.g., 101593). The start of care (SOC) date is the first Medicare billable visit. This date remains the same on subsequent plans of treatment until the patient is discharged. Home health care may be suspended and later resumed under the same start of care date in accordance with your internal procedures.

3.   Certification Period.--Enter the 2 digit month, day, year, MMDDYY (e.g., 101593-121593), which identifies the period covered by the physician's plan of care. The "From" date for the initial certification must match the start of care date. The "To" date can be up to, but never exceed, two calendar months and mathematically never exceed 62 days. Always repeat the "To" date on a subsequent recertification as the next sequential "From" date. Services delivered on the "To" date are covered in the next certification period.

EXAMPLE: Initial certification "From" date 101593
               Initial certification "To" date 121593

               Recertification "From" date 121593
               Recertification "To" date 021594

4.   Medical Record Number.--Enter the patient's medical record number that you assign. This is an optional item. If not applicable, enter "N/A."

5.   Provider Number.--Enter your 6-digit number issued by Medicare. It contains 2 digits, a hyphen, and 4 digits (e.g., 00-7000).

6.   Patient's Name and Address.--Enter the patient's last name, first name, and middle initial as shown on the health insurance card followed by the street address, city, State, and ZIP code.

7.   Provider's Name, Address, and Telephone No.--Enter your name and/or branch office (if applicable), street address (or other legal address), city, State, ZIP code, and telephone number.

8.   Date of Birth.--Enter the date (6 digit month, day, year) in numerics (MMD-DYY, e.g., 040120).

9.   Sex.--Check the appropriate box.

10.   Medications: Dose/Frequency/Route.--Enter all physician orders for all medications, including the dosage, frequency, and route of administration for each.

> o   Use an Addendum for drugs which cannot be listed on the plan of treatment.
>
> o   Use the letter "N" after the medication(s) which are "new" orders.
>
> o   Use the letter "C" after the medication(s) which are "change" orders either in dose, frequency, or route of administration.

"New" orders refer to medications which the patient has not taken recently, i.e., within the last 30 days. "Change" orders for medications include dosage, frequency, or route of administration changes within the last 60 days.

11.   Principal Diagnosis, ICD-9-CM Code and Date of Onset/Exacerbation.--Enter the principal diagnosis on all HCFA-485 forms. The principal diagnosis is the diagnosis most related to the current plan of treatment. It may or may not be related to the patient's most recent hospital stay, but must relate to the services you rendered. If more than one diagnosis is treated concurrently, enter the diagnosis that represents the most accurate condition and requires the most intensive services.

Enter the appropriate ICD-9-CM code in the space provided. The code must be the full ICD-9-CM diagnosis code including all digits. V codes are acceptable as both primary and secondary diagnosis. In many instances, the V code more accurately reflects the care provided. However, do not use the V code when the acute diagnosis code is more specific to the exact nature of the patient's condition. A list of V codes is in Exhibit III.

EXAMPLES: Patient is surgically treated for a subtrochanteric fracture (code 820.22). Admission to home care is for rehabilitation services (V57.1). Use 820.22 as the primary diagnosis since V57.1 does not specify the type or location of the fracture.

Patient is surgically treated for a malignant neoplasm of the colon (code 153.2) with exteriorization of the colon. Admission to home care is for instruction in care of colostomy (V55.3). Use V55.3 as the primary diagnosis since it is more specific to the nature of the services.

The principal diagnosis may change on subsequent forms only if the patient develops an acute condition or an exacerbation of a secondary diagnosis requiring intensive services different than those on the established plan of care.

List the actual <u>medical</u> diagnostic term next to the ICD-9-CM code. DO not describe in narrative format any symptoms or explanations. Do not use surgical procedure codes.

The <u>date</u> is always represented by six digits (MMDDYY); if the exact day is not known, use 00. The date of onset is specific to the medical reason for home health care services. If a condition is chronic or long term in nature, use the date of exacerbation. Use one or the other, not both. Always use the latest date. Enter all dates as close as possible to the actual date, to the best of your knowledge.

     12.   <u>Surgical Procedure, Date, ICD-9-CM Code</u>.--Enter the surgical procedure relevant to the care rendered. For example, if the diagnosis in Item 11 is "Fractured Left Hip," note the ICD-9-CM Code, the surgical procedure, and date (e.g., 81.62, Insertion of Austin Moore Prosthesis, 100293). If a surgical procedure was not performed or is not relevant to the plan of care, do not leave the box blank. Enter N/A. Use an addendum for additional relevant surgical procedures. At a minimum, the month and year must be present for the date of surgery. Use 00 if the day is unknown.

     13.   <u>Other Pertinent Diagnoses: Dates of Onset/Exacerbation, ICD-9-CM Code</u>.-- Enter all pertinent diagnoses, both narrative and ICD-9-CM codes, relevant to the care rendered. Other pertinent diagnoses are all conditions that coexisted at the time the plan of care was established or which developed subsequently. Exclude diagnoses that relate to an earlier episode which have no bearing on this plan of care. These diagnoses can be changed to reflect changes in the patient's condition.

In listing the diagnoses, place them in order to best reflect the seriousness of the patient's condition and to justify the disciplines and services provided. If there are more than four pertinent diagnoses, use an addendum to list them. Enter N/A if there are no pertinent secondary diagnoses.

Part Nine: Excerpts from Medicare *Home Health Agency Manual*   325

234.7 (Cont.)   COVERAGE OF SERVICES   02-98

The date reflects either the date of onset if it is a new diagnosis or the date of the most recent exacerbation of a previous diagnosis. Note the date of onset or exacerbation as close to the actual date as possible. If the date is unknown, note the year and place 00s in the month or day if not known.

14. <u>DME and Supplies</u>.--All nonroutine supplies must be specifically ordered by the physician or the physician's order for services must require the use of the specific supplies. Enter in this item, nonroutine supplies that you are billing to Medicare that are not specifically required by the order for services. For example, an order for foley insertion requires specific supplies, i.e., foley catheter tray. Therefore, these supplies are not required to be listed. Conversely, an order for wound care may require the use of nonroutine supplies which would vary by patient. Therefore, list the nonroutine supplies.

If you use a commonly used commercially packaged kit, you are not required to list the individual components. However, if there is a question of cost or content, the intermediary can request a breakdown of kit components.

Refer to the Provider Reimbursement Manual, Part I, §2115 for a definition of nonroutine supplies.

List DME ordered by the physician that will be billed to Medicare. Enter N/A if no supplies or DME are billed.

15. <u>Safety Measures</u>.--Enter the physician's instructions for safety measures.

16. <u>Nutritional Requirements</u>.--Enter the physician's order for the diet. This includes specific therapeutic diets and/or any specific dietary requirements. Record fluid needs or restrictions. Total Parenteral Nutrition (TPN) can be listed, and if more room is needed, place additional information under medications.

17. <u>Allergies</u>.--Enter medications to which the patient is allergic and other allergies the patient experiences (e.g., foods, adhesive tape, iodine). "No known allergies" may be an appropriate response.

18A. <u>Functional Limitations</u>.--Check all items which describe the patient's current limitations as assessed by the physician and you.

18B. <u>Activities Permitted</u>.--Check the activity(ies) which the physician allows and/or for which physician orders are present.

19. <u>Mental Status</u>.--Check the block(s) most appropriate to describe the patient's mental status. If you check "Other," specify the conditions.

20.   <u>Prognosis</u>.--Check the box which specifies the most appropriate prognosis for the patient: poor, guarded, fair, good, or excellent.

21.   <u>Orders for Discipline and Treatments (Specify amt/freq/dura)</u>.--The physician must specify the frequency and the expected duration of the visits for each discipline. The duties/treatments to be performed by each discipline must be stated. A discipline may be one or more of the following: skilled nursing (SN), physical therapy (PT), speech therapy (ST), occupational therapy (OT), medical social service (MSS), or home health aide (AIDE).

Orders must include all disciplines and treatments, even if they are not billable to Medicare. In general, the narrative explanation for applicable treatment codes is acceptable to the order when that narrative is sufficiently descriptive of the services to be furnished. However, additional explanation is required in this item to describe specific services, i.e., (See §234.9) A1, A4, A5, A6, A7, A22, A23, A28, A29, A32, B15, C9, D11, E4, E6, and F15. Refer to treatment codes in Exhibit II. Additional explanation is also required where the physician has ordered specific treatment, medications, or supplies. When aide services are needed to furnish personal care, an order for "personal care" is sufficient. See example of orders below.

Frequency denotes the number of visits per discipline to be rendered, stated in days, weeks, or months. Duration identifies the length of time the services are to be rendered and may be expressed in days, weeks, or months.

A range of visits may be reflected in the frequency (e.g., 2 to 4 visits per week). When a range is used, consider the upper limit of the range as the specific frequency. An agency may use ranges if acceptable to the physician without regard to diagnosis or other limits.

EXAMPLE OF PHYSICIAN'S ORDERS: Certification period is from 101593 to 121593.

OT -   Eval., ADL training, fine motor coordination 3x/wk x 6 wks

ST -   Eval., speech articulation disorder treatment 3x/wk x 4 wks

SN -   Skilled observation and assessment of C/P and neuro status instruct meds and diet/hydration, instruct 3x/wk x 2 wks

MSS -   Assessment of emotional and social factors 1x/mo x 2 mos

AIDE -   Assist with personal care, catheter care 3x/wk x 9 wks

Specific services rendered by physical, speech, and occupational therapists may involve different modalities. The "AMOUNT" is necessary when a discipline is providing a specific modality for therapy. Modalities usually mentioned are for heat, sound, cold, and electronic stimulation.

EXAMPLE: PT - To apply hot packs to the C5-C6 x <u>10 minutes</u> 3x/wk x 2 wks

PRN visits may be ordered on a plan of care only where they are qualified in a manner that is specific to the patient's potential needs. Both the nature of the services and the number of PRN visits to be permitted for each type of service must be specified. Open-ended, unqualified PRN visits do not constitute physician orders since neither their nature nor their frequency is specified.

EXAMPLE: Skilled nursing visits 1xmx2m for Foley change and PRNx2 for emergency Foley irrigations and/or changes.

               Skilled nursing visits 1xmx2m to draw blood sugar and PRNx2 to draw emergency blood sugar if blood sugar level is above 400.

          22.   <u>Goals/Rehabilitation Potential/Discharge Plans</u>.--Enter information which reflects the physician's description of the achievable goals and the patient's ability to meet them as well as plans for care after discharge.

Examples of realistic goals:

          o   Independence in transfers and ambulation with walker.

          o   Healing of leg ulcer(s).

          o   Maintain patency of Foley catheter. Decrease risk of urinary infection.

          o   Achieve optimal level of cardiovascular status. Medication and diet compliance.

          o   Ability to demonstrate correct insulin preparation and administration.

Rehabilitation potential addresses the patient's ability to attain the goals and an estimate of the time needed to achieve them. This information is pertinent to the nature of the patient's condition and ability to respond. The words "Fair" or "Poor" alone are not acceptable. Add descriptors.

EXAMPLE: Rehabilitation potential good for partial return to previous level of care, but patient will probably not be able to perform ADL independently.

Where daily care has been ordered, be specific as to the goals and when the need for daily care is expected to end.

EXAMPLE: Granulation of wound with daily wound care is expected to be achieved in
4 weeks. Skilled nursing visits will be decreased to 3 x week at that time.

Discharge plans include a statement of where, or how, the patient will be cared for once home
health services are not provided.

23.   Nurse's Signature and Date of Verbal Start of Care.--This verifies for surveyors, HCFA representatives, and intermediaries that a registered nurse, qualified therapist, social
worker, or any health professional responsible for furnishing or supervising the patient's care
spoke to the attending physician and has received verbal authorization to visit the patient. This
date may precede the SOC date in Item 2 and the "from" date in Item 3.

This field may be used to document receipt of verbal orders when services are furnished prior
to the physician's written orders, SOC, or recertification. If this field is used, the order must
be written on Form HCFA-485 and signed and dated with the date of receipt by the nurse,
qualified therapist, social worker, or qualified health professional to begin or modify care or
continue care at recertification.

The item is signed by the nurse, qualified therapist, social worker, or health professional responsible for the completion of the Form HCFA-485, or by non-clerical personnel authorized to do
so by applicable State and Federal laws and regulation as well as internal policies.

Enter N/A if the physician has signed and dated Form HCFA-485 on or before the SOC or recertification date or has submitted a written order to start, modify, or continue care on a document
other than Form HCFA-485.

The item is signed by the nurse receiving the verbal orders, by the nurse responsible for completion of the form, or by a nonclerical agency representative responsible for review. The date
is necessary. If the nurse who received the orders does not prepare the HCFA-485, then the
orders must be transcribed to a form, signed and dated by her/him, and retained in your files.
Document the initial and ongoing communications with the physician.

24.   Physician's Name and Address.--Print the physician's name and address. The
attending physician is the physician who establishes the plan of care and who certifies and recer-
tifies the medical necessity of the visits and/or services. The physician must be qualified to sign
the certification and plan of care in accordance with 42 CFR 424, Subpart B. Physicians who
have significant ownership interest in or a significant financial or contractual relationship with
an HHA may not establish or review a plan of care or certify or recertify the need for home
health services. (See §234.6 for information about physician certification/recertification.)

25.   Date HHA Received Signed POC.--Enter the date you received the signed POC
from the attending/referring physician. Enter N/A if Item 27 (DATE) is completed.

26.   Physician Certification.--This statement serves to verify that the physician has reviewed the plan of care and certifies to the need for the services.

27.   Attending Physician's Signature and Date Signed.--The attending physician signs and dates the plan of care/certification prior to you submitting the claim. Rubber signature stamps are not acceptable. The form may be signed by another physician who is authorized by the attending physician to care for his/her patient in his/her absence.

While the regulations specify that documents must be signed, they do not prohibit the transmission of the plan of care or oral order via facsimile machine. You are not required to have the original signature on file. However, you are responsible for obtaining original signatures if an issue surfaces that would require verification of an original signature. If you maintain patient records by computer rather than hard copy, you may use electronic signature. However, all such entries must be appropriately authenticated and dated. Authentication must include signatures, written initials, or computer secure entry by a unique identifier of a primary author who has reviewed and approved the entry. You must have safeguards to prevent unauthorized access to the records and a process for reconstruction of the records upon request from the intermediary, State surveyor, or other authorized personnel or in the event of a system breakdown.

Do not predate the orders for the physician, nor write the date in this field. If the physician left it blank, enter the date you received the signed POC under Item 25. Do not enter "N/A." Submit an unsigned copy of the HCFA-485. Retain the signed copy.

28.   Penalty Statement.--This statement specifies the penalties imposed for misrepresentation, falsification, or concealment of essential information on the HCFA-485.

234.8   Treatment Codes for Home Health Services.--The agency may use the narrative explanation for the treatment codes which represent the services to be furnished. The narrative is entered in Item 21 of the HCFA-485. Additional narrative is required under Item 21 of the HCFA-485 to describe specific services, i.e., A1, A4, A5, A6, A7, A22, A23, A28, A29, A32, B15, C9, D11, E4, E6, and F15. (See asterisked items/services in Exhibit II.) Non-asterisked items/services do not require additional narrative unless the physician has ordered specific treatment and/or use of prescription medications and/or nonroutine supplies.

Listing of a code for a particular service is not intended to imply coverage. The codes are to ease identification of services ordered by the physician whether or not these services are payable individually by Medicare. Physician's orders reflect a narrative description of treatment and services to be furnished.

A.   Skilled Nursing.--These represent the services to be performed by the nurse. Services performed by the patient or other person in the home with the teaching or supervision of the nurse are not coded. The following is a further explanation for each service.

o   A1. Skilled Observation and Assessment (Inc. V.S., Response to Med., etc.) -Includes all skilled observation and assessment of the patient where the physician determines that the patient's condition is such that a reasonable probability exists that significant changes may occur which require the skills of a licensed nurse to supplement the physician's personal contacts with the patient.

o   A2. Foley Insertion - Insertion and/or removal of the Foley catheter by nurse.

o   A3. Bladder Instillation - Instilling medications into the bladder.

o   A4. Wound Care/Dressing - Includes irrigation of open, postsurgical wounds, application of medication, and/or dressing changes. Does not include decubitus care. Describe dimension of wound (size and amount and type of drainage) on an addendum. See Treatment Code A28 for observation of uncomplicated surgical incision.

o   A5. Decubitus Care - Includes irrigation, application of medication, and/or dressing changes to decubitus. The agency describes size (depth and width) on the addendum. Use this code only if the decubitus being treated presents the following characteristics:

— Partial tissue loss with signs of infection such as foul odor or purulent drainage;

— Full thickness tissue loss that involves exposure of fat or invasion of other tissue such as muscle or bone.

For care of decubitus not meeting this definition, see Treatment Code A29.

o   A6. Venipuncture - The HHA specifies the test and frequency to be performed under physician's orders.

o   A7. Restorative Nursing - Includes exercises, transfer training, carrying out of restorative program ordered by the physician. This may or may not be established by a physical therapist. This code is not used to describe nonskilled services (e.g., routine range of motion exercises).

o   A8. Post Cataract Care - Includes observation, dressings, teaching, etc. of the immediate postoperative cataract patient.

Part Nine: Excerpts from Medicare *Home Health Agency Manual*   331

234.8 (Cont.)   COVERAGE OF SERVICES   02-98

o   <u>A9. Bowel/Bladder Training</u> - Includes training of patients who have neurological or muscular problems or other conditions where the need for bowel or bladder training is clearly identified.

o   <u>A10. Chest Physio (Inc. postural drainage)</u> - Includes breathing exercises, postural drainage, chest percussion, conservation techniques, etc.

o   <u>A11. Adm. of Vitamin B/12</u> - Administration of vitamin B-12 preparation by injection for conditions identified in Medicare guidelines.

o   <u>A12. Prep/Adm. Insulin</u> - Preparation of insulin syringes for administration by the patient or other person or the administration by the nurse.

o   <u>A13. Adm. Other IM/Subq.</u> - Administration of any injection other than vitamin B/12 or insulin ordered by the physician.

o   <u>A14. Adm. IV's/Clysis</u> - Administration of intravenous fluids or clysis or intravenous medications.

o   <u>A15. Teach. Ostomy or Ileo Conduit Care</u> - Teaching the patient or other person to care for a colostomy, ileostomy or ileoconduit, or nephrostomy.

o   <u>A16. Teach. Nasogastric Feeding</u> - Teaching the patient or other person to administer nasogastric feedings. Includes teaching care of equipment and preparation of feedings.

o   <u>A17. Reinsertion Nasogastric Feeding Tube</u> - Includes changing the tube by the nurse.

o   <u>A18. Teach. Gastrostomy Feeding</u> - Teaching the patient or other person to care for gastrostomy and administer feedings. Includes teaching care of equipment and preparation of feedings.

o   <u>A19. Teach. Parenteral Nutrition</u> - Teaching the patient and/or family to administer parenteral nutrition. Includes teaching aseptic technique for dressing changes to catheter site. Agency documentation must specify that this service is necessary and does not duplicate other teaching.

o   <u>A20. Teach. Care of Trach.</u> - Teaching the patient or other person to care for a tracheostomy. This includes care of equipment.

o   <u>A21. Adm. Care of Trach.</u> - Administration of tracheostomy care by the nurse, including changing the tracheostomy tube and care of the equipment.

o   <u>A22. Teach. Inhalation Rx</u> - Teaching patient or other person to administer therapy and care for equipment.

o   <u>A23. Adm. Inhalation Rx</u> - Administration of inhalation treatment and care of equipment by the nurse.

o   <u>A24. Teach. Adm. of Injection</u> - Teaching patient or other person to administer an injection. Does not include the administration of the injection by the nurse (see Treatment Code A11, A13) or the teaching/administration of insulin. (See Treatment Codes A12, A25).

o   <u>A25. Teach. Diabetic Care</u> - Includes all teaching of the diabetic patient (i.e., diet, skin care, administration of insulin, urine testing).

o   <u>A26. Disimpaction/Follow-up Enema</u> - Includes nursing services associated with removal of an impaction. Enema administration in the absence of an impaction only if a complex condition exists, e.g., immediate postoperative rectal surgery.

o   <u>A27. Other (Spec. Under Orders)</u> - Includes any SN or teaching ordered by the physician and not identified above. The agency specifies what is being taught in Item 21 (HCFA-485).

o   <u>A28. Wound Care/Dressing</u> - Skilled observation and care of surgical incision/suture line including application of DSD. (See Treatment Code A4).

o   <u>A29. Decubitus Care</u> - Includes irrigation, application of medication, and/or dressing changes to decubitus/other skin ulcer or lesion, other than that described in Treatment Code A5. The HHA describes size (depth and width) and appearance on the addendum.

o   <u>A30. Teaching Care of Any Indwelling Catheter</u> - Teaching patient or other person to care for indwelling catheter.

o   <u>A31. Management and Evaluation of a Patient Care Plan</u> - The complexity of necessary unskilled services require skilled management of a registered nurse to ensure that these services achieve their purpose and to promote the beneficiary's recovery and medical safety.

o   <u>A32. Teaching and Training (Other)</u> - Specify under physician orders.

B.   Physical Therapy (PT).--These codes represent all services to be performed by the physical therapist. If services are provided by a nurse, they are included under Treatment Code A7. The following is a further explanation of each service:

o   B1. Evaluation - Visit(s) made to determine the patient's condition, physical therapy plans, and rehabilitation potential; to evaluate the home environment to eliminate structural barriers; and to improve safety to increase functional independence (ramps, adaptive wheelchair, bathroom aides).

o   B2. Therapeutic Exercise - Exercise designed to restore function. Specific exercise techniques (e.g., Proprioceptive Neuromuscular Facilitation (PNF), Rood, Brunstrom, Codman's, William's) are specified. The exercise treatment is listed in the medical record specific to the patient's condition, manual therapy techniques which include soft tissue and joint mobilization to reduce joint deformity, and increase functional range of motion.

o   B3. Transfer Training - To evaluate and instruct safe transfers (bed, bath, toilet, sofa, chair, commode) using appropriate body mechanics and equipment (sliding board, Hoyer lift, trapeze, bath bench, wheelchair). Instruct patient, family, and caregivers in appropriate transfer techniques.

o   B4. Establish or Upgrade Home Program - To improve the patient's functional level by instruction to the patient and responsible individuals in exercise which may be used as an adjunct to PT programs.

o   B5. Gait Training - Includes gait evaluation and ambulation training of a patient whose ability to walk has been impaired. Gait training is the selection and instruction in use of various assistive devices (orthotic appliances, crutches, walker, cane, etc.)

o   B6. Pulmonary Physical Therapy - Includes breathing exercises, postural drainage, etc., for patients with acute or severe pulmonary dysfunction.

o   B7. Ultra Sound - Mechanism to produce heat or micro-massage in deep tissues for conditions in which relief of pain, increase in circulation, and increase in local metabolic activity are desirable.

o   B8. Electro Therapy - Includes treatment for neuromuscular dysfunction and pain through use of electrotherapeutic devices (electromuscular stimulation, TENS, Functional Electrical Stimulation (FES), biofeedback, high voltage galvanic stimulation (HVGS), etc.)

o   B9. Prosthetic Training - Includes stump conditioning (shrinking, shaping, etc.) range of motion, muscle strengthening, and gait training with or without the prosthesis and appropriate assistive devices.

    o   <u>B10. Fabrication Temporary Devices</u> - Includes fabrication of temporary prostheses, braces, splints, and slings.

    o   <u>B11. Muscle Reeducation</u> - Includes therapy designed to restore function due to illness, disease, or surgery affecting neuromuscular function.

    o   <u>B12. Management and Evaluation of a Patient Care Plan</u> - The complexity of necessary unskilled services require skilled management by a qualified physical therapist to ensure that these services achieve their purpose and to promote the beneficiary's recovery and medical safety.

    o   <u>B13. through B14</u> - Reserved.

    o   <u>B15. Other (Spec. Under Orders)</u> - Includes all PT services not identified above. Specific therapy services are identified under physician's orders (HCFA-485, Item 21).

    C.   <u>Speech Therapy (ST)</u>.--These codes represent the services to be performed by the speech therapist. Following is a further explanation of each.

    o   <u>C1. Evaluation</u> - Visit made to determine the type, severity, and prognosis of a communication disorder, whether speech therapy is reasonable and necessary, and to establish the goals, treatment plan, and estimated frequency and duration of treatment.

    o   <u>C2. Voice Disorders Treatments</u> - Procedures and treatment for patients with an absence or impairment of voice caused by neurologic impairment, structural abnormality, or surgical procedures affecting the muscles of voice production.

    o   <u>C3. Speech Articulation Disorders Treatments</u> - Procedures and treatment for patients with impaired intelligibility (clarity) of speech - usually referred to as anarthria or dysarthria and/or impaired ability to initiate, inhibit, and/or sequence speech sound muscle movements - usually referred to as apraxia/dyspraxia.

    o   <u>C4. Dysphagia Treatments</u> - Includes procedures designed to facilitate and restore a functional swallow.

    o   <u>C5. Language Disorders Treatments</u> - Includes procedures and treatment for patients with receptive and/or expressive aphasia/dysphasia, impaired reading comprehension, written language expression, and/or arithmetical processes.

    o   <u>C6. Aural Rehabilitation</u> - Procedures and treatments designed for patients with communication problems related to impaired hearing acuity.

o   C7. Reserved

o   C8. Nonoral Communications - Includes any procedures designed to establish a nonoral or augmentive communication system.

o   C9. Other (Spec. Under Orders) - Speech therapy services not included above. Specify service to be rendered under physician's orders (HCFA-485, Item 21).

D.   Occupational Therapy.-- These codes represent the services to be rendered by the occupational therapist. Following is a further explanation:

o   D1. Evaluation - Visit made to determine occupational therapy needs of the patient at the home. Includes physical and psychosocial testings, establishment of plan of care, rehabilitation goals, and evaluating the home environment for accessibility and safety and recommending modifications.

o   D2. Independent Living/Daily Living Skills (ADL training) - Refers to the skills and performance of physical cognitive and psychological/emotional self care, work, and play/leisure activities to a level of independence appropriate to age, life-space, and disability.

o   D3. Muscle Re-education - Includes therapy designed to restore function lost due to disease or surgical intervention.

o   D4. Reserved

o   D5. Perceptual Motor Training - Refers to enhancing skills necessary to interpret sensory information so that the individual can interact normally with the environment. Training designed to enhance perceptual motor function usually involves activities which stimulate visual and kinesthetic channels to increase awareness of the body and its movement.

o   D6. Fine Motor Coordination - Refers to the skills and the performance in fine motor and dexterity activities.

o   D7. Neurodevelopmental Treatment - Refers to enhancing the skills and the performance of movement through eliciting and/or inhibiting stereotyped, patterned, and/or involuntary responses which are coordinated at subcortical and cortical levels.

o   D8. Sensory Treatment - Refers to enhancing the skills and performance in perceiving and differentiating external and internal stimuli such as tactile awareness, stereognosis, kinesthesia, proprioceptive awareness, occular control, vestibular awareness, auditory awareness, gustatory awareness, and olfactory awareness necessary to increase function.

o   D9. Orthotics/Splinting - Refers to the provision of dynamic and static splints, braces, and slings for relieving pain, maintaining joint alignment, protecting joint integrity, improving function, and/or decreasing deformity.

o   D10. Adaptive Equipment (fabrication and training) - Refers to the provision of special devices that increase independent functions.

o   D11. Other - Occupational therapy services not quantified above.

E.   Medical Social Services (MSS).--These codes represent the services to be rendered by the medical social service worker. Following is a further explanation:

o   E1. Assessment of Social and Emotional Factors - Skilled assessment of social and emotional factors related to the patient's illness, need for care, response to treatment, and adjustment to care; followed by care plan development.

o   E2. Counseling for Long-Range Planning and Decision Making - Assessment of patient's needs for long term care including: evaluation of home and family situation; enabling patient/family to develop an inhome care system; exploring alternatives to in-home care; arrangement for placement.

o   E3. Community Resource Planning - The promotion of community centered service(s) including education, advocacy, referral, and linkage.

o   E4. Short Term Therapy - Goal oriented intervention directed toward management of terminal illness; reaction/adjustment to illness; strengthening family/support system; conflict resolution related to chronicity of illness.

o   E5. Reserved

o   E6. Other (Specify Under Orders) - Includes other medical social services related to the patient's illness and need for care. Problem resolution associated with high risk indicators endangering patient's mental and physical health including: abuse/neglect, inadequate food/medical supplies; high suicide potential. The service to be performed must be written under doctor's orders (HCFA-485, Item 21).

F.   Home Health Aide.--These codes represent the services to be rendered by the home health aide. Specific personal care services to be provided by the home health aide must be determined by a registered professional nurse. Services are given under the supervision of the nurse, and if appropriate, a physical, speech, or occupational therapist. Following is a further explanation:

o   <u>F1. Tub/Shower Bath </u>- Assistance with tub or shower bathing.

o   <u>F2. Partial/Complete Bed Bath</u> - Bathing or assisting the patient with bed bath.

o   <u>F3. Reserved</u>

o   <u>F4. Personal Care </u>- Includes shaving of patient or shampooing the hair.

o   <u>F5. Reserved</u>

o   <u>F6. Catheter Care</u> - Care of catheter site and/or irrigations under nursing supervision.

o   <u>F7. Reserved</u>

o   <u>F8. Assist with Ambulation</u> - Assisting the patient with ambulation as determined necessary by the nurse care plan.

o   <u>F9. Reserved</u>

o   <u>F10. Exercises</u> - Assisting the patient with exercises in accordance with the plan of care.

o   <u>F11. Prepare a Meal</u> - May be furnished by the aide during a visit for personal care.

o   <u>F12. Grocery Shop</u> - May be furnished as an adjunct to a visit for personal care to meet the patient's nutritional needs in order to prevent or postpone the patient's institutionalization.

o   <u>F13. Wash Clothes</u> - This service may be provided as it relates to the comfort and cleanliness of the patient and the immediate environment.

o   <u>F14. Housekeeping</u> - Household services incidental to care and which do not substantially increase the time spent by the home health aide.

o   <u>F15. Other (Specify Under Orders)</u> - Includes other home health aide services in accordance with determination made by a registered professional nurse. Specified in Item 21 of the HCFA-485.

234.9   Addendum to Form HCFA-485, Plan of Care.--When additional space is needed to complete Form HCFA-485 fields, use an addendum identifying items 1-9.

To provide additional documentation of items on the plan of care or medical information, check the appropriate block. Identify the item being addressed on the addendum. For example, if the plan of treatment block is checked and Item 10 (medications) requires additional space, specify Item 10 in the addendum. Upon completion of Item 10, note the next item number, e.g., Item 14 (DME), then complete that item.

1.   Patient's HICN.--See §234.7, Item 1.

2.   Start of Care Date.--See §234.7, Item 2.

3.   Certification Period.--See §234.7, Item 3.

4.   Medical Record Number.--See §234.7, Item 4.

5.   Provider Number.--See §234.7, Item 5.

6.   Patient's Name and Address.--See §234.7, Item 6.

7.   Provider Name, Address, and Telephone Number.--See §234.7, Item 7.

8.   Signature of Physician.--If the certification/plan of treatment block is checked, the physician's signature or an annotation is required on the HCFA-485 which indicates that the physician is aware that he/she is signing for information contained on additional pages (e.g., page 1 of 2). Retain the signed copy in your files.

9.   Date.--The physician enters the date he/she signed the addendum in this space.

234.10   Coverage Compliance Review.--The intermediary performs coverage compliance reviews by reviewing medical records onsite or in-house. The purpose of the review is to assure that services meet Medicare program requirements and to verify that the information on Form 485 matches that in the medical record and claim.

A.   Selection of HHAs.--The intermediary may select HHAs for review based on a number of factors (e.g., denial rates, provider profiling, problem areas identified during prepayment review, failure on prior compliance review, new HHAs).

B.   Coverage Compliance Review.--

1.   Sample Selection.--Claims are selected with recent service dates or those reviewed and paid within the last 120 days.

The intermediary selects enough beneficiaries (a minimum of 15) to review a minimum of 100 visits or a maximum of 5 percent of your average monthly visits billed. Visits can be reduced if your volume is low.

Claims that have been fully denied are excluded.

       2.   File Compilation.--The intermediary establishes an audit trail which identifies the claims and beneficiaries selected, sample size, the period of review for medical records, the records reviewed, and the review findings.

       3.   HHA Onsite vs. In-House (at the Intermediary) Reviews.--The intermediary determines whether to conduct a review onsite at the HHA or in-house at the intermediary.

       4.   Notification of Selection for Coverage Compliance Review.--

       a.   In-House.--You are notified in writing when an in-house coverage compliance review is scheduled. The intermediary furnishes a list of beneficiaries for whom medical documentation is needed. Submit documentation within 30 days of the notification.

       b.   On-site at HHA.--You are advised by telephone of the visit 24 working hours in advance, followed with a written confirmation. The intermediary advises you which records will be reviewed at the start of the review.

       5.   Review.--Points which are addressed:

       o   Was the physician certification requirement met?

       o   Were the services rendered medically necessary?

       o   Were visits billed only when appropriate?

       o   Were visits billed actually furnished?

       o   Did skilled nursing and aide visits meet part-time or intermittent requirements?

       o   Were medical appliances and/or medical supplies appropriately ordered and/or supplied?

       o   Do the records support the evidence submitted originally? What information, or lack thereof, influenced the prepayment coverage decision?

o   Is the certifying physician qualified to establish and certify a plan of care? (See 42 CFR §424.22.)

o   Is the patient homebound?

o   Is the patient's residence an §1819(a)(1) facility?

o   Were the services furnished under a plan of care?

o   Was the plan put into writing timely?

o   Is the plan complete?

o   Were plan of care changes or extensions made in accord with policy?

o   Compare home health aide tasks ordered with those furnished to assure tasks are accomplished.

NOTE: If you have obviously omitted a part of the data needed for review, e.g., home health aide notes, the intermediary alerts you to correct the problem.

Services prior to the period of the selected claims are not reviewed unless the issue is homebound status. Where that question is raised, all previous records are reviewed to determine when the patient ceased to meet that criterion. Where applicable, you are asked to submit the actual hours spent in the home for all skilled nursing and aide visits. Coverage criteria in effect at the time services were rendered are applied if changes have occurred in the interim which make coverage more restrictive.

6.   Special On-Site Requirements.--

a.   Staff.--Only intermediary staff who have authority to deny claims perform the review. This process intends that if denials occur, they occur during the onsite review. The pertinent records are photocopied for the physician's review only where a question arises which requires physician consultation. In these cases, the final decision to deny the claim is made by the physician reviewer, based upon information gathered at the onsite review.

b.   Copying Records.--The intermediary photocopies the pertinent records when the on-site reviewer has denied services, where physician consultation is needed, or where records may have been altered.

c.   Entrance and Exit Interviews.--The intermediary holds both entrance and exit interviews. It explains in the entrance interview the scope and purpose of the review. You are given an opportunity to produce documents during the review process.

Part Nine: Excerpts from Medicare *Home Health Agency Manual*   341

234.10 (Cont.)   COVERAGE OF SERVICES   02-98

The tentative findings of the review are discussed during the exit interview. You are provided with sufficient information to enable you to provide comments on the cases involved.

Physician review is completed within 7 days of the date of the interview. You are notified in writing of any additional services which are noncovered.

You may submit written comments on the denied services within 2 weeks of the exit conference, or receipt of the letter regarding the physician's findings, whichever is later.
The intermediary must finalize its findings within 6 weeks after the exit conference.

      d.   Beneficiary Home Visits.--Home visits may occur. This is decided by the intermediary with RO approval.

      7.   Distribution of Findings.--The intermediary advises you in writing of the results within 6 weeks after the on-site review including:

        o   Written findings of the review;

        o   Specifics of denied care for educational purposes;

        o   Impact on prepayment review or documentation requirements; and

        o   Overpayments resulting from denials that are not payable under waiver of liability.

For denied services, the intermediary sends the beneficiary a notice if one would have been sent in the course of prepayment review. The intermediary sends you a copy of these denial notices since the beneficiary will be contacting you about the letter(s).

For in-house reviews, 14 days from the date of the report of findings are allowed for your rebuttal or response.

      8.   Impact of Adverse Review Findings.--

      a.   Impact Upon Payment.--The intermediary applies the waiver of liability provision where applicable. (See §§262-265 where you are determined to be liable.)

Where care is not covered for a reason for which waiver of liability provisions do not apply (e.g., lack of physician certification), the claim is denied. In these cases, the amount of overpayment is determined and recovered. (See §§262-265.) Payment is made for cases which were previously denied and now covered. The intermediary credits the denial rate for these visits.

b.   Impact on Prepayment Review.--Where appropriate, prepayment review is intensified until identified problems are corrected. A denial rate exceeding 15 percent, calculated by the total number of visits denied (medical and technical), divided by the total number of visits reviewed for this audit, may indicate a need for intensified review. When looking at denial rates, the reasons for denials are considered. For example, denial of dependent services may disproportionately increase the denial rate and may not be indicative of a problem. The level and length of intensified review is determined by the RHHI in consultation with the RO.

10.   Other Impact.--As a result of the coverage compliance audit, your intermediary may implement actions to improve your performance. For example, if the audit identifies problems with the accuracy of the information, i.e., you did not include pertinent information on Form HCFA-485, the intermediary advises you of corrective action to be taken. In another example, where cases contain erroneous or insufficient information, but the coverage decision remains the same, they discuss this with you. If a trend is noted where the documentation does not support the information submitted on the forms, corrective action is indicated. This could include an additional coverage compliance review within 3 months to determine if the problems have been corrected. Training is provided to HHA staff on identified problem areas through bulletins, correspondence, and teleconferences, etc.

When the lack of documentation or inaccurate information results in inappropriate payment, the intermediary identifies the reason, conducts educational training, usually on coverage and documentation, and evaluates the further need for intensified review. The intermediary pursues corrective action where the audit results in inappropriate payment. At a minimum, it must recoup the inappropriate payments.

234.11   Documentation of Skilled Nursing and Home Health Aide Hours.--To document that SN and aide services are part-time or intermittent, you must maintain records which show the entrance and exit times of skilled nurse's and aide's visits and total hours spent in the home by each discipline. Exclude travel time.

Intermediaries may request this information when a question arises as to whether services are part-time or intermittent under §206.7.

o   When actual hours per day are full-time (up to and including 8 hours per day) 7 days per week, document their need. Document the medical complications, safety needs, condition of the beneficiary, and reasons for the intensive full-time care. Document the specific services provided.

o   Extension beyond 21 days of full-time services for a finite and predictable period of time may be approved on an exception basis only when you have clearly documented the need, or the justification, for this frequency. Document the medical complications, safety needs, and/or other individual care needs that warrant your services. Stress the inherent complexity of services provided, the medical condition of the patient, functional losses, and/or other reasons that confirm that the service(s) can only be safely and effectively provided through skilled nursing care.

EXHIBIT I

Department of Health and Human Services
Health Care Financing Administration

Form Approved
OMB No. 0938-0357

HOME HEALTH CERTIFICATION AND PLAN OF CARE

1. Patient's HI Claim No.	2. Start Of Care Date	3. Certification Period		4. Medical Record No.	5. Provider No.
		From:	To:		

6. Patient's Name and Address

7. Provider's Name, Address and Telephone Number

8. Date of Birth		9. Sex	M	F	10. Medications: Dose/Frequency/Route (N)ew (C)hanged
11. ICD-9-CM	Principal Diagnosis		Date		
12. ICD-9-CM	Surgical Procedure		Date		
13. ICD-9-CM	Other Pertinent Diagnoses		Date		

14. DME and Supplies

15. Safety Measures:

16. Nutritional Req.

17. Allergies:

18.A. Functional Limitations

1	Amputation	5	Paralysis	9	Legally Blind
2	Bowel/Bladder (Incontinence)	6	Endurance	A	Dyspnea With Minimal Exertion
3	Contracture	7	Ambulation	B	Other (Specify)
4	Hearing	8	Speech		

18.B. Activities Permitted

1	Complete Bedrest	6	Partial Weight Bearing	A	Wheelchair
2	Bedrest BRP	7	Independent At Home	B	Walker
3	Up As Tolerated	8	Crutches	C	No Restrictions
4	Transfer Bed/Chair	9	Cane	D	Other (Specify)
5	Exercises Prescribed				

19. Mental Status:

| 1 | Oriented | 3 | Forgetful | 5 | Disoriented | 7 | Agitated |
| 2 | Comatose | 4 | Depressed | 6 | Lethargic | 8 | Other |

20. Prognosis:

| 1 | Poor | 2 | Guarded | 3 | Fair | 4 | Good | 5 | Excellent |

21. Orders for Discipline and Treatments (Specify Amount/Frequency/Duration)

22. Goals/Rehabilitation Potential/Discharge Plans

23. Nurse's Signature and Date of Verbal SOC Where Applicable:

25. Date HHA Received Signed POT

24. Physician's Name and Address

26. I certify/recertify that this patient is confined to his/her home and needs intermittent skilled nursing care, physical therapy and/or speech therapy or continues to need occupational therapy. The patient is under my care, and I have authorized the services on this plan of care and will periodically review the plan.

27. Attending Physician's Signature and Date Signed

28. Anyone who misrepresents, falsifies, or conceals essential information required for payment of Federal funds may be subject to fine, imprisonment, or civil penalty under applicable Federal laws.

Form 3485R/4P BRIGGS, Des Moines, IA 50306 (800) 247-2343

PROVIDER

Form HCFA-485 (C-4) (02-94) (Print Aligned)

EXHIBIT II
TREATMENT CODES
FOR PROFESSIONAL SERVICES REQUIRED

Skilled Nursing

A1*	Skilled Observation and Assessment (Inc. V.S., Response to Med., etc.)	A15	Teach Ostomy or Ileo conduit care
A2	Foley Insertion	A16	Teach Nasogastric Feeding
A3	Bladder Instillation	A17	Reinsertion Nasogastric Feeding Tube
A4	Open Wound Care/Dressing	A18	Teach Gastrostomy Feeding
A5*	Decubitus Care (Partial tissue-loss with signs of infection or full thickness tissue loss, etc.)	A19	Teach Parenteral Nutrition
		A20	Teach Care of Trach
A6*	Venipuncture	A21	Adm. Care of Trach
A7*	Restorative Nursing	A22*	Teach Inhalation Rx
A8	Post Cataract Care	A23*	Adm. Inhalation Rx
A9	Bowel/Bladder Training	A24	Teach Adm. of Injection
A10	Chest Physio (Inc. Postural drainage)	A25	Teach Diabetic Care
		A26	Disimpaction/F.U. Enema
A11	Adm. of Vitamin B/12	A27*	Other (Spec. under Orders)
A12	Adm. Insulin	A28*	Wound Care/Dressing-Closed Incision/Suture Line
A13	Adm. Other IM/Subq.	A29*	Decubitus Care (Other than A4 A5)
A14	Adm. IV/s/Clysis	A30	Teaching Care of Any Indwelling Catheter
		A31	Management and Evaluation of Patient Care Plan
		A32*	Teaching and Training (other) (spec. under order)

Physical Therapy

B1	Evaluation	B7	UltraSound
B2	Therapeutic Exercise	B8	Electrotherapy
B3	Transfer Training	B9	Prosthetic Training
B4	Home Program	B10	Fabrication Temporary Devices
B5	Gait Training	B11	Muscle Re-education
B6	Pulmonary Physical Therapy	B12	Management and Evaluation
		B13-14	Reserved
		B15*	Other (Specify under orders)

* Code which requires a more extensive descriptive narrative for physician's orders.

EXHIBIT II (Cont.)

Speech Therapy

C1	Evaluation	C6	Aural Rehabilitation
C2	Voice Disorders Treatments	C7	Reserved
C3	Speech Articulation Disorders Treatments	C8	Nonoral Communication
C4	Dysphagia Treatments	C9*	Other (Specify under C4
C5	Language Disorders Treatments		Orders)

Occupational Therapy

D1   Evaluation
D2   Independent Living/Daily Living Skills (ADL Training)
D3   Muscle Re-education
D4   Reserved
D5   Perceptual Motor Training
D6   Fine Motor Coordination
D7   Neuro-developmental Treatment
D8   Sensory Treatment
D9   Orthotics/Splinting
D10   Adaptive Equipment (fabrication and training)
D11* Other (Specify Under Orders)

Medical Social Services

E1   Assessment of Social and Emotional Factors
E2   Counseling for Long Range Planning and Decision Making
E3   Community Resource Planning
E4*   Short Term Therapy
E5   Reserved
E6*   Other (Specify Under Orders)

Home Health Aide

F1	Tub/Shower Bath	F8	Assist with Ambulation
F2	Partial/Complete Bath	F9	Reserved
F3	Reserved	F10	Exercises
F4	Personal Care	F11	Prepare Meal
F5	Reserved	F12	Grocery Shop
F6	Catheter Care	F13	Wash Clothes
F7	Reserved	F14	Housekeeping
		F15*	Other (Spec. under orders)

* Code which requires a more extensive descriptive narrative for physician's orders.

EXHIBIT III

ACCEPTABLE V CODES

V45.6	States following surgery of eye and adnexa
V45.81	Postsurgical status, aortocoronary bypass status
V45.89	Postsurgical status, presence of neuropacemaker or other electronic device
V46.0	Dependence on Aspirator
V46.1	Dependence on Respirator
V52.0	Fitting and adjustment of artificial arm
V52.1	Fitting and adjustment of artificial leg
V53.5	Fitting and adjustment ileostomy or other intestinal appliance
V53.6	Fitting and adjustment urinary devices
V54.0	Orthopedic aftercare involving removal of internal fixation device
V54.8	Orthopedic aftercare kirschner wire, plaster cast, external splint, external fixation device or traction device
V54.9	Unspecified orthopedic aftercare
V55.0	Attention to tracheostomy
V55.1	Attention to gastrostomy
V55.2	Attention to ileostomy
V55.3	Attention to colostomy
V55.4	Attention to other artificial opening of digestive tract
V55.5	Attention to cystostomy
V55.6	Attention to other artificial opening of urinary tract
V58.3	Attention to surgical dressing and sutures
V58.4	Other aftercare following surgery

PART TEN
Resources

Abbreviation List

ABD	Abdomen
AC	Before Meals
ADL	Activities of Daily Living
ADR	Adverse Drug Reaction
ADR	Additional Development Request
ad lib	As Desired
AHCPR	Agency for Health Care Policy and Research
AIDS	Acquired Immune Deficiency Syndrome
AKA	Above Knee Amputation
ALJ	Administrative Law Judge
ALS	Amyotrophic Lateral Sclerosis
AM	Morning
AMB	Ambulatory
AMI	Acute Myocardial Infarction
AOTA	American Occupational Therapy Association
APHA	American Public Health Association
APTA	American Physical Therapy Association
ASCVD	Arteriosclerotic Cardiovascular Disease
ASD	Atrial Septal Defect
ASHA	American Speech-Language-Hearing Association
ASHD	Arteriosclerotic Heart Disease
BBA	Balanced Budget Act (of 1997)
BID	Twice a Day
BKA	Below Knee Amputation
BM	Bowel Movement
BP	Blood Pressure
BPH	Benign Prostatic Hypertrophy
BR	Bathroom
BRP	Bathroom Privileges
BS	Blood Sugar
C (centigrade)	Celsius
CA	Cancer
CABG	Coronary Artery Bypass Graft
CAP	Correction Action Plan
CARF	Commission on Accreditation of Rehabilitation Facilities

CBC	Complete Blood Count
cc	Cubic Centimeter
CDC	Centers for Disease Control (and Prevention)
CHAP	Community Health Accreditation Program
CHF	Congestive Heart Failure
CHHA	Certified Home Health Aide
CLIA	Clinical Laboratory Improvement Act
cm	Centimeter
CNS	Clinical Nurse Specialist
CO_2	Carbon Dioxide
COPD	Chronic Obstructive Pulmonary Disease
COPs	(Medicare) Conditions of Participation
COTA	Certified Occupational Therapy Assistant
CPAP	Continuous Positive Airway Pressure
CPM	Continuous Passive Motion
CPR	Cardiopulmonary Resuscitation
CQI	Continuous Quality Improvement
C/S	Cesarean Section
C & S	Culture and Sensitivity
CVA	Cerebral Vascular Accident
CVC	Central Venous Catheter
CWF	Common Working File
CXR	Chest X Ray
DC	Discharge/Discontinue
DJD	Degenerative Joint Disease
DM	Diabetes Mellitus
DME	Durable Medical Equipment
DMERC	Durable Medical Equipment Regional Carriers
DNI	Do Not Intubate
DNR	Do Not Resuscitate
DOE	Dyspnea on Exertion
DRG	Diagnosis Related Group
DVT	Deep Vein Thrombosis
DX	Diagnosis
ECG (EKG)	Electrocardiogram
ED	Emergency Department
EOC	Episode of Care
ER	Emergency Room
ESRD	End-Stage Renal Disease
ET	Enterostomal Therapist
F	Fahrenheit

FBS	Fasting Blood Sugar
FHR	Fetal Heart Rate
FI	Fiscal Intermediary
FMR	Focused Medical Review
FX	Fracture
GI	Gastrointestinal
G-tube (GT)	Gastronomy Tube
gtts.	Drops
GU	Genitourinary
H2O	Water
HCFA	Health Care Financing Administration
HCPCS	HCFA Common Procedure Coding System
HEP	Home Exercise Program
HHA	Home Health Aide (or Home Health Agency)
HHC	Home Health Care
HHS	Health and Human Services
HICN	Health Insurance Claim Number
HIM	Health Insurance Manual
HME	Home Medical Equipment
HMO	Health Maintenance Organization
HOB	Head of Bed
HOH	Hard of Hearing
HR	Heart Rate
@hs	At Bedtime
hs	Hour of Sleep
HTN	Hypertension
IADL	Instrumental Activities of Daily Living
IDDM	Insulin Dependent Diabetes Mellitus
IDG	Interdisciplinary Group
IDT	Interdisciplinary Team
IG	Inspector General
IM	Intramuscular
I & O	Intake and Output
IPPB	Intermittent Positive Pressure Breathing
IPS	Interim Payment System
IV	Intravenous
JCAHO	Joint Commission on Accreditation of Healthcare Organizations
L	Left
LLE	Left Lower Extremity
LLL	Left Lower Lung

LLQ	Left Lower Quadrant
LOC	Level of Consciousness
LOS	Length of Stay
LPN	Licensed Practical Nurse
LUE	Left Upper Extremity
LUQ	Left Upper Quadrant
LVN	Licensed Vocational Nurse
MBS	Modified Barium Swallow
MI	Myocardial Infarction
MNT	Medical Nutrition Therapist
MOW	Meals on Wheels
MS	Multiple Sclerosis
MSS	Medical Social Services
MSW	Medical Social Work
MT	Massage Therapist
NG Tube	Nasogastric Tube
NHP	Nursing Home Placement
NICU	Neonatal Intensive Care Unit
NIDDM	Non-insulin Dependent Diabetes Mellitus
NOC	Night Time
NIH	National Institutes of Health
NPO	Nothing By Mouth
NSAIDS	Nonsteroidal Antiinflammatory Drugs
NTG	Nitroglycerine
O2	Oxygen
OASIS	Outcome and Assessment Information Set
OBRA	Omnibus Budget Reconciliation Act
OBG	OASIS Based Grouping
OBS	Organic Brain Syndrome
OD	Right Eye
OIG	Office of the Inspector General
OOB	Out of Bed
ORT	Operation Restore Trust
OS	Left Eye
OSHA	Occupational Safety and Health Administration
OT	Occupational Therapist
OTA	Occupational Therapy Assistant
P	Pulse
PCA	Patient-Controlled Analgesia
PERLA	Pupils Equal, React to Light and Accommodation
PI	Performance Improvement

PICC (line)	Peripherally Inserted Central Catheter
PKU	Phenylketonuria
PM	Afternoon
PO	By Mouth (orally)
POC	Plan of Care
POS	Point of Service
POT	Plan of Treatment
PPO	Preferred Provider Organization
PPS	Prospective Payment System
PRE	Progressive Resistive Exercises
PRN	As Needed
PT	Physical Therapy
PTA	Physical Therapist Assisant
PVD	Peripheral Vascular Disease
q	Every
qhs	Every Bedtime
QD	Every Day
QID	Four Times a Day
QOD	Every Other Day
qs	Quantity Sufficient
qt	Quart
R	Right or Respirations
Rehab	Rehabilitation
RHHI	Regional Home Health Intermediary
RLE	Right Lower Extremity
RLL	Right Lower Lung
RO	Regional Office
R/O	Rule Out
ROM	Range of Motion
RN	Registered Nurse
RR	Respiratory Rate
RSDS	Reflex Sympathetic Dystrophy Syndrome
RUE	Right Upper Extremity
Rx	Prescription
SL (sl)	Sublingual
SLP	Speech-Language Pathology (or Pathologist)
SNF	Skilled Nursing Facility
SNV	Skilled Nursing Visit
SOB	Shortness of Breath
SOC	Start of Care
SOM	State Operations Manual

S/P	Status Post
SQ	Subcutaneous
SR	Side Rail
SSA	Social Security Administration
ST	Speech Therapist
STAT	Immediately
STD	Sexually Transmitted Disease
SX	Symptoms
T	Temperature
TB	Tuberculosis
TBS	Tablespoon
TC	Telephone Call
TENS	Transcutaneous Electrical Nerve Stimulation
TF	Tube Feeding
TIA	Transient Ischemic Attack
TID	Three Times a Day
Title XVIII	The Medicare Section of the Social Security Act
Title XIX	The Medicaid Section of the Social Security Act
Title XX	The Social Services Section of the Social Security Act
TKR	Total Knee Replacement
TO	Telephone Order
TPN	Total Parenteral Nutrition
TPR	Temperature, Pulse, Respirations
TSP	Teaspoon
TURP	Transurethral Resection of Prostate
TX	Treatment
UA/C&S	Urinalysis/Culture and Sensitivity
UB	Universal Billing (form)
UE	Upper Extremity
up ad lib	Up as Desired
UPIN	Unique Physician Identification Number
URI	Upper Repiratory Infection
UTI	Urinary Tract Infection
VAD	Vascular Access Devices
VF	Video fluoroscopy
VO	Verbal Order
VS	Vital Signs
WFL	Within Functional Limits
WIC	Women, Infants, and Children Program
WNL	Within Normal Limits

Glossary of Terms

Access The ability of an individual to receive health care, encompassing cost, location, and transportation.

Accreditation A rigorous and labor-intensive process that examines various components of home care, hospice or other site operations and clinical practice and meets predetermined standards as measured by on-site survey team members. It is a process that an organization or program undertakes to demonstrate it has met established standards or requirements (e.g., the Joint Commission on Accreditation of Health Care Organizations [JCAHO] Standards or the Home Health and the Community Health Accreditation Program [CHAP]).

Activities of Daily Living (ADL) Basic, usually self-care directed activities that must be performed daily to care for bodies and overall health. These activities include personal hygiene tasks such as bathing, grooming, dressing, and eating/feeding, obtaining and preparing food. Other ADL include toileting and transfers. They are important indicators because they demonstrate or show the patient's functional status or health care needs relative to the patient's level of functional independence.

Acuity The degree of disease or injury before a patient receives treatment. The measurement of this degree determines the amount of health care resources projected to be expended on this patient (e.g., nursing care or placement in a specialized care unit).

Adaptive Devices Equipment designed to modify a patient/client's environment to improve their ability to perform a movement or activity. Examples of adaptive devices include an elevated commode seat, an adaptive spoon/fork, and elastic shoe laces.

Adjusted Average Per Capita Cost (AAPCC) An estimate of the total payment for services a managed care payer would make for a unique category of services, divided by the number of beneficiaries eligible for the services. This estimate is usually used in negotiating capitated agreements.

Admission/Evaluation/Assessment Visit The initial evaluation or admission visit is the visit that essentially determines the patient/client course of care and the decision to admit to the organization. The roles of the professional nurse or therapist at this visit includes the explanation of the organization's unique program and services and explanations of various important information including the Patient/Client Bill of Rights, Advanced Directive status, and others.

Advance Directive(s) A legal document that allows an individual to give directions about future medical care or to designate another person(s) to make such medical decisions if he/she has lost his/her decision-making abilities. Advance directives may include living wills, durable powers of attorney for health care, or similar documents relaying the patient's wishes. The Patient Self-Determination Act of 1990 mandates that certain health care providers query patients, at the time of admission to the specific agency or facility, regarding their status with advance directives and whether or not they need assistance in generating one.

Advocacy A role assumed by a health care professional designed to maximize patient self-determination through education, support, and affirmation of patient health care decisions.

Agency for Health Care Policy and Research (AHCPR) An agency of the U.S. Department of Health and Human Services that sponsors research projects and develops clinical practice guidelines related to the delivery of health care services. Topics include pain, wound care, sickle cell disease, and others. This free information can be accessed by calling (800) 358-9295.

Alaryngeal Speech Referring to speech techniques achieved without the larynx (or voice box), post-laryngectomy speech.

Alternative Delivery Systems Organizations where health care services are provided, other than acute care settings or hospitals.

Aphasia Absence or impairment of the ability to communicate through verbal or written language or signing, due to neurological lesion(s). Aphasia may be expressive, referring to impairment in conveying information, or receptive, referring to impairment in receiving and understanding information.

Apraxia Inability to perform purposeful motor skills, caused by damage to the central nervous system.

Arthroplasty Surgical correction of a joint, as in hip or knee joint replacement.

Assessment The systematic review and analysis of data from a multitude of sources, assisting in the identification of needs, abilities, and available resources.

Assistive Devices Equipment designed to improve or increase a client/patient's ability to perform a movement or activity. Examples of assistive devices are wheelchairs, walkers, canes, reachers, adaptive eating utensils, splints, electro-larynx, communication boards/picture boards, etc.

Autonomy   The ability of individuals who are capable of sound decision-making to outline their own choices about health care and lifestyle options. Respect for clients as individuals who are capable of making their own choices about health care and lifestyle options.

Availability   The degree to which appropriate care and services are available to meet a patient's assessed need(s).

Balance   The ability to recognize and control body motion/equilibrium. Static balance refers to the ability to maintain equilibrium while stationary. Dynamic balance refers to the ability to maintain equilibrium while moving (i.e. walking, transferring, etc.)

Balanced Budget Act of 1997   The legislation passed that made numerous changes and budget cuts to the Medicare program, including the implementation of a prospective payment system (PPS) for home care.

Barium Swallow   A procedure utilizing radiographic examination of the esophagus during and after introduction of a contrast medium (barium). Structural abnormalities of the esophagus and vessels may be diagnosed during this procedure using videofluoroscopic techniques. See also Modified Barium Swallow Study (MBS).

Benchmark   A systematic process to measure or quantify; a standard for comparing two similar types of products and services when trying to identify areas for improvement in an organization.

Beneficiary   A Medicare patient or the consumer of Medicare care or services.

Capitated Risk   The financial risk involved in not being able to accurately estimate the cost of and contract appropriately for care or services to a capitated population.

Capitation   A set dollar amount established to cover the cost of health care services delivered to an individual as part of a larger beneficiary group. The cost is based on the number of members in the plan and budgeted use of services. It is usually expressed as per member per month PMPM. Calculation: Annual Utilization Rate X Unit Cost/12 = Cost PMPM.

Care Coordination   The process utilized by the multidisciplinary clinical team and the patient/client and/or caregivers in the development of a viable, realistic, outcome-based plan of care. Care coordination may be formalized in a care planning conference or be informal between two or more individuals and documented in the clinical record.

Caregiver Anyone who provides or assists in the care or services to or for a patient.

Care Plan A plan of action for care that is developed, delivered, and evaluated by a nurse, therapist, or other team member. This may also be called the plan of care, and its format may vary among organizations.

Case Management The supervision of the care given to a specific patient or caseload population. A system for overseeing patient care and resource utilization across health care systems. For example, a nurse or therapist case manager may coordinate care and services from the hospital, to the nursing home, and to the patient's home. A system of patient care delivery that focuses on the achievement of outcomes within effective and appropriate time frames and use of resources. Case management attempts to control the quality and cost of patient care and focuses on an entire episode of illness, crossing all settings in which the patient receives care. Case management incorporates the principles of managed care. In home health care, this is often a care model with the nurse or therapist case manager rendering the skilled care, supervising, or collaborating with other ordered professional services. Communication among the services and disciplines involved in the care must be documented in the clinical record.

Case (Care) Manager One person who is responsible for the overall care of the patient and for the use of resources for that care. The case (or care) manager may be a nurse, a social worker, or a therapist and is the primary person responsible for developing patient care outcomes for his or her case load. A case manager is accountable for meeting outcomes within an appropriate length of stay, effective use of resources, and pre-established standards, and he or she collaborates with the health care team and the patient to accomplish those outcomes.

Case Mix The distribution of different types of patients seen at a health care setting; a collection of case types.

Case Mix Adjustment A methodology to ensure that agencies are not penalized for serving a mix of patients whose care needs are more expensive than those of the group on which the predetermined payment rate is based, and to eliminate the incentive for agencies to reject patients who may require unusual or higher resource utilization (e.g., visits, services, etc.)

Case Mix Report A graphical or tabular document that provides average values for patient attributes at start of care. Comparative data are provided for either 1) agency case mix for a prior time period, 2) case mix for a reference sample of patients from other agencies, or 3) both of the above.

Case Type A system that groups patients based on the different types (mix) of diagnoses (cases) for which its patients are treated.

Chronic A slow or persistent illness or health problem that must be cared for throughout life. Examples include diabetes, congestive heart failure, glaucoma, and some chronic lung conditions.

Claims Denials Payment for services is refused by the insuring organization. Reasons for this may be due to the frequency of service, providing a noncovered service, use of an invalid procedure code, lack of physician signature, failure to document homebound status of patient, and many others.

Classification System A system of categorizing elements of similar groups using pre-established criteria.

Client The one who receives care and who may be called the patient, customer, or consumer of health care services or products.

Clinical Care All of the events that encompass the diagnosis and treatment of illness and the attainment of specific patient outcomes; it is also the interaction of the health care team members and the physician working with the patient and the patient's family to meet predetermined clinical outcomes.

Clinical (Critical) Path(way) (CP) A clinical management tool that organizes, sequences, and times the major interventions of nursing staff, physicians, rehabilitation therapists, and other health professionals for a particular case type, condition or functional diagnosis. They identify and standardize tools and information, interventions, and processes for achieving pre-determined outcomes and quantifiable goals of care. Their development is similar to project management wherein certain key processes are mapped out on a diagram that can be used to monitor the effectiveness of the plan and determine the progress of the project through a process of quality improvement to positively impact and improve patient care. The pathways may structure a plan for care and describe a standard of practice and are, in essence, a clinical budget.

Clinical Record The record that chronicles the patient/client's stay throughout the course of care while on the home care organization's service roster. The importance of the home care clinical record is that it is the one source that houses the specific clinical information and entries that is used to make payment (or denial) determinations, facilitate regulatory compliance, for examples, Medicare certification or coverage compliance reviews, and is the source for communication among team members to help assure the safe provision of patient/client centered care.

Coinsurance The amount of percentage of the cost of services that beneficiaries may be required to pay under a cost-sharing agreement with their insurance plan or program. It may also be called a copayment.

Collaboration The active process of team members working together and valuing each other's input toward reaching common patient goals. In health care, collaboration is a joint effort of staff from many disciplines who work together to improve the processes, leading to improved patient care.

Competency The quantifiable ability of an individual to perform a task to established criteria.

Conditions of Participation (COPs) The framework and standards used to survey home care, hospice or other Part A organizations. Organizations must be in compliance with these standards or face sanctions, penalties and risk losing their Medicare certification. The ongoing demonstration of compliance with the COPs is the challenge for the entire team. Many of the conditions are related to the clinical information, such as forms, housed in the home care clinical record.

Continuous Passive Motion (CPM) A therapeutic technique involving use of a machine (CPM machine) which supports one or more body parts and provides continuous passive motion to one or more joints. CPM use for early post-operative knee rehabilitation is common in home care.

Continuous Quality Improvement (CQI) An ongoing process that seeks to continuously improve patient care, delivery of services, staff education, and other important segments of an organization's operations or other parts of an organization. Accreditation and Medicare requirements demand continuous quality improvement. It is a conceptual framework for evaluating the quality of care emphasizing an analytical approach to understanding the contributions of all components of the health care system in achieving results and constantly incorporating improvements into the system.

Continuum of Care The array of health care services available to an individual based on the assessed need of the patient and provided at the most appropriate level of care.

Contracture A permanent shortening or tightening of a muscle, resulting from spasm, atrophy due to paralysis or immobility, resulting in abnormal, reduced range of motion and fixed position of one or more joints.

Coordination The systematic and efficient function of various muscles and/or systems which produces controlled, purposeful and intended movement. Often relates or refers to fine-motor skills of the hand.

Cost-Based Reimbursement Historical method of reimbursement to health care providers based on the aggregation of allowable costs, up to a certain limit (e.g., cost caps.)

Cost Reimbursement The methodology historically used by the Health Care Financing Administration to pay providers for Medicare home health benefits. The reimbursement is based on the cost of care, and profit is not included. Settlement is accomplished through the submission of a cost report to the organization's fiscal intermediary.

Cost Shifting The act of increasing rates to one segment of the patient population to offset losses incurred by another segment, such as Medicaid recipients.

Criteria Established standards that performance or any other measure is judged against.

Daily Medicare defines daily as 7 days a week. The only exception to daily is insulin injections, and other patients who receive daily care must have a realistic, projected end date.

Data Products of measurement (singular form: datum) compiled in such a fashion that discussion can be formulated or inference can be obtained.

Data Entry Entry of data from a paper (clinical record) form into a software package that contains the appropriate data entry fields for the form. Data entry ("encoding") of OASIS items typically consists of entering a single numeric value corresponding to the response selected on the form.

Data Editing After an OASIS record has been entered, it is possible to detect various types of errors and edit (or update) the contents of the record. Editing is normally done only if errors are discovered in the data. Edit-checking software provides the most convenient method for determining whether errors exist in an OASIS data file.

Data Tracking Refers to the process of keeping track of the various records that comprise an episode of care for an individual patient according to the OASIS data collection protocol. In order to compute outcome measures, it is necessary to have complete data from start of care until discharge. This includes such intervening time points as assessments performed at 60-day intervals, transfer to an inpatient facility, and resumption of care after an in-patient stay. Tracking systems (whether paper- or computer-based) rely on key patient identifying information to match the records that form an episode of care. Key identifying information in the OASIS includes patient ID number, Medicare number, last name, date of birth, and start of care date.

Decubitus Ulcer An area of redness or skin breakdown possibly affecting surrounding tissues, usually over a bony prominence and related to immobility. The revised, new term is pressure ulcer.

Dementia A progressive disorder of changes in brain function that cause memory loss, confusion, personality changes, disorientation, impaired judgment and/or the loss of ability to safely function independently.

Deviation In mathematics, deviation is an abnormality or departure from the norm; statistically, a deviation is the difference in absolute numbers between one number in the set and the calculated mean of the set.

Diagnoses The identification of problems or diseases.

Diagnostic-Related Groups (DRGs) A code of classifying patient illnesses according to principal diagnosis and treatment requirements. Under Medicare, each DRG has its own price (weight) that a hospital is paid regardless of the actual cost of treatment.

Dialysis The process of artificially cleansing the blood when the patient has renal or kidney failure. There are two kinds of dialysis, hemodialysis and peritoneal dialysis.

Dietitian A member of the health care team who promotes optimal nutrition, based on the patient's individual needs. The dietitian may be called a registered dietitian (RD) or a licensed dietitian (LD). The dietitian may make home visits or teach the other team members about dietary related issues such as effective nutrition, meal preparation, and special diets.

The role of the professional, registered dietitian in home care is expanding as more patients are cared for in the community setting. Many home health agencies and hospices have professional dietitians available to make home visits and provide consultative services to promote optimal patient nutrition. Another important component of the dietitian's role is an in-service educator for the home health and hospice team.

Distal Away from the center or medial line. The opposite of proximal.

Documentation The writing of clinical notes that contain information needed for patient status communication reflecting clinical, legal, and/or other issues.

Dysarthria Impaired control of muscles of speech, reduced breath support, weakness in the speech articulators, resulting in decreased speech intelligibility caused by damage to the central or peripheral nervous system usually caused by neurological damage.

Dysnomia Word finding difficulties. A form of expressive aphasia caused by damage to the central nervous system.

Dysphagia Impaired swallowing.

Dysphasia Impaired speech resulting from a neurological lesion.

Dyspraxia A motor sequencing problem caused by damage to the central nervous system; less severe than apraxia.

Edema An abnormal accumulation of fluid causing swelling in a particular part of the body. For example, the patient with swelling in the ankles or feet has edema.

Edit Checks The OASIS items define a set of rules (both explicit and implicit) for what can be considered logical responses to individual items or a set of related items. Edit checks are the formal specification of these rules. Some common types of edit checks are range checks (to determine if a response falls within the range of acceptable values for a given item), missing data checks, and checks for logical inconsistencies (both within an individual item and between two or more items). Edit-checking software runs a large number of edit checks on an OASIS data file and generates a report listing any data collection rules that have been violated for each specific patient.

Effective Management A health care management style that shares the focus of patient care with administration of the program and effectively seeks improvement through the simplification and review of all systems involved in care or service delivery.

Electrotherapeutic Modalities A broad group of treatment procedures which utilize electricity to produce a therapeutic effect. Examples include electrical muscle stimulation and ultrasound.

Encounter Data Data on the use of products or services (usually expressed in units or a dollar value) by a given population.

End-Result Feedback A review of a specific process or series of processes; the end results are integrated into the input information to effect a change in the ongoing process.

Enteral Nutrition Provision of nourishment via a tube inserted either through the nose and into the stomach or through a surgical site and into the stomach. A G-tube is an example of a device used to deliver enteral nutrition.

Enterostomal Therapy (ET) A nurse specialist with special education and training who cares for patients with wounds or who assists other nurses and team members to care for these patients. The ET nurse may also visit patients who have an ostomy, a urinary or fecal diversion from usual function, or other skin challenges.
   Some HHAs have an ET nurse available to their nurses as a consultant and clinical specialist. This role is particularly important in the HHA and in hospice settings with a high volume of patients with ostomy and wound problems. The clinical specialist role is also important in that the educational needs of the clinical visiting staff and community are served.

Environmental Barriers Physical obstacles that practically or potentially limit client/patient function in a given setting. In the home, environmental barriers may include pets, narrow doorways, inadequate lighting, unsafe flooring, etc.

Equity of Care A health care system that differentiates levels of care based on assessed patient needs, not on individual or group characteristics (e.g., ability to pay).

Evaluation Visit (Assessment Visit) This is the first or initial home visit to determine whether the patient meets the organization's criteria for admission. In home care, it is oftentimes the first skilled visit, made when the therapist or nurse already has specific physician's orders and is providing a skilled service to the patient.

Extended Care Services Patient care services provided as an alternative to inpatient hospitalization, either in a skilled nursing facility, rehabilitation facility, or subacute facility after an acute illness or injury.

Fee for Service A health plan in which beneficiaries choose their health care provider and the health plan pays the provider's charge for services. This type of plan usually includes some element of utilization review or prior approval by the plan for certain, if not all, services.

Flaccidity A lack of normal muscle tone resulting in weak or flabby tone and usually due to neurological lesion(s).

Focused Medical Review (FMR) This is the targeting or directing of medical review efforts by the regional home health intermediary (RHHI) in an attempt to identify providers who may be providing inappropriate or noncovered care. Often this review takes place long after the care has been provided; hence a paid claim is not necessarily a covered claim. *That is why the documentation must be accurate and complete and support covered care.*

Fraud Medicare defines fraud as making false statements or representations of material facts in order to obtain some benefit or payment for which no entitlement would otherwise exist. Fraud is the intentional deception or misrepresentation to the government, including incorrect reporting of diagnoses or procedures to maximize benefits, billing for beneficiaries who do not qualify for benefits (e.g., beneficiaries who are not homebound) and falsifying records to meet or continue to meet the Medicare Conditions of Participation. The number for the Medicare fraud hotline is (800) 447-8477.

Functional Communication The ability to convey and receive information, regardless of the method or mode.

Functional Limitation A restriction or impairment in the ability to perform a motion or activity in an efficient, independent, safe or typical manner.

G-Tube A stomach or gastrostomy tube used to place nutrients into the stomach when the patient cannot safely swallow or eat.

Gatekeeper The one who has the overall responsibility for a patient's course of care and reviews and approves or disapproves all requests for health care services. This role has traditionally been held by a physician but may be a managed care provider, a payer, or a subcontracted utilization review group.

Geriatrics Services or care related to or provided to the elderly; related to the process of aging.

Goals The endpoint of care or the desired results for care of an action or series of actions an individual or organization might strive for. For example, if the goal is to provide safe mobility, everything done should support that goal. Team members work together to achieve patient goals. A goal is different from an objective in that a goal is more broad-based. Objectives are more quantifiable and specific and are derived from a goal statement.

Goniometric Measurements A method of assessing the degree of joint range of motion using a calibrated measurement device called a goniometer.

Health Care Financing Administration (HCFA) An agency of the U.S. Government under the Department of Health and Human Services (HHS) responsible for the Medicare and Medicaid programs. This direction includes various requirements, policies, payment for services, and many other operational aspects of the programs. HCFA sets the coverage policy and payment and other guidelines and directs the activities of government contractors (e.g., carriers and fiscal intermediaries).

Health Education Training or education activities provided to patients to encourage lifestyle modifications, thereby reducing behavioral risk factors and improving health activities.

Health Maintenance Organization (HMO) A health care provider organization that offers a comprehensive health service plan to its beneficiaries through an established network of primary care physicians, specialists, clinics, and hospitals. It provides these services on a prepaid, fixed-cost basis.

Hemiplegia Paralysis or loss of motor ability to move one side of the body.

Health and Human Services (HHS) The United States Department of Health and Human Services that oversees the Health Care Financing Administration and the Medicare (federal) and Medicaid (state) programs.

Hip Precautions Medically imposed restrictions to the hip joint to prevent positions and stresses which would promote hip dislocation. Typical restrictions for hip precautions include avoidance of excessive hip flexion, hip adduction, and hip internal rotation.

Homebound A term used in the Medicare home care program that means the patient cannot leave the home without assistance. It means that leaving the home is a considerable and taxing effort that occurs infrequently and lasts for a short duration. Homebound means primarily confined to the home for medical reasons. "Homebound" is one of the eligibility criteria for Medicare-reimbursed home care, such as patients admitted to a home care program. For this reason, when patients are "no longer homebound," they are discharged from Medicare home care.

Home Care/Home Health The provision of a range of health services, products, supplies, and equipment to patients in their homes. Medicare currently reimburses skilled nursing, speech-language pathology, physical and occupational therapy, medical social work, and home health aide services.

Home Exercise Program (HEP) A series of activities, exercises, and/or tasks designed to achieve desired therapeutic and functional outcomes. The home exercise program is designed to be carried out by the patient, possibly with the assistance of a caregiver, on a regular and predetermined basis, to supplement the skilled treatment plan, or in an effort to extend or maintain therapeutic benefit after discontinuation of skilled services.

Home Health Agency (HHA) An organization that provides care to patients in their homes. The organization may or may not be licensed, depending on the state and its requirements. Medicare-certified agencies must have a survey or a special review in order to be certified to accept Medicare reimbursement. These agencies may or may not be licensed by a governmental health care organization (e.g., the department of health), depending on state statute. Medicare-certified organizations need additional review to be certified to accept Medicare patients and receive government payment for those services.

Home Health Aide (HHA) An individual trained specifically to provide personal care services and ADL assistance to a patient in his or her place of residence on an intermittent basis (by visit or by hour). This role and the associated functions are very important to the patient and family. The HHA usually spends more actual time with the patient and family than any other team member. The HHA's contribution is invaluable to both the team process and in achieving positive patient outcomes. The Medicare Conditions of Participation outline the specific competency criteria for home health aides that need to be adhered to in order to maintain compliance.

Hospice A special way of caring for patients with a terminal illness or a limited life expectancy. Hospice team members provide care for patients and their family members and try to make every remaining day the best that it can be. Hospice team members may include specially trained hospice volunteers, bereavement counselors, certified nursing assistants (CNAs) or hospice aides, spiritual counselors, nurses, therapists, and social workers. Hospice is a philosophy, not a place; most hospice care is provided at home but can be provided in any setting, such as in a skilled nursing facility or an inpatient hospice unit. Services are provided to patients with a documented terminal illness for whom the focus changes from curative intervention to palliative care. The service implies patient knowledge and acceptance of disease prognosis and life expectancy. Medicare coverage includes nursing care under the supervision of a registered nurse, medical social services under the direction of a physician, physician services, counseling services for the individual and caregivers, medical supplies, home health aide and homemaker services, and physical, occupational, and speech-language pathology therapy services. Other important hospice services include volunteer support, spiritual support, and bereavement counseling.

ICD-9 Code A coding methodology developed to identify specific clinical diagnoses for the purpose of data collection and payment.

Indemnity Insurance Plan An insurance plan that allows members to choose their own health care providers who are paid on a fee-for-service basis and are not usually controlled through prior authorization or utilization controls.

Interdisciplinary Approach An approach to clinical care requiring representatives from various disciplines (i.e. occupational therapy, nursing, speech-language pathology, physical therapy, social work, dietitian) to work collaboratively within a holistic and integrated treatment plan.

International Normalized Ratio (INR) The International Normalized Ratio is a mathematical "correction" of the results of the one-stage prothrobin time (PT). It is a common scale that standardizes PT ratio determinations worldwide.

Instrumental Activities of Daily Living (IADLs) Activities including shopping, cooking home cleaning and maintenance, financial management, and community access which require cognitive and physical abilities beyond the level of basic ADLs (bathing, dressing, eating, transfers). The level of independence in IADL is an important factor in determining a client/patient's ability to live alone.

Instrumental Care (Instrumental Activities of Daily Living [IADLs]) The provision of assistance with instrumental activities of daily living, such as shopping, cooking, transportation, financial management, homemaking, and home maintenance.

Integrated Delivery Network A provider of health care services that offers a wide continuum of services to its customer population. It usually comprises one or more acute care hospital(s), skilled and intermediate nursing facilities, outpatient and ambulatory surgery centers, home health care agency(ies), and physicians who are either employees of the group or are tightly controlled by utilization management techniques.

Interim Payment System (IPS) A cost-based reimbursement system enacted by the Balanced Budget Act of 1997. Under these guidelines, home care agencies are paid the lowest amount of 1) actual, allowable costs; 2) aggregate cost limit; or 3) aggregate per beneficiary annual limit.

Intermediate Care Facility (ICF) An organization licensed by state law and recognized under the Medicaid program to provide care to those individuals whose treatment regimen does not require the degree or skills necessary to justify placement in an acute or skilled care facility.

Intervention Any happening or event that interrupts or changes events in progress.

Iontophoresis A therapeutic procedure involving the introduction of ions into tissues by means of electric current, performed by a therapist.

Laryngeal Mirror A small (00) dental mirror used in thermal stimulation, a technique to improve or trigger a reflexive swallow. Used in swallowing therapy.

Laryngectomy Surgical removal of the voicebox resulting in the loss of normal speech ability.

Larynx A musculocartilaginous structure located at the upper end of the trachea. The organ of voice.

Length of Stay (LOS) The number of hospital or home care days for each patient. Each patient's hospitalization is subject to review to determine the appropriateness of the length of stay (ALOS - average length of stay).

Licensure A legal right granted by a government agency complying with state statute allowing an individual (e.g., registered nurse, licensed vocational nurse, physical therapist) and/or an organization (e.g., hospital, skilled nursing facility, home health agency) the ability to practice or operate in a certain specialty or geographic area.

Long-Term Care A variety of health services provided to individuals with physical or mental disabilities needing assistance on a continuing basis. These services can be provided in a multitude of settings (e.g., homes, subacute skilled nursing facilities, retirement facilities, assistive living centers, intermediate care facilities, and senior day care).

Maintenance Continued services or activities provided to a patient/client with a chronic condition in efforts to avoid or minimize deterioration.

Managed Care A system of health care that has been designed and implemented to manage the delivery of services in such a way that limited resources are controlled. Care that is organized to achieve specific patient outcomes within fiscally responsible timeframes (length of stay) using resources that are appropriate in amount and sequenced to the specific case type and population of the individual patient. Care may be structured by case management care plans and clinical paths that are based on knowledge by case type regarding usual length of stay, critical events and their timing, anticipated outcomes, and resource use.

Managed Care Plan or Organization (MCP or MCO) Any organization providing a network of patient care services, including physician and clinic or hospital care, for a set, agreed-upon payment, using cost-containment measures.

Management and Evaluation of the Plan of Care (POC) This Medicare service is called various things, including skilled management, skilled planning and assessment, skilled management and planning, case management, and M and E of the patient POC. This is a Medicare-reimbursable program for home health patients (Part A) whose unskilled care needs are an inherent part of their medical treatment. The unskilled care needs are so complex that the involvement of skilled nursing and/or therapy services to monitor the outcomes of the provision of that care are deemed necessary to promote the patient's recovery and medical safety.

Massage Therapy   A hands-on therapeutic intervention characterized by massaging, rubbing or kneading parts of the body. Massage therapy focuses on increasing circulation, normalizing muscle tone and promoting relaxation.

Master Capitation   The primary holder of a capitated contract who may subcontract to other providers for services but remains financially at risk for the capitated contract.

Medicaid A health program that is administered at the state level for patients who qualify. The qualification is financial. Medicaid coverage varies by state, and sometimes even the name is different. For example, in California it is called MediCal.

Medical Social Worker (MSW) The medical social worker (MSW) provides services to support maximization of patient health and function through identification of financial or community access needs and referral to appropriate resources. Referral to social work services should be considered whenever a barrier to implementation of the care plan is present.

Medical Social Services (MSS) Social services in home health care and hospice are directly related to the patient's medical condition and support to the patient and family. When social concerns impede the effective implementation of the POC, a social worker may be appropriate. This may include finances, grief work, housing, and caregiver concerns. The services must be documented to focus on the patient, even though the social worker also assists the family, in conjunction with the patient in HHC. The social worker has an important role in assisting hospice patients and families through their unique situation and journey.

Medicare A federal program for people who are over the age of 65, disabled, or have end-stage renal disease (ESRD). Medicare has two parts, Part A and Part B, that cover different services such as inpatient hospitalization (after the Medicare beneficiary pays a deductible), home care, hospice, and other services. Medicare is a medical insurance program, and like all insurance programs there are exclusions, eligibility criteria, and specific coverage rules.

Medicare Health Maintenance Organization (HMO) (Senior Risk Program)
An alternative insurance product for Medicare beneficiaries that allows commercial insurers to contract with the Health Care Financing Administration to provide similar Medicare-covered services. Providers must have a contract with such insurers to provide beneficiary care. The advantages of such a program are that beneficiaries do not have to submit paperwork for payment, do not have to pay a co-payment or deductible, and may appear to have a richer benefit package, such as medications are "covered." However, beneficiaries are limited in the number of providers they may go to for services and in the number or types of services allowed.

Modified Barium Swallow Study A video radiographic examination utilizing barium mixed with different food textures to access the oral and pharyngeal stages of the swallow and to assist in evaluating aspiration.

OASIS (Outcome and ASsessment Information Set) A set of data items developed largely for purpose of measuring (and risk adjusting) patient outcomes in home health care. OASIS items include sociodemographic, physiologic, and mental/behavioral/emotional health status, functional status, and service utilization information. Since the OASIS is used for measuring outcomes, most data items are obtained at start of care and follow-up time points (i.e., recertification and discharge). The OASIS in not a comprehensive assessment but is intended to be integrated into agency clinical record forms. OASIS is a compilation of patient-related data items to be used for outcomes-based quality improvement (OBQI) activities and in creating the basis for PPS reimbursement in home health. The original pilot selected 50 Medicare-certified home care organizations across the nation. HCFA mandated the OASIS use in rules published in the January and June 1999 *Federal Registers.*

Occupational Safety and Health Administration (OSHA) The department of the U.S. Government that regulates employee or worker safety. OSHA requires that various standards be maintained related to health care.

Occupational Therapy (OT) Occupational therapy is one of the six Medicare-covered home health services. OT focuses on quality of life and helping the patient to function more independently. Areas of expertise include fine motor coordination, perceptual-motor skills, sensory testing, adaptive/assistive equipment, ADLs, and specialized upper extremity/hand function. The occupational therapist may be called in for a home safety assessment, to identify needed adaptive or assistive devices that make the patient safer at home, teach energy conservation techniques to patients with shortness of breath, teach adaptive transfers, and many other reasons. The kinds of problems frequently addressed by the OT include CVAs, amputations, arthritis, joint replacements, and pulmonary and cardiac limitations. In the Medicare home care program, OT is not a qualifying skilled service that can initiate services. However, when a patient has already been receiving another skilled service, such as nursing or physical therapy, and the patient no longer needs these services, the occupational therapist can continue to provide covered OT services.

Office of the Inspector General (OIG) By law, the OIG's mission is to protect the integrity of the U.S. Department of Health and Human Services programs and the health and welfare of beneficiaries served by these programs. This is done through a nationwide program of audits, investigations, surveys, inspections, sanctions, and fraud alerts. The Inspector General informs the Secretary of Health and Human Services of program and management problems and recommends legislative, regulatory, and operational approaches to correct them.

Operation Restore Trust (ORT) This is an effort by the government to combat and identify health care fraud. Activities may include on-site and intensive chart reviews to see if patients admitted and billed to Medicare or Medicaid met (or did not meet) coverage or program requirements. This includes whether patients were homebound or needed skilled care. In this environment it is imperative that clinicians practicing in home and hospice care know the rules related to care, coverage, and documentation requirements.

Orthotic Devices Mechanical appliances designed to support and position weak, injured, or ineffective joints and/or muscles. Examples of orthotics include casts, splints, and braces.

Outcome-Based Quality Improvement (OBQI)   A framework for demonstrating quantifiable quality to payers, consumers and others. The OASIS data elements are a component of HCFA's OBQI initiative. OBQI is a two-stage improvement approach, premised on the principle that patient outcomes are central to continuous quality improvement. The first stage begins with collecting uniform patient health status data and culminates with an outcome report that reflects agency performance by comparing the agency's outcomes to those of a reference group of patients (which could be patients from a prior period at the same agency). The second state (or the outcome enhancement stage) consists of selecting target outcomes for follow up. It entails conducting an investigation to determine key care behaviors that influence these target outcomes, culminating with the development and implementation of a plan of action to remedy substandard care practices or reinforce exemplary care practices. The effects of implementing the plan of action are evaluated in the next outcome report.

Outcome Criteria   The ends to be achieved. From a knowledge of the usual course of events and the factors relevant to the patient group involved, the clinician should be able to determine the desired results that, in a given patient at the end of a program or service of care, were based on knowledge about the needs of this group of patients and carried out in a fashion adequate to achieve its purpose.

Outcome Measure   A quantification of a change in health status between two or more time points. In OBQI, outcomes measures are computed utilizing OASIS data from start of care and from subsequent time points or discharge. Two common types of outcome measures used in OBQI pertain to improvement in or stabilization of a specific health status attribute.

Outcome Report   A graphical or tabular document that compares an agency's patient outcomes for a given time period to either 1) analogous agency-level outcomes for a prior time period, 2) outcomes for a reference sample of patients from other agencies, or 3) both of the above. An outcome report contains information on selected outcome measures for all patients in the agency, or for patients with specific conditions.

Outcomes   The effects of services provided to patients. Outcomes are quantifiable or measurable goals of care, measuring changes in the patient health status (including functional, physiologic, emotional and cognitive) between two or more time points, such as those on admission and discharge.

Outcomes, Clinical The results or effects of clinical processes on patients. The results may be described by outcome criteria.

Palliative Care Palliative care is the active total care of patients whose disease is not responsive to curative treatment. The goal of palliative care is to achieve the best quality of life for terminally ill patients. It is medically directed care with interdisciplinary care plan development and implementation, coordination with community services, family involvement, and use of volunteers.

Paraplegia Paralysis or loss of motor ability to move the lower extremities or legs.

Parenteral Nutrition The provision of nourishment via an intravenous (IV) route.

Patient The patient is the central member of the home care team. Effort should be made by the clinical staff to include the patient and family members in every appropriate facet of the care planning and delivery process. The level of involvement will vary, based on the individual patient's personality, desire and ability to participate in the process.

Payer The payer or insurance company financially responsible for the services or care provided to patients. Examples include Medicare and other insurance companies. The organization responsible for paying a health care provider for the health care products and/or services provided to a patient or beneficiary.

Pediatric or Pediatrics Services or care related to children. Pediatrics is a specialty that involves the development, care, and problems or diseases of children and childhood. This includes newborns, infants, toddlers, and all ages of children through adolescence.

Performance Improvement (PI) The ongoing review and revision of functions and processes within an organization focused on the improvement of those processes related to the provision of patient care and/or services.

Performance Measure Quantifiable standards or measurements to determine how successful a health care provider has been in meeting established outcomes or goals of care.

Personal Emergency Response System (PERS) A technology that links the frail, elderly, or homebound person to community resources, neighbors, or a friend in the case of a fall or other emergency. PERS may be appropriate for single patients returning home after surgery, patients who live alone or spend many hours at home alone, or for patients at risk from falls. PERSs usually have a personal help button that calls for help when activated. To be effective, the PERS personal help button must be worn by the person or be within reach at all times. Home care and hospice nurses and therapists are in a unique position to identify this safety need in the community setting, so a referral can be initiated.

Pharmacist The role of the clinical pharmacist in hospice and home care is growing, as the emphasis on quality and addressing patient needs from an inter-disciplinary model continues. In practice, clinicians are acutely aware of many patients who are inappropriately or overmedicated.

Many patients arc elderly and have multiple risk factors for therapeutic problems, secondary to drug therapy. They may have multiple pathologies, different prescribers, exhibit polypharmacy (both prescription and nonprescription medications), and are at a greater risk for adverse effects from medications due to altered physiology, secondary to aging and disabilities (i.e., poor eyesight, impaired hearing, arthritic fingers).

Physical Therapy (PT) A specialty of the rehabilitative services that focuses on optimal mobility and function of patients due to illness or injury and is one of the six Medicare-covered home health services. Physical therapist services usually are based on patient need and diagnosis. PT, like OT and SLP, should have a restorative or safety focus. The PT documentation must show progression toward a goal. PTs work with stroke patients, muscular dystrophy patients, and others who need home exercises or home exercise programs to restore safe mobility and function.

Physician The physician provides services of care-plan oversight for the home care patient, including initial certification of the plan of care, ongoing super-vision, modification, and recertification of the plan as needed. Throughout the home care admission, the physician is the formal "director" of the patient's care, utilizing direct assessment and verbal and written communication from the patient, family and home care staff to initiate changes in diagnoses, medications, and the treatment regimen.

Plan of Care (POC) The Plan of Care can be the 485 form, entitled the "Home Health Certification and Plan of Treatment." The *Home Health Agency Manual* (HCFA Pub.-11), uses the term "plan of care" to refer to the medical plan of treatment established by the physician with the assistance of home care clinicians.

Point of Service Clinical Documentation Software   Refers to software that permits paperless collection of assessment information such as OASIS. Such software runs on a laptop, hand-held, or other type of portable computer to provide a means for clinical staff to enter assessment information in the patient's home. Once entered, data are then transferred (or uploaded) to a central computer system that houses a master database. Information that will be needed for upcoming visits may also be downloaded to the portable computer prior to the visits. Data editing and tracking are needed even when using such software. Ideally, editing and tracking functions should be integrated with the data entry software (either on the portable or central computer system).

Policies   The formal description of how an organization defines, organizes, and carries out patient care functions. They are approved by the Governing Body of an organization.

Preferred Provider Organization (PPO)   A health services program that provides its members with services from contracted providers of care. Beneficiaries receive better cost coverage by using a contracted provider; they can use a noncontracted provider but will be responsible for a co-payment or an additional fee or service.

Pressure Ulcer   An area of redness or skin breakdown possibly affecting surrounding tissues, usually over a bony prominence and related to immobility.

Primary Prevention   Measures that actively promote health, prevent illness, and provide specific protection.

Process   A series of activities or events that are related and sequenced in such a way as to result in a prescribed or established patient outcome.

Professional Care   Home health services in which the boundaries of practice are determined by professional standards with a basis in scientific theory, research, or evidenced-based practice.

Proprioception   A sensation within the body which identifies the body or body parts regarding position in space and muscular activity.

Prospective Payment System (PPS)   The third-party payment system that establishes certain payment rates for services regardless of the actual cost of care provided. The Medicare diagnostic-related group system for inpatient acute care services is the most widely known example of this type of payment.

Prosthesis An artificial replacement of a missing body part used to promote and improve function or cosmesis. Examples of prostheses include artificial limbs, heart valves, total joint replacements or dentures.

Proximal Nearest to the center, or point of attachment. The opposite of distal.

Prothrobin Time (PT) Laboratory measurement of the time (in seconds) required for blood to clot.

Quadriplegia Paralysis or loss of motor ability to move all upper and lower extremities, i.e., both arms and legs.

Quality A degree of excellence that is organizationally defined. The achievement of individualized outcomes.

Quality Assessment/Improvement (QA/QI) The measurement or assessment of care that is provided to an individual or group.

Quality Improvement (QI) The implementation of an organized, continuous, data-driven evaluation and systems change process that focuses on patient rights, outcomes of care; patient, physician and provider satisfaction; and performance improvement.

Quality Indicator A specific, valid, and reliable measure of access, care outcomes, or satisfaction, or a measure of a process of care that has been empirically shown to be predictive of access, care outcomes, or satisfaction.

Range of motion (ROM) The degree or distance of available movement/motion in a joint or series of joints. Range of motion can be passive (PROM) meaning performed by something or someone other than the patient, active (AROM) meaning performed by the patient, assisted (AAROM) meaning performed by the patient with additional assistance provided, or resisted (RROM) meaning performed by the patient in the presence of externally applied resistance to motion and requires increased strength.

Ratio of Cost to Charges (RCC) Method of estimating the cost of care. Cost includes fixed (administrative) and variable (supplies). Ratio = cost/charges.

Rehabilitative Services/Rehabilitation Care The term used to describe the care and results of team members to restore function and mobility after illness or injury. Members of the rehabilitation team include the physical therapist, occupational therapist, and speech-language pathologist. When any of these services are indicated, based on patient need, diagnosis, and patient rehabilitation potential status, there must be sufficient documentation and communication among all services. This interdisciplinary case conferencing or care coordination should be reflected in the clinical record on an ongoing basis. The aide may have assignments related to the patient's rehabilitation program that the therapist or nurse may assign, based on the patient's individualized rehabilitation program and other assessed needs.

Resource Utilization The use of assets; the kinds and number of items (e.g., nursing hours, visits, supplies) used in performing patient care.

Respiratory Therapist The respiratory therapist (RT) administers services related to the patient's respiratory care and treatments. The RT services often include assessment (i.e., evaluation of airway disturbances), direct care and intervention activities (i.e., breathing exercises or inhalation treatments) and patient and family teaching (i.e., instruction in the use of devices such as nebulizers or ventilators).

Risk Adjustment The process of minimizing the effects of risk-factor differences when comparing outcome findings between two groups of patients. Two common risk adjustment methods are grouping/stratification and (multivariate) statistical procedures.

Risk Factor A patient condition or circumstance that (positively or negatively) influences the likelihood of a patient attaining the outcome.

Risk Pool An incentive pool of monies, over and above the direct payment made to a service provider, that is distributed to a determined number of providers if certain predetermined financial outcomes are met.

Secondary Care Early diagnosis measures and prompt interventions to limit disabilities.

Sentinel Event A significant or serious patient event or outcome that needs to be evaluated immediately. Sentinel events are commonly legal and risk management concerns.

Skilled Nursing Specialized services that, to be safe and effective, must be provided by a registered nurse or by a licensed vocational/practical nurse under the supervision of a registered nurse. Skilled nursing occurs when the nurse uses knowledge as a professional nurse to execute skills, render judgments, and evaluate process and outcome. The inherent complexity of the service or care to be provided, the condition of the patient, and the accepted standards of clinical practice must be considered when determining what is or is not skilled nursing care. If a nonprofessional can perform a particular function, it is probably not a skilled function. Teaching, assessment, and evaluation skills are some of the many areas of expertise that are classified as skilled services.

Social Work Services (SWS) Social work services, also called medical social services (MSS), is one of the six Medicare-reimbursed home health services and is a valuable service to patients and their families for a number of reasons. The social worker may be involved when there are problems that prevent the plan of care from being implemented. For example, if the patient has diabetes and cannot afford food or insulin or if there are family or other problems that are causing the patient to fail to improve or be in unsafe circumstances this may trigger a referral.

Speech-Language Pathology (SLP) Speech-language pathology involves working primarily with patients who have swallowing or communication problems following surgery or due to other problems, such as a stroke. Other patients that may need SLP services may have a tracheostomy, laryngectomy, or various neuromuscular diseases. Progress must be noted in the clinical documentation, and case conferencing must occur. It is important that the reason for homebound status be clearly and regularly identified in the clinical record.

Standards A level of performance or a set of conditions considered acceptable by some authority or by the individual or individuals. A *clinical standard of practice* may include generally-accepted interventions associated with specific patient conditions or diagnoses.

Structure The framework of an organization that supports and defines how the components of a process are bound together to meet or achieve a given outcome (e.g., in home health agencies, the policies, procedures, and clinical competency checklists and standards define in part how patient care will be delivered).

Sub-Capitation A subset of capitated monies set aside for a particular group of services (e.g., home care services under a hospital plan or home medical equipment as a sub-capitator to a home care organization).

Supervisory Visit   Supervisory visits are requirements of the Medicare home health program. The nurse or other designated clinician may visit the patient's home during the HHA's visit or when the aide is not at the home. Supervision is a standard practice in home and hospice care. This supervision helps to ensure quality of care for patients, and currently must be performed at least once every 2 weeks, as noted in the Medicare conditions of participation. This is not a covered service and may be an administrative expense. A supervisory visit becomes billable when a skilled service is performed during the course of a supervisory visit. For example, a bedridden patient has a pressure ulcer and the nurse changes the dressing after observing the HHA completing the bed/bath and reviewing the HHA assignment sheet. Where allowed by law, therapists may supervise HHAs. Similarly, where allowed by law, therapists may also supervise therapy assistants utilizing supervisory visits as one method of supervision.

Tertiary Prevention   Rehabilitative activities and measures that reduce impairments and disabilities, minimize suffering caused by departures from good health, and promote the patient's adjustment to immediate conditions.

Therapy Assistants   The home care team may include therapy assistants, who provide patient care under the direction and delegation of a supervising therapist. The physical therapist assistant (PTA) and the certified occupational therapy assistant (COTA) administer therapeutic treatments, in accordance with the physician's ordered care, the supervising therapist's instruction, agency policy, state regulation, professional scope of practice, payer requirements, and individual clinician competence.

Thermal Stimulation   A technique used in dysphagia (swallowing) therapy to stimulate and trigger a reflexive swallow. A small laryngeal mirror is dipped in ice water for this procedure.

Time Line   Identifies when an event or a series of events should occur and follows a preestablished and agreed upon framework for those events to happen or specific outcomes to be achieved.

Tracheostomy   Surgical creation of an opening in the skin to the trachea, the breathing tube.

Transcutaneous Electrical Nerve Stimulation (TENS)   A therapeutic technique utilizing electrical energy applied via skin surface electrodes to provide stimulation to cutaneous and peripheral nerves in efforts to modify pain perception.

Transfer The process of moving a body/person from one surface or location to another. Examples of transfers include moving from supine to sit, moving from a wheelchair to a bed, getting into a tub, or getting out of a car.

Ultrasound A therapeutic procedure utilizing high-frequency sound waves to produce heat, thus promoting circulation and healing.

Uniform Clinical Data Set A mandate from the Health Care Financing Administration (HCFA) that is a part of the peer review organization's (PRO) scope of work to ultimately provide HCFA with the data necessary to start defining Medicare research activities. This information is aggregated into 1800 data fields and provides health care data that are not currently being gathered or evaluated on a national level.

Utilization Management (UM) A program established by health care providers to assess efficiency and quality of patient care based on established criteria.

Validity The amount or degree to which an observed or measured outcome or event correlates with the criteria or event it was intended to measure.

Variance The difference between what is expected and what actually happens. Variances are differentiated by system (internal or external), practitioner, and patient.

STATE LICENSING INFORMATION

STATE	PT	SLP	OT
Alabama	Alabama Board of PT 400 S Union St., Ste 315 Montgomery, AL 36104 (334) 242-4064 Fax (334) 240-3288	Alabama Board of Examiners for Speech Pathology and Audiology 400 S. Union St. Montgomery, AL 36104 (334) 269-1434 Fax (334) 409-0680	Alabama Board of OT 64 Union St., Ste 734 Montgomery, AL 36130 (334) 353-4466
Alaska	State PT Board 333 Willoughmy Ave.- - 9th Floor Juneau, AK 99811 (907) 465-2551 Fax (907) 465-2974	Division of Occupational Licensing PO Box 110806 Juneau, AK 99811 (907) 465-2695 Fax (907) 465-2974	State of Alaska Dept of Commerce and Economic Development Div of Occupational Licensing State OT and PT Board PO Box D Juneau, AK 99811 (907) 465-2551 Fax (907) 465-2974
Arizona	Arizona State Board of PT Examiners 1400 W. Washington, Ste 230 Phoenix, AZ 85007 (602) 542-3095 Fax (602) 542-3093	Audiologists and Speech-Language Pathologists Licensing Program 1647 E Morten Ave., Ste 160 Phoenix, AZ 85020 (602) 255-1177 ext 4307 Fax (602) 255-1109	Arizona Board of OT Examiners 1400 W Washington St., Ste 240 Phoenix, AZ 85007 (602) 542-6784 Fax (602) 542-5469
Arkansas	Arkansas Board of PT 9 Shackleford Plaza Ste 1 Little Rock, AR 72211 (501) 228-7100 Fax (501) 228-5535	Arkansas Board of Examiners in Speech Pathology and Audiology 101 E Capitol, Ste 211 Little Rock, AR 72201 (501) 682-9180 Fax (501) 682-9181	Arkansas State Medical Medical Board 2100 Riverfront Drive Ste 200 Little Rock, AR 72202 (501) 296-1802 Fax (501) 296-1805
California	PT Board of California 1418 Howe Ave., Ste 16 Sacramento, CA 95825 (916) 263-2550 Fax (916) 263-2560	Speech Pathology and Audiology Examining Committee 1434 Howe Ave., Ste 86 Sacramento, CA 95825 (916) 263-2666 Fax (916) 263-2668	OT Associations of CA 2150 River Plaza Dr Ste 125 Sacramento, CA 95833 (916) 567-7000

STATE LICENSING INFORMATION

STATE	PT	SLP	OT
Colorado	PT Licensure 1560 Broadway, Ste 680 Denver, CO 80202 (303) 894-2440 Fax (303) 894-2821	Audiologists and Hearing Aid Dealers Registration 1560 Broadway, Ste 680 Denver, CO 80202 (303) 894-2464 Fax (303) 894-2821	Div of Registration Dept of Regulatory Agencies 1560 Broadway, Ste 1300 Denver, CO (303) 894-7690 Fax (303) 894-7692
Connecticut	Dept of Public Health PT Licensure 410 Capital Ave., MS#12HSR PO Box 340308 Hartford, CT 06134 (860) 509-7407 Fax (860) 509-7539	SLP and Audiology Licensure Dept of Health PO Box 340308 Hartford, CT 06134 (860) 509-7560	Dept of Public Health OT Licensure 410 Capital Ave. Mail Stop #12APP Hartford, CT 06134
Delaware	Examining Board of PTs Cannon Bldg., Ste 203 861 Silver Lake Blvd. Dover, DE 19904 (302) 739-4522 Fax (302) 739-2711	Board of Audiology, SLPs and HAD PO Box 1401 Cannon Bldg, Ste 203 Dover, DE 19903 (302) 739-4522, ext 215 Fax (302) 739-2711	DE State Board of OT Div of Professional Regulation Cannon Bldg, Ste 203 Dover, DE 19903 (302) 739-4522, ext 203 Fax (302) 739-2711
District of Columbia	DC Board of PT 825 N. Capital St. Washington, DC 20002 (202) 442-4778 Fax (202) 442-4830		DC Board of OT Dept of Consumer and Regulatory Affairs, OPLA-BCSD PO Box 37200 Washington, DC 20013 (202) 727-9794 Fax (202) 727-4087
Florida	PT State Board Dept. of Health, Medical Therapies, Psychology 2020 Capital Circle SE Bin #CO5 Tallahassee, Fl 32399 (850) 488-0595 Fax (850) 414-6860	Board of SLP and Audiology Dept of Health 1940 North Monroe Tallahassee, FL 32399 (850) 487-1129 Fax (850) 921-5389	Dept of Business and Professional Regulation OT Council Northwood Center 1940 N Monroe St. Tallhassee, FL 32399 (904) 488-0595 (904) 921-7865
Georgia	Georgia State Boar of PT State Examining Boards 166 Pryor St., SW Atlanta, GA 30303 (404) 657-2002 Fax (404) 651-9532	Georgia Board of Examiners for SLP and Audiology 166 Pryor St., SW Atlanta, GA 30303 (404) 656-3933 Fax (404) 651-9532	GA Board of OT Examining Board Division 166 Pryor St., SW Atlanta, GA 30303 (404) 656-3921 Fax (404) 651-9532

STATE LICENSING INFORMATION

STATE	PT	SLP	OT
Hawaii	Dept of Commerce and Consumer Affairs Professional and Vocational Licensing Div Board of PT 1010 Richards St. PO Box 3469 Honolulu, HI 96801 (808) 586-2696 Fax (808) 586-2874	Board of Speech Pathology and Audiology PO Box 3469 Honolulu, HI 96801 (808) 586-2693 Fax (808) 586-2689	Professional and Vocational Licensing Division Commerce and Consumer Affairs Dept PO Box 3469 Honolulu, HI 96801 (808) 586-3000 Fax (808) 586-2877
Idaho	Idaho Board of Medicine 280 N 8th St. Ste. 202 PO Box 83720 Boise, ID 83720 (208) 334-2822 Fax (208) 334-2801		ID State Board of Medicine PO Box 83720 280 N 8th St., Ste. 202 Boise, ID 83720 (208) 334-2822 Fax (208) 334-2801
Illinois	Dept of Professional Regulation 320 W. Washington, 3rd Fl. Springfield, IL 62786 (217) 782-0218 Fax (217) 782-7645	Illinois Dept of Professional Regulations 320 W Washington St. Springfield, IL 62786 (217) 782-8556 Fax (217) 782-7645	Dept of Professional Regulation 320 W Washington St., 3rd Fl. Springfield, IL 62786 (217) 782-1663 Fax (217)782-7645
Indiana	Health Professions Bureau 402 W Washington St. Rm 041 Indianapolis, IN 46204 (317) 232-2960 Fax (317) 233-4236	Indiana Speech-Language Pathology and Audiology Board 402 W Washington St., Rm 041 Indianapolis, IN 46204 (317) 233-4407 Fax (317) 233-4236	Health Professions Bureau 402 W Washington St., Rm 041 Indianapolis, IN 46204 (317) 232-2960 Fax (317) 233-4236
Iowa	Dept. of Public Health, Bureau of Professional Licensure Board of PT and OT Examiners 4th Fl., Lucas Bldg. Des Moines, IA 50319 (515) 281-7074 Fax (515) 281-3121	State Board of SLP and Audiology Examiners Bureau of Professional Licensure Lucas State Office Bldg, 4th Fl Des Moines, IA 50319 (515) 281-4408 Fax (515) 281-3121	Professional Licensure Office PT and OT Board of Examiners Lucas State Office Bldg. Des Moines, IA 50319 (515) 281-7074 Fax (515) 281-3121

STATE LICENSING INFORMATION

STATE	PT	SLP	OT
Kansas	Kansas State Board of Health Arts 235 SW Topeka Blvd. Topeka, KS 66603 (785) 296-7413 Fax (785) 296-0852	Speech-Language Pathology/Audiology Advisory Board 109 SW 9th St. Topeka, KS 66612 (913) 296-0056 Fax (913) 296-7025	KS State Board of Healing Arts 235 S Topeka Blvd Topeka, KS 66603 (913) 296-7413 Fax (913) 296-0852
Kentucky	Kentucky State Board of PT 9110 Leesgate Road, #6 Louisville, KY 40222 (502) 327-8497 Fax (502) 423-0934	Board of Examiners of SLP and Audiology PO Box 456 Frankfort, KY 40602 (502) 564-3296 Fax (502) 564-4818	KY OT Board PO Box 456 Frankfort, KY 40602 (502) 564-3296 Fax (502) 564-4818
Louisiana	Louisiana State Board of PT Examiners 2014 W Pinhook, #701 Lafayette, LA 70508 (318) 262-1043 Fax (318) 262-1054	Louisiana Board of Examiners for SLP and Audiology 11930 Perkins Road, Ste. B Baton Rouge, LA 71108 (504) 763-5480 Fax (504) 673-3085	LA State Board of Medical Examiners 630 Camp Street New Orleans, LA 70130 PO Box 30250 New Orleans, LA 70190 (504) 524-6763 Fax (504) 568-8893
Maine	Board of Examiners in PT Dept of Professional and Financial Regulation 35 State House Station Augusta, ME 04333 (207) 624-8600 Fax (207) 624-8637	Board of Examiners on Speech Pathology and Audiology 35 State House Station Augusta, ME 04333 (207) 624-8603 ext 48609 Fax (207) 624-8637	Dept of Professional and Financial Regulation Board of OT Practice State House Station #35 Augusta, ME 04333 (207) 624-8626 Fax (207) 582-5415
Maryland	Board of PT Examiners 4201 Patterson Ave., Ste. 318 Baltimore, MD 21215 (410) 764-4752 Fax (410) 358-1183	Maryland Board of Examiners for Audiology, HADs and SLPs 4201 Patterson Ave. Baltimore, MD 21215 (410) 764-4725 Fax (410) 764-5987	Metro Exec. Office Bldg. State Board of OT 3rd Fl, Rm 314 4201 Patterson Ave. Baltimore, MD 21215
Massachusetts	Board of Allied Health 100 Cambridge St. Rm 1513 Boston, MA 02202 (617) 727-3071 Fax (617) 727-2197	Board of Registration for Speech-Language Pathology and Audiology 100 Cambridge St., Rm 1513 Boston, MA 02202 (617) 727-1747	Board of Allied Health Professions Div of Registration 100 Cambridge St., Rm 1516 Boston, MA 02202 (617) 727-3071 Fax (617) 727-2197

STATE LICENSING INFORMATION

STATE	PT	SLP	OT
Michigan	PT State Board Dept of Consumer and Industry Services Office of Health Services PO Box 30670 Lansing, MI 48909 (517) 373-9102 Fax (517) 373-2179		MI Dept of Licensing and Regulation PO Box 30018 Lansing, MI 48909 (517) 335-0918
Minnesota	Board of Medical Practice PT Advisory Council 2829 University Ave. SE, Ste. 400 Minneapolis, MN 55414 (612) 617-2130 Fax (612) 617-2166	Minnesota Dept of Health 121 E Seventh Place PO Box 64975 St Paul, MN 55164 (612) 282-5629 Fax (612) 282-3839	Minnesota Dept of Health 121 E Seventh Place PO Box 64975 St Paul, MN 55164 (612) 282-6319 Fax (612) 282-5629
Mississippi	Mississippi State Dept of Health Professional Licensure Div PO Box 1700 Jackson, MS 39215 (601) 987-4153 Fax (601) 987-3784	Mississippi State Dept of Health Professional Licensure Div PO Box 1700 Jackson, MS 39215 (601) 987-4153 Fax (601) 987-3784	Mississippi State Dept of Health Professional Licensure 2423 N State St PO Box 1700 Jackson, MS 39215 (601) 987-4153 Fax (601) 987-3784
Missouri	Missouri Board of Healing Arts 3605 Missouri Blvd. Jefferson City, MO 65109 (573) 751-0096 Fax (573) 751-3166	Missouri Board of Registration for the Healing Arts 3605 Missouri Blvd Jefferson City, MO 65102 (573) 751-0098 Fax (314) 751-3166	Office of Health Care Providers Box 1335 Jefferson City, MO 65102 (573) 751-0877
Montana	Dept of Commerce, Div of Public Safety Board of PT Examiners 111 N Jackson, PO Box 200513 Helena, MT 59620 (406) 444-3728 Fax (406) 444-1667	Board of SLPs and Audiology Bureau of Professional Licensing 111 North Jackson St. Helena, MT 59620 (406) 444-3091 Fax (406) 444-1667	Dept of Commerce MT Board of OT 111 N Jackson PO Box 200513 Helena, MT 59620 (406) 444-3091 Fax (406) 444-1667

STATE LICENSING INFORMATION

STATE	PT	SLP	OT
Nebraska	Dept of Health and Human Services Regulation and Licensure Credentialing Div 301 Centennial Mall S PO Box 94986 Lincoln, NE 68509 (402) 471-0547 Fax (402) 471-3577	Board of Examiners in Audiology and SLP Dept of Health 301 Centennial Mall St. Lincoln, NE 68509 (402) 471-0547 Fax (402) 471-3577	Division of Professional Licensing Rehabilitation and Community Services Section Dept of Health PO Box 95007 Lincoln, NE 68509 (402) 471-0547 Fax (402) 471-0383
Nevada	Nevada State Board of PT Examiners PO Box 81467 Las Vegas, NV 89180 (702) 876-5535 Fax (702) 876-2097	Nevada State Board of Examiners for Audiology and Speech Pathology PO Box 70550 Reno, NV 89570 (702) 857-3500 Fax (702) 857-2121	State of Nevada Board of OT PO Box 70220 Reno, NV 89570 (702) 857-1700
New Hampshire	Board of Registration in Medicine 2 Industrial Park Dr., Ste. 8 Concord, NH 03301 (603) 271-1203 Fax (603) 271-6702	Board of Speech Language Pathologists 2 Industrial Park Dr, Ste. 8 Concord, NH 03301 (603) 271-1203 Fax (603) 271-6702	NH Board of Medicine OT Licensure Health and Welfare Bldg 2 Industrial Park Dr. Concord, NH 03301 (603) 271-1203 Fax (603) 271-6702
New Jersey	New Jersey State Board of PT 124 Halsey St., 6th fl. PO Box 45014 Newark, NJ 07101 (973) 504-6455 Fax (973) 648-3536	Audiology and SLP Advisory Committee New Jersey Division of Consumer Affairs 124 Halsey St., 6th Fl Newark, NJ 07102 (973) 504-6390 Fax (973) 648-3355	Advisory Council of OT PO Box 45005 Newark, NJ 07101 (201) 504-6395 Fax (201) 648-3355
New Mexico	New Mexico PT Licensing Board 2055 S. Pacheco, Ste.. 400 Santa Fe, NM 87505 (505) 827-7117 Fax (505) 827-7095	SLP, Audiology and AUD Practices Board Regulation and Licensing Dept PO Box 25101 Santa Fe, NM 87504 (505) 827-7554, ext 24 Fax (505) 827-7548	NM Board of OT Practice PO Box 25101 Santa Fe, NM 87504 (505) 827-7162 Fax (505) 827-7095

STATE LICENSING INFORMATION

STATE	PT	SLP	OT
New York	State Board for PT State Education Dept Cultural Education Ctr, Rm 3019 Albany, NY 12230 (518) 474-6374 Fax (518) 474-6375	State Board for SLP and Audiology Room 3013 CEC Empire State Plaza Albany, NY 12230 (518) 473-0221 Fax (518) 473-6995	NY State Board of OT Rm 3013 CEC Empire State Plaza Albany, NY 12230 (518) 473-0221 Fax (518) 473-6995
North Carolina	NC Board of PT Examiners 18 W Colony Pl, Ste. 120 Durham, NC 27705 (919) 490-6393 Fax (919) 490-5106	North Carolina Board of Examiners for SLP and Audiology PO Box 16885 Greensboro, NC 27416 (910) 272-1828 Fax (910) 272-4353	NC Board of OT PO Box 2280 Raleigh, NC 27602 (919) 832-1380 Fax (919) 833-1059
North Dakota	ND State Examining Committee for PT 115 Westwood Dr. Grafton, ND 58237 (701) 352-4553 Fax (701) 352-1270	Board of Examiners on Audiology and SLP Bureau of Educational Services and Applied Research PO Box 7189 Grand Forks, ND 58202 (701) 777-4421 Fax (701) 777-4365	ND State Board of OT Practice 1837 S 15th St. Fargo, ND 58103 (701) 293-7971
Ohio	Ohio OT, PT, and Athletic Trainers Board 77 S High St., 16th Fl Columbus, OH 43266 (614) 466-3774 Fax (614) 644-8112	Board of SLP and Audiology 77 S High St., 16th Fl Columbus, OH 43266 (614) 466-3145 Fax (614) 644-8112	Ohio OT, PT, and AT Board 77 S High St., 16th Fl Columbus, OH 43226 (614) 848-6841 Fax (614) 644-8112
Oklahoma	Oklahoma State Board of Medical Licensure and Supervision 5104 N Francis, Ste. C Oklahoma City, OK 73118 (405) 848-6841 Fax (405) 848-8240	State Board Examiners for SLP and Audiology PO Box 53592 Oklahoma City, OK 73152 (405) 840-2774 Fax (405) 840-2774	Board of Medical Licensure & Supervision PO Box 18256 Oklahoma City, OK 73154 (405) 848-6841 Fax (405) 848-8240
Oregon	Oregon PT Licensing Board 800 NE Oregon Ave., Ste. 407 Portland, OR 97232 (503) 731-4047 Fax (503) 731-4207	Board of Examiners for SLP and Audiology 800 NE Oregon St., #21 Portland, OR 97232 (503) 731-4050 Fax (503) 731-4207	OR OT Licensing Board 800 NE Oregon #21 Ste. 407 Portland, OR 97232 (503) 731-4084 Fax (503) 731-4207

STATE LICENSING INFORMATION

STATE	PT	SLP	OT
Pennsylvania	Pennsylvania State Board of PT PO Box 2649 Harrisburg, PA 17105 (717) 783-7134 Fax (717) 787-7769	Board of Examiners in Speech, Language and Hearing PO Box 2649 Harrisburg, PA 17105 (717) 783-1389 Fax (717) 787-7769	State Board of OT Education and Licensure PO Box 2649 Harrisburg, PA 17105 (717) 783-1389 Fax (717) 787-7769
Rhode Island	Rhode Island Board of Examiners in PT Three Capitol Hill 104 Cannon Bldg Providence, RI 02908 (401) 277-2827 Fax (401) 277-1272	Board of Examiners in SLP and Audiology Rhode Island Dept of Health Three Capitol Hill, Rm 104 Providence, RI 02908 (401) 277-2827 Fax (401) 277-1272	Division of Professional Regulation Three Capitol Hill, Rm 104 Providence, RI 02908 (401) 277-2827 Fax (401) 277-1272
South Carolina	State Board of PT Examiners 110 Centerview Drive PO Box 11329 Columbia, SC 29211 (803) 896-4655 Fax (803) 896-4719	South Carolina Board of Examiners in Speech Pathology and Audiology PO Box 11329, Ste. 101 Columbia, SC 29211 (803) 734-4253 Fax (803) 734-4248	SC Board of OT 110 Centerview Dr PO Box 11329 Columbia, SC 29211 (803) 896-4683 Fax (803) 896-4719
South Dakota	South Dakota State Board of Medical and Osteopathic Examiners 1323 S. Minnesota Ave. Sioux Falls, SD 57105 (605) 334-8343 Fax (605) 336-0270		SD Board of Medical & Osteopathic Examiners 1323 S Minnesota Ave. Sioux Falls, SD 57105 (605) 336-1965
Tennessee	Tennessee Board of OT/PT Examiners 1st Floor Cordell Hull Bldg 426 5th Ave. N Nashville, TN 37247 (615) 532-5136 Fax (615) 532-5164	State Board of Communication Disorders and Sciences Speech Pathology and Audiology 426 5th Ave., N Floor 1 Nashville, TN 37214 (615) 532-5160 Fax (615) 532-5164	TN Board of OT and PT Examiners 426 5th Ave. N Cordell Bldg, Fl 1 Nashville, TN 37247 (615) 532-5135 Fax (615) 532-5164

STATE LICENSING INFORMATION

STATE	PT	SLP	OT
Texas	Texas State Board of PT Examiners 333 Guadalupe, Ste. 2-510 Austin, TX 78701 (512) 305-6900 (512) 305-6951	State Board of Examiners for SLP and Audiology 1100 W 49th St. Austin, TX 78756 (512) 834-6627 Fax (512) 834-6677	Coordinator of OT Programs Executive Council of PT and OT Texas Board of OT Examiners 333 Guadalupe, Ste. #2-510 Austin, TX 78701 (512) 305-6900 Fax (512) 305-6951
Utah	Div of Occupational and Professional Licensing 160 E 300 S PO Box 45805 Salt Lake City, UT 84145 (801) 530-6621 Fax (801) 530-6511	Div of Occupational and Professional Licensing 160 E 300 S Salt Lake City, UT 84114 (801) 530-6632 Fax (801) 530-6511	Div of Occupational and Professional Licensing PO Box 45805 Salt Lake City, UT 84145 (801) 530-6632 Fax (801) 530-6511
Vermont	Office of Professional Regulation Office of the Secretary of State Licensing and Registration Div 109 State St. Montpelier, VT 05609 (802) 828-2390 Fax (802) 828-2496		Secretary of State's Office 109 State St. Montpelier, VT 05609 (802) 828-2390 Fax (802) 828-2496
Virginia	Licensing Dept of Health Professions Board of Medicine 6606 W Broad St., 4th Fl Richmond, VA 23230 (804) 662-9073 Fax (804) 662-9943	State Board of Audiology and Speech Pathology 6606 W Broad St., 4th Fl Richmond, VA 23230 (804) 662-7390 Fax (804) 662-9943	VA Board of Medicine 6606 W Broad St., 4th Fl Richmond, VA 23230 (804) 662-7664

STATE LICENSING INFORMATION

STATE	PT	SLP	OT
Washington	Dept of Health 1300 SE Quince St. PO Box 47868 Olympia, WA 98504 (360) 753-3132 Fax (360) 753-0657	Board of Audiology, Speech and Hearing Instrument Fitters Dept of Health Health Service Unit Two 1300 SE Quince St. Olympia, WA 98504 (360) 586-0205 Fax (360) 586-7774	Dept of Health, OT Board PO Box 47868 Olympia, WA 98504 (360) 664-8662 Fax (360) 753-0657
West Virginia	West Virginia Board of PT JW Davis Government Bldg 153 W Main St., Ste. 103 Clarksburg, WV 26301 (304) 627-2251 Fax (304) 627-2253	West Virginia Board of Examiners for SLP and Audiology PO Box 854 Dunbar, WV 25064 (304) 766-1096	WV Board of OT 119 S Price St. Kingwood, WV 26537 (304) 329-0480
Wisconsin	Dept of Regulation and Licensing Medical Examining Board PO Box 8935 Madison, WI 53708 (608) 266-0483 Fax (608) 267-0644	Council on SLP and Audiology Dept of Regulation and Licensing PO Box 8935 Madison, WI 53708 (608) 266-1396 Fax (608) 267-0644	State of WI Dept of Regulation and Licensing PO Box 8935 Madison, WI 53703 (608) 267-9377
Wyoming	Wyoming State Board of PT 2020 Carey Ave., Ste. 201 Cheyenne, WY 82002 (307) 777-3507 Fax (307) 777-3508	State Board of Examiners in SLP and Audilogy 2020 Carey Ave., Ste. 201 Cheyenne, WY 82002 (307) 777-7780 Fax (307) 777-3508	Wyoming Board of OT First Bank Plaza 2020 Carey Ave., Ste. 201 Cheyenne, WY 82002 (307) 777-6313 Fax (307) 777-3508

STATE LICENSING INFORMATION

STATE	PT	SLP	OT
Puerto Rico	Office of Regulation and Certification of the Profession of Health Call Box 10200 Santurce, PT 00908 (787) 725-8161 Fax (787) 725-7903		Dept of Health Office of Regulations and Certification of Health Professions Call Box 10200 San Juan PR 00908 (787) 725-8121 Fax (787) 725-7903
Virgin Islands	Virgin Islands Board of PT Examiners Dept of Health 48 Sugar Estate St Thomas, VI 00802 (809) 774-0117 Fax (809) 777-4001		

DIRECTORY OF RESOURCES

ACCREDITATION

Joint Commission on Accreditation of Healthcare Organizations (JCAHO)
One Renaissance Boulevard
Oakbrook, IL 60181
(630)792-5000
www.jcaho.org

Community Health Accreditation Program (CHAP)
61 Broadway, 33rd Floor
New York, NY 10006
(800) 669-1656

The Rehabilitation Accreditation Commission (CARF)
4891 E. Grant Rd.
Tucson, AZ 85712
(520) 523-1044
www.carf.org

AMPUTATION

Amputee Coalition of America (ACA)
900 East Hill Ave., Suite 285
Knoxville, TN 37915-2568
(888) 358-9295, (423) 524-8772
www.amputee-coalition.org

National Amputee Foundation, Inc.
AMP Newsletter
38-40 Church Street
Malverne, NY 11565
(516) 887- 3600

Parents of Amputee Children Together
W. Kessler Rehabilitation Institute
1199 Pleasant Valley Way
West Orange, NJ 07052
(201) 731-3600

AMYOTROPHIC LATERAL SCLEROSIS

Amyotrophic Lateral Sclerosis Association
21021 Ventura Blvd., Suite 321
Woodland Hills, CA 91364
(818) 340-7500, (800) 782-4747

ARTHRITIS

National Arthritis Foundation
1314 Spring Street
Atlanta, GA 30309
(404) 872-7100, (800) 284-7800
www.arthritis.org

ASSESSMENT

Dittmar, SS and Gresham, GE: *Functional assessment and outcome measures for the rehabilitation health professional*, Gaithersburg. MD, 1997, Aspen Publishers.

Emlet, C and Crabtree, J, et al: *In-home assessment of older adults: an interdisciplinary approach*, Gaithersburg, MD, 1996, Aspen Publishers.

COMMUNICATION

Alexander Graham Bell Association for the Deaf
3417 Volta Place, NW
Washington, DC 20007
(202) 337-5220

American Speech-Language Hearing Association
10801 Rockville Pike
Rockville, MD 20852
(301) 897-5700

AT&T National Special Needs Center
5 Woodhollow
Parsippany, NJ 07054
(800) 233-1222

National Association for the Deaf
814 Thayer Ave.
Silver Spring, MD 20910
(301) 587-1788

National Information Center on Deafness (NICD) Gallaudet University
800 Florida Ave., NE
Washington, DC 20002
(202) 651-5051 (voice), (202) 651-5052 (TDD)

National Institute of Deafness and Other Communication Disorders
National Institute of Health
Bethesda, MD 20892
(800) 241-1044

National Institute of Neurological and Communicative Disorders and Stroke
National Institute of Health
Bethesda, MD 20892
(301) 496-9746

The Orton Dyslexia Society
Chester Building, Suite 382
8600 LaSalle Road
Baltimore, MD 21286-2044
(410) 296-0232, (800) 223-3123

Stuttering Foundation of America
P.O. Box 11749
Memphis, TN 38111-0749

Matthews-Flint, Lenora J and Lucas, Linda J: "Telecommunication Relay Services: Linking Nurses to Patient with Communication Disorders," *Home Healthcare Nurse*, 17(5): 301-5, 1999.

DISABLED PERSONS

Clearinghouse on Disability Information Office on Special Education & Rehabilitative Services
Switzer Bldg., Room 3132
330 C Street, SW
Washington, DC 20202-2524
(202) 732-1723

National Easter Seal Society
70 East Lake Street
Chicago, IL 60601
(312) 726-6200

EMERGENCY RESPONSE SYSTEM

Lifeline Systems Inc.
1 Arlenal Marketplace
Watertown, MA 02172
(800) 543-3546

Medic Alert Foundation
2323 Colorado Ave.
Turlock, CA 95382
(800) 432-5378

EQUIPMENT COMPANIES

AliMed Inc.
297 High Street
Dedham, MA 02026
(800) 337-2400

Invacare Corporation
899 Cleveland St.
Elyria, OH 44036
(800) 333-6900

Jay Medical
PO Box 18656
Boulder, CO 80308
(800) 300-7502

North Coast Medical, Inc.
187 Stauffer Boulevard
San Jose, CA 95125
(800) 821-9319

Sammons Preston, Inc.
PO Box 5071
Bolingbrook, IL 60440
(800) 323-5547

Smith & Nephew Rolyan, Inc.
One Quality Drive, PO Box 1005
Germantown, WI 53022
(800) 558-8633

FALL PREVENTION

Fall Prevention Project For Older Adults
Dr. Roberta Newton
Dept. of Physical Therapy
Temple University
3307 N. Broad Street
Philadelphia, PA 19140
(215) 707-8913
www.temple.edu/older_adult

FORMS

Briggs Forms & Supplies
P.O. Box 1698
Des Moines, IA 50306-1698
(515) 327-6400, (800) 247-2343

Home Therapy Services
www.oasisanswers.com

HEAD INJURY

Brain Injury Association, Inc.
1776 Massachusetts Ave., NW, Suite 100
Washington, DC 20036-1904
(800) 444-6443

HEALTH CARE FINANCING ADMINISTRATION
(See Medicare)

Health Care Financing Administration (HCFA) has many publications available for downloading on its website at www.hcfa.gov/pubforms/progman.htm.
These publications include: Pub 11: *Home Health Agency Manual*, Pub 21:
Hospice Manual, and the *OASIS User's Manual*. HCFA also has OASIS
software available for downloading. To download the OASIS User's Manual
or the Home Assessment Validation and Entry (HAVEN) software go to:
www.hcfa.gov/medicare/hsqb/oasis/oasishmp.htm. For help with OASIS
or to order the CD-ROM version of the software call the OASIS help desk
at (877) 201-4721.

HOME HEALTH CARE

American Medical Association: *Guidelines for the medical management of the home care patient*, Chicago, 1994, American Medical Association.

Emlet C, Crabtree J, Condon V, Treml L: *In-home assessment of older adults: an interdisciplinary approach*, Gaithersburg, MD, 1996, Aspen Publishers.

Kosta JC, Mitchell CA: "Current procedures for diagnosis dysphagia in elderly clients," *Geriatric Nursing*, 19(4): 195-9, 1998.

Krulish L: "Optimizing clinical and financial outcomes in home care: a niche program approach," *Topics in Geriatric Rehabilitation*, 14(4), 1999.

Marrelli T: *Handbook of home health orientation*, St. Louis, 1998, Mosby.

Marrelli T: *Handbook of home health standards and documentation guidelines for reimbursement*, ed 3, St. Louis, 1998, Mosby.

Marrelli T, Hilliard L: "Documentation and effective patient care planning," *Home Care Provider*, 1(4): 198, 1996.

Marrelli T, Hilliard L: *Manual of home health practice: guidance for effective clinical operations*, St. Louis, 1998, Mosby.

Marrelli T, Whittier S: *Home health aide: guidelines for care*, Englewood, FL 1996, Marrelli and Associates.

Marrelli T, Friend L: *Home health aide: guidelines for care instructor manual*, Englewood, FL, 1997, Marrelli and Associates.

Marrelli T: *Mosby's home care & hospice drug handbook*, St. Louis, 1999, Mosby.

May BJ: *Home health and rehabilitation: concepts of care*, Philadelphia, F.A. Davis Company.

Zakrajsek, Darlene: "Home care therapist as case manager," *Topics in Geriatric Rehabilitation*, 15(1): 1999.

HOSPICE

Hospice Foundation of America

777 17th St., # 401
Miami Beach, FL 33139
(800) 854-3402

2001 S St., NW, Suite 300
Washington, DC 20009
(202) 638-5419

Hospice and Palliative Nurses Association (HPNA)
Medical Center East, Suite 375
211 North Whitfield St.
Pittsburgh, PA 15206-3031
(412) 361-2470

National Hospice Organization
1901 North Moore St., Suite 901
Arlington, VA 22209
(703) 243-5900
www.nho.org

NHO Standards and Accreditation Committee: *Standards of a hospice program of care*, Arlington, VA, 1999, National Hospice Organization.

Hospice Care: A Physician's Guide, published by the National Hospice Organization (NHO), this 96-page book provides in-depth information for physician's dealing with patients in hospice care. Copices of this book and many other useful publications can be obtained through the NHO store at 1901 North Moore Street, Suite 901, Arlington, VA 22209; phone: (703) 243-5900; or visit the website at www.nho.org.

Marrelli T: *Hospice and palliative care handbook*, St. Louis, 1999, Mosby.

Marrelli T: *Mosby's home care & hospice drug handbook*, St. Louis, 1999, Mosby.

Scotece GG: "Restoring dignity: rehab's role in hospice pain management," *Advance for Directors in Rehabilitation*, November, 1997: 18-9, 1997.

Sheehan DC, Forman WB: *Hospice and palliative care: concepts and practice*, Boston, 1996, Jones and Bartlett.

INDEPENDENT LIVING

National Council on Independent Living
2111 Wilson Blvd., Suite 405
Arlington, VA 22201
(703) 525-3409

INTERNET RESOURCES

Agency for Health Care Policy and Research (AHCPR)
www.ahcpr.gov

Alzheimer's Disease Education and Research
www. alzheimers.org/adear

American Academy of Hospice and Palliative Medicine
www.aahpm.org

American Academy of Private Practice in Speech Pathology and Audiology (AAPPSPA)
www.aappspa.org

American Dietetic Association (ADA)
www.eatright.org

American Occupational Therapy Association (AOTA)
www.aota.org

American Physical Therapy Association (APTA)
www.apta.org

American Speech-Language-Hearing Association (ASHA)
www.asha.org

Atlanta Voice and Swallowing Center
www.mindspring.com/~newvoice/

Dysphagia Research Society
www.als.uiuc.edu/drs/

Evaluation and Interpretation of Acute Dysphagia Disorders and Dysphagia Rehabilitation/EMG Biofeedback Assisted Treatment
www.speechpaths.com/pms9.htm

Food and Drug Administration
www.fda.gov

Government Printing Office (GPO)
www.access.gpo.gov

Health and Human Services, Department of (DHHS)
www.dhhs.gov

Health Care Financing Administration
www.hcfa.gov

Hospice Hands
www.hospice-care.com

House of Representatives
www.house.gov

Library of Congress
www.loc.gov

Map Quest (internet directions site)
www.mapquest.com

Marrelli and Associates, Inc.
www.marrelli.com

National Committee for Quality Assurance (HMOs)
www.ncqa.org

National Institutes of Health (NIH)
www.nih.gov

NIH Speech Pathology
www.cc.nih.gov/rm/sp

OASIS Answers
www.oasisanswers.com

Occupational Safety and Health Administration
www.osha.gov

Rehab Central
www.rehabcentral.com

Social Security Administration
www.ssa.gov

Swallowing Disorders
www.webpages.marshall.edu/~lynch4/swallow.html

Swallowing Disorders Program
www.stjosephs.org/iv_k_6.htm

Temple University Fall Prevention Project For Older Adults
www.temple.edu/older_adult

White House
www.whitehouse.gov

MEDICARE (See Health Care Financing Administration)

Health Care Financing Administration (HCFA) manuals are available through the National Technical Information Services (NTIS) at 5285 Port Royal Road, Springfield, VA 22161, (800) 553-6847.

Medicare Conditions of Participation (COPs) are available through the National Technical Information Services (NTIS) at 5285 Port Royal Road, Springfield, VA 22161, (800) 553-6847.

Medicare A Newsline Forum, Medicare A Newsline Forum-Station 56, Wellmark, Inc., P.O. Box 9175, Des Moines, IA 50306-9175, (fax) (515) 235-4411.

Medicare Fraud Hotline, Office of Inspector General, Department of Health and Human Services, HHS-TIPS Hot Line, P.O. Box 23489, Washington, DC 20026, (800) HHS-TIPS (447-8477).

Medicare Handbook: HCFA publication detailing Medicare program benefits, free, contact the Health Care Financing Administration (HCFA) (800) 638-6833.

OASIS User's Manual, this 600+ page publication from HCFA can be downloaded via the HCFA website at www.hcfa.gov/medicare/hsqb/oasis/oasishmp.htm , or ordered by mail through the National Association for Home Care (NAHC), (202) 547-7424.

MEDICATIONS

Marrelli T: M*osby's home care & hospice drug handbook*, St. Louis, 1999, Mosby.

Pharmacology Home Study Course, Orthopaedic Section, APTA, Inc., 2920 East Avenue South, Suite 200, La Crosse, WI 54601, (800) 444-3982.

Prescription Medicines and You: A Consumer's Guide, a brochure available from the National Council on Patient Information and Education (NCPIE). For 10 or fewer free copies, contact the Agency for Health Care Policy and Research (AHCPR) Publications Clearinghouse, P.O. Box 8547, Silver Spring, MD 20907, (800) 358-9295. For larger orders contact the NCPIE, 666 Eleventh St., NW, Suite 810, Washington, DC 20001-4542, (202) 347-6711.

Using Your Medicines Wisely: A Guide for the Elderly, a booklet developed by the National Institute on Drug Abuse. For free copies contact the National Clearinghouse for Alcohol and Drug Information, P.O. Box 2345, Rockville, MD 20852, (800) 729-6686.

When Medicine Hurts Instead of Helps is a booklet designed to help prevent medication problems in older persons it can be ordered through the Alliance for Aging Research at (202) 293-2856.

MULTIPLE SCLEROSIS

National Multiple Sclerosis Society
733 3rd Ave., 6th Floor
New York, NY 10017
(800) 344-4867, (212) 986-3240

MUSCULAR DYSTROPHY

Muscular Dystrophy Association
3300 E. Sunrise Drive
Tuscon, AZ 85718-3208
(602) 529-2000, (800) 572-1717
www.mdausa.org

NATIONAL ORGANIZATIONS

Alzheimer's Association
919 N Michigan, Suite 1000
Chicago, IL 60611
(800) 621-0379

American Association for Respiratory Care
11030 Ables Lane
Dallas, TX 75229
(972) 243-2272

American Association of Retired Persons (AARP)
601 E Street NW
Washington, DC 20049
(202) 434-2277

American Board for Certification in Orthotics & Prosthetics, Inc.
1650 King Street, Suite 500
Alexandria, VA 22314
(703) 836-7114

American Diabetes Association
1660 Duke Street, PO Box 25757
Alexandria, VA 22314
(800) 232-3472

American Federation of Home Care Providers, Inc.
1320 Fenwick Lane, Suite 100
Silver Spring, MD 20910
(301) 588-1454
Website: http://www.his.com/~afhha/usa.html

American Heart Association
7272 Greenville Ave.
Dallas, TX 75231
(800) 242-8721

American Lung Association
6160 Central Ave.
St. Petersburg, FL 33707
(800) 586-4872

American Occupational Therapy Association (AOTA)
Home and Community Health Special Interest Section
4720 Montgomery Lane, PO Box 31220
Bethesda, MD 20854-1220
(301) 652-2682
(800) 701-7735 (automated fax on demand service)
www.aota.org

American Parkinson Disease Association
1250 Highland Blvd., Suite 4B
Staten Island, NY 10305
(800) 223-2732

American Physical Therapy Association (APTA)
Home Health Section
1111 North Fairfax Street
Alexandria, VA 22314-1488
(703) 684-2782
(800) 399-2782 (automated fax on demand service)
www.apta.org

American Speech-Language-Hearing Association (ASHA)
10801 Rockville Pike
Rockville, MD 20852-3279
(301) 897-5700
www.asha.org

Amyotrophic Lateral Sclerosis Association
21021 Ventura Blvd., Suite 321
Woodland Hills, CA 91364
(818) 340-7500, (800) 782-4747

Arthritis Foundation
1330 W Peachtree St.
Atlanta, GA 30309
(404) 872-7100

Association of Rehab Nurses
4700 W. Lake Ave.
Glenview, IL 60025-1485
(847) 375-4710, (800) 229-7530
www.rehabnurse.org

Association of Academic Physiatrists
5987 E. 71st St., Suite 112
Indianapolis, IN 46220-4056
(317) 845-4200
www.physiatry.org/what.html

Case Management Society of America (CMSA)
8201 Cantrell, Suite 230
Little Rock, AR 72227-2448
(501) 225-2229

Home Care Association of America (HCAA)
9570 Regency Square Blvd.
Jacksonville, FL 32225
(800) 386-4222
www.hcaa-homecare.com

Home Health Services & Staffing Association (HHSSA)
1875 Eye Street, NW, 12th Floor
Washington, DC 20006
(202) 296-3800

Hospice Association of America
228 Seventh St., SE
Washington, DC 20003
(202) 547-7424
www.nahc.org

Hospice Foundation of America
777 17th St., # 401   2001 S St., NW, Suite 300
Miami Beach, FL 33139   Washington, DC 20009
(800) 854-3402   (202) 638-5419

Hospice and Palliative Nurses Association (HPNA)
Medical Center East, Suite 375
211 North Whitfield St.
Pittsburgh, PA 15206-3031
(412) 361-2470

International Association of Cystic Fibrosis Adults
82 Ayer Rd.
Harvard, MA 01451

Intraveneous Nurses Society
10 Fawcett St.
Cambridge, MA 02138
(617) 441-3008

Myasthenia Gravis Foundation of America, Inc.
222 South Riverside St., Suite 1540
Chicago, IL 60606
(312) 258-0522, (800) 541-5454

National Association for Home Care (NAHC)
228 Seventh St., SE
Washington, DC 20003
(202) 547-7424
www.nahc.org

National Association for Medical Equipment Services (NAMES)
625 Slaters Lane, Suite 2000
Alexandria, VA 22314-1171
(703) 836-6263

National Association for the Deaf
814 Thayer Ave.
Silver Spring, MD 20910
(301) 587-1788

National Council on Patient Information and Education
666 11th Street, NW, Suite 810
Washington, DC 20001-4542
(202) 347-6711

National Family Caregivers Association (NCFA)
9621 East Bexhill Drive
Kensington, MD 20895-3104
(301) 942-6430
www.nfcacares.org

National Hospice Organization (NHO)
1901 North Moore St. Suite 901
Arlington, VA 22209
(703) 243-5900
www.nho.org

National Institute of Neurological and Communicative Disorders and Stroke
National Institute of Health
Bethesda, MD 20892
(301) 496-9746

National Institute on Aging
PO Box 8057
Gaithersburg, MD 20898-8057
(800) 222-2225
www.nih.gov/nia www.niainfo@access.diges.com

National Osteoporosis Foundation
1150 17th St. NW, Suite 500
Washington, DC 20036
(800) 223-9994

National Multiple Sclerosis Society
733 3rd Ave., 6th Floor
New York, NY 10017
(212) 986-3240, (800) 344-4867

National Organization on Disability
910 Sixteenth Street, NW
Washington, DC 20006
(202) 293-5968

National Osteoporosis Foundation
1150 17th St., NW, Suite 500
Washington, DC 20036
(800) 223-9994

National Stroke Association
96 Inverness Dr., E., Suite I
Englewood, CO 80112
(800) STROKES, (303) 649-9299

Occupational Safety and Health Administration (OSHA)
(202) 219-6463

Parkinson's Disease Foundation
710 W 168 St. 3rd Floor
New York, NY 10032
(212) 923-4700

Spina Bifida Association of America (SBAA)
4590 MacArthur Blvd., NW, Suite 250
Washington, DC 20007
(800) 621-3141
www.sbaa.org

United Cerebral Palsy Association
1660 L Street NW, Suite 700
Washington, DC 20036
(800) 872-5827

Visiting Nurse Association of America
11 Beacon St., Suite 910
Boston, MA 02108
(800) 426-2547

OASIS

OASIS User's Manual, this 600+ page publication from HCFA can be downloaded via the HCFA website at www.hcfa.gov, or ordered by mail through the National Association for Home Care (NAHC), (202) 547-7424.

Heatherly D: "OASIS implementation (the who, what, when, why, and how," *Home Care Nurse News*, 6(3): 5, 1999.

Heatherly D: "OASIS implementation: policies and procedures impacted by OASIS data collection," *Home Care Nurse News*, 6(2): 5-7, 1999.

Krulish L: Home therapy OASIS assessment forms, Powell, OH, 1999, Home Therapy Services.

Krulish L: "Integrating OASIS into your organization's therapy documentation," *Home Care Nurse News*, 6(5): 5-7, 1999.

Krulish L: "OASIS and the home care physical therapist," *The Quarterly Report of the Community Home Health Section*, 34(1): 9-10, 1999, American Physical Therapy Association.

Krulish L: "OASIS regulation published: regulatory review with therapy impacts," *The Quarterly Report of the Community Home Health Section*, 34(1): 9-10, 1999, American Physical Therapy Association.

Sperling, Randa L. and Humphrey, Carolyn: *OASIS and OBQI: a guide for education and implementation*, Philadelphia, PA, 1998, Lippincott, Williams & Wilkins.

OCCUPATIONAL THERAPY

American Occupational Therapy Association (AOTA)
Home and Community Health Special Interest Section
4720 Montgomery Lane, P.O. Box 31220
Bethesda, MD 20854-1220
(301) 652-2682
(800) 701-7735 (automated fax on demand service)
www.aota.org

American Occupational Therapy Association: *Guidelines for occupational therapy practice in home health*, Bethesda, MD, 1995, American Occupational Therapy Association.

American Occupational Therapy Association: "Occupational therapy and hospice: a position paper," *American Journal Occupational Therapy*, 40:839, 1986.

American Occupational Therapy Association: "Occupational therapy roles," *American Journal of Occupational Therapy*, Vol 47: 1087-99, 1993.

American Occupational Therapy Association: Standards of practice for occupational therapy, Bethesda, Md, 1998, *American Occupational Therapy Association*.

American Occupational Therapy Association, "Statement of occupational therapy referral," *American Journal Occupational Therapy*, 48(11): 1034, 1994.

American Occupational Therapy Association, "Position paper: purposeful activity," *American Journal Occupational Therapy*, 47(12):1081-2, 1993.

Seibert, Carol: "Meeting the challenge of new home health care mandates," *OT Practice*, 4(2): 25-29, American Occupational Therapy Association.

Touchard BM, Berthelot K: "Collaborative home practice: nursing and occupational therapy ensure appropriate medication administration," *Home Healthcare Nurse*, 17(1): 45-51, 1999.

Walker, V: "Assessment and documentation guidelines for the COTA," *OT Week*, Nov. 7, 1996: 9-10, American Occupational Therapy Association.

Walker, V: "Can COTAs work in a home health setting?" *OT Week*, Aug. 10, 1995, American Occupational Therapy Association.

Walker, V: "COTA and the evaluation process," *OT Week*, Sept. 14, 1995: 13, American Occupational Therapy Association.

Zahoransky, Missi: "Teamwork in home care: fundamental to survival" *OT Practice*, 3(11): 29-31, American Occupational Therapy Association.

PAIN

International Association for the Study of Pain
909 NE 43rd St., Suite 306
Seattle, WA 98105
(206) 547-6409

International Association for the Study of Pain: "Physical therapy for chronic pain," *Pain Clinical Updates*, VI: 3.

PATIENT EDUCATION RESOURCES

Agency for Health Care Policy and Research
Free clinical practice guidelines (800) 358-9295

Aging with Ease: A Positive Approach to Pain Management, is a helpful booklet which provides a brief overview of how to recognize, understand, and safely treat pain. It uses information from the American Geriatrics Society's clinical practice guidelines for controlling recurring pain in older people. This booklet can be ordered through the Alliance for Aging Research at (202) 293-2856.

PEDIATRICS

Children's Hospice International
2202 Mount Vernon Ave., Suite 3 C
Alexandria, VA 22301
(800) 242-4453 (24-CHILD)

Easter Seals
(800) 221-6827
www.easterseals.org
Offers publications: "Understanding Occupational Therapy, Understanding
Physical Therapy, Understanding Speech-Language Pathology and Audiology,"
"Understanding Rehabilitation," and others.

National Information Center for Children and Youth with Disabilities
P.O. Box 1492
Washington, DC 20013-1492
(800) 695-0285

Battshaw, Mark L. and Perret, Yvonne M.: *Children with handicaps: a medical primer*, Paul H. Brookes, 1986.

Finnie, Nancie, et al: *Handling the young child with cerebral palsy at home,* Butterworth-Heinemann, 1997.

Fraiberg, Selma H.: *The magic years: understanding and handling the problems of early childhood*, Fireside, 1996 (reissue).

Long, Toby M. and Cintas, Holly L.: *Handbook of pediatric physical therapy*, Williams & Wilkins, 1995.

Pearson, Paul H., Williams, Carol, et al: *Physical therapy services in the developmental disabilities*, Charles C. Thomas, 1972.

Shepherd, Roberta: *Physiotherapy in paediatrics*, Butterworth-Heinemann, 1995.

Sher, Barbara: *Extraordinary play with ordinary things: recycling everyday materials to build motor skills*, Academic Press Inc., 1992.

Tecklin, Jan S.: *Pediatric physical therapy*, Lippincott-Raven, 1998.

PERSONAL EMERGENCY RESPONSE SYSTEMS

Lifeline Systems, Inc.
1 Arlenal Marketplace
Watertown, MA 02172
(800) 543-3546

Medic Alert Foundation
2323 Colorado Ave.
Turlock, CA 95382
(800) 432-5378

PHYSICAL THERAPY

American Physical Therapy Association
1111 N. Fairfax Street
Alexandria, VA 22314
(800) 999-2782, (703) 684-APTA
www.apta.org

American Physical Therapy Association: *Guidelines for the provision of physical therapy in the home*, Alexandria, Va, 1996, American Physical Therapy Association Community Home Health Section.

American Physical Therapy Association: *Guide to physical therapist practice*, Alexandria, Va, 1997, American Physical Therapy Association.

SPEECH-LANGUAGE PATHOLOGY

American Speech-Language Hearing Association (ASHA)
10801 Rockville Pike
Rockville, MD 20852-3279
(301) 897-5700
www.asha.org

American Speech-Language-Hearing Association: "Position statement. delivery of speech-language pathology and audiology services in home care," ASHA, 30, 77-9, 1998.

American Speech-Language-Hearing Association: *Preferred practice patterns for the profession of speech-language pathology*, ASHA, Rockville, Md, 1997.

American Speech-Language-Hearing Association: "Scope of practice in speech-language pathology," ASHA, Vol. 38, (Suppl. 16), 16-20, 1996.

Diagnosis and treatment of swallowing disorders (dysphagia) in acute-care stroke patients, a clinical findings report from the Agency for Health Care Policy and Research is available by calling (800) 358-9295.

Kosta JC and Mitchell CA, "Current procedures for diagnosing dysphagia in elderly clients," *Geriatric Nursing*, 19(4): 195-9, 1998.

Nelson, Gloria Bartholomew: "Assessment and intervention for communication problems in home health care," *Journal of Home Health Care Practice*, 1(1): 61-76, 1998.

SPINAL CORD

American Association of Spinal Cord Injury Nurses
75-20 Astoria Blvd.
Jackson Heights, NY 11370-1177

**American Association of Spinal Cord Injury
Psychologists and Social Workers**
75-20 Astoria Blvd.
Jackson Heights, NY 11370-1177

American Paralysis Association
500 Morris Ave.
Springfield, NJ 07081
(800) 225-0292

"In Touch with Kids," a special support network of the National Spinal Cord Injury Association, offers a pen-pal directory (which is also available to the child's siblings and parents). The members range in age from one to 18. All members have a spinal cord injury, spina bifida, or other spinal cord illnesses. These services are **free** by calling (800) 962-9629.

National Spinal Cord Injury Association
8300 Colesville Road, Suite 551
Silver Spring, MD 20910
(800) 962-9629

Rebecca Finds a New Way: How Kids Learn, Play, and Live with Spinal Cord Injuries and Illnesses. This 56-page booklet was written for children aged three to eight. This resource can be obtained by calling the Paralyzed Veterans of America at (888) 860-7244, or (202) 872-1300.

Spinal Cord Information Network
Sponsored by the University of Alabama at Birmingham,
Department of Physical Medicine and Rehabilitation
www.spinalcord.uab.edu

Spinal Cord Injury Resources: *Constipation and Spinal Cord Injury: A Guide to Symptoms and Treatment, Follow Your Dreams, Inform Yourself: Alcohol, Drugs, and Spinal Cord Injury,* and *Tell It Like it Is.* Free booklets available by calling the Paralyzed Veterans of America (888) 860-7244, or (202) 872-1300.

STROKE

National Stroke Association
96 Inverness Dr. E., Suite I
Englewood, CO 80112
(800) STROKES, (303) 649-9299

VISION

American Council of the Blind
1155 15th Street, NW
Washington, DC 20005
(202) 467-5081

American Foundation for the Blind
15 West 16th Street
New York, NY 10011
(800) 232-5463

National Association for Visually Handicapped
22 W. 21st Street, 6th Floor
New York, NY 10010
(212) 889-3141

NEWSLETTERS / MAGAZINES / JOURNALS

Caring Magazine
National Association for Home Care
228 Seventh St., SE
Washington, DC 20003
(202)547-7424

Home Care Nurse News
Marrelli and Associates
PO Box 629
Boca Grande, FL 33921-0629
(800) 993-NEWS (6397)

Home Care Provider
Mosby-Year Book, Inc.
11830 Westline Industrial Drive
St. Louis, MO 63146
(800) 340-3356

Home Health Aide Digest
Stonerock & Associates
404 Parkwood
Kalamazoo, MI 49001
(616) 344-4593, (800) 340-3356

Home Health Care Management and Practice
Aspen Publishers Inc.
200 Orchard Ridge DR
Gaithersburg, MD 20878
(800) 638-8437

Home Healthcare Nurse
Lippincott Williams & Wilkins
12107 Insurance Way
Hagerstown, MD 21740
(800) 638-3030

Home Health Digest
Aspen Publishers Inc.
7201 McKinney Circle
Frederick, MD 21701
(800) 234-1660

Home Health Line
11300 Rockville Pike #1100
Rockville, MD 20852
(800) 929-4824

APPENDICES
APPENDIX A: OASIS-(B1)
Outcome and Assessment Information Set (OASIS-B1)

This data set should not be reviewed or used without first reading the accompanying narrative prologue that explains the purpose of the OASIS and its past and planned evolution.

Items to be Used at Specific Time Points

Start or Resumption of Care -- M0010-M0820

    Start of care—further visits planned
    Start of care—no further visits planned
    Resumption of care (after inpatient stay)

Follow-Up --- M0010-M0100, M0150, M0200-M0220, M0250,
M0280-M0380, M0410-M0840

    Recertification (follow-up) assessment
    Other follow-up assessment

Transfer to an Inpatient Facility --------------------------------- M0010-M0100, M0830-M0855, M0890-M0906

    Transferred to an inpatient facility—patient not discharged from an agency
    Transferred to an inpatient facility—patient discharged from agency

Discharge from Agency — Not to an Inpatient Facility

    Death at home--- M0010-M0100, M0906
    Discharge from agency ------------------------------------ M0010-M0100, M0150, M0200-M0220, M0250,
M0280-M0380, M0410-M0880, M0903-M0906

    Discharge from agency—no visits completed
    after start/resumption of care assessment ------------------- M0010-M0100, M0906

Note: For items M0640-M0800, please note special instructions at the beginning of the section.

CLINICAL RECORD ITEMS

(M0010) Agency Medicare Provider Number: _ _ _ _ _ _

(M0012) Agency Medicaid Provider Number: _ _ _ _ _ _ _ _ _ _ _ _ _ _

> **Branch Identification** (Optional, for Agency Use)
>
> **(M0014) Branch State:** _ _
>
> **(M0016) Branch ID Number:** _ _ _ _ _ _ _ _ _ _
>   (Agency-assigned)

(M0020) Patient ID Number: _ _ _ _ _ _ _ _ _ _ _ _ _ _ _ _ _ _

(M0030) Start of Care Date: _ _ / _ _ / _ _ _ _
                    month day   year

(M0032) Resumption of Care Date: _ _ / _ _ / _ _ _ _   ☐ **NA – Not Applicable**
                            month day   year

(M0040) Patient Name:

(First) _ _ _ _ _ _ _ _ _ _ _ _ (MI) (Last) _ _ _ _ _ _ _ _ _ _ _ _ _ _ (Suffix)

Reprinted with permission from the Center for Health Services and Policy Research, Denver, 1998.

(M0050) **Patient State of Residence:** _ _

(M0060) **Patient Zip Code:** _ _ _ _ _   _ _ _ _

(M0063) **Medicare Number:** _ _ _ _ _ _ _ _ _ _ _   ☐ **NA – No Medicare**
                                                    (including suffix)

(M0064) **Social Security Number:** _ _ _ - _ _ - _ _ _ _   ☐ **UK – Unknown or Not Available**

(M0065) **Medicaid Number:** _ _ _ _ _ _ _ _ _ _ _ _   ☐ **NA – No Medicaid**

(M0066) **Birth Date:**   _ _ / _ _ / _ _ _ _
                          month day   year

(M0069) **Gender:**

   ☐   1 - Male
   ☐   2 - Female

(M0072) **Primary Referring Physician ID:**

   _ _ _ _ _ _ _ _ _   ☐ **UK – Unknown or Not Available**

(M0080) **Discipline of Person Completing Assessment:**

   ☐ 1-RN   ☐ 2-PT   ☐ 3-SLP/ST   ☐ 4-OT

(M0090) **Date Assessment Completed:**   _ _ / _ _ / _ _ _ _
                                         month day   year

(M0100) **This Assessment is Currently Being Completed for the Following Reason:**

   Start/Resumption of Care
   ☐   1 – Start of care—further visits planned
   ☐   2 – Start of care—no further visits planned
   ☐   3 – Resumption of care (after inpatient stay)

   Follow-Up
   ☐   4 – Recertification (follow-up) reassessment **[Go to *M0150*]**
   ☐   5 – Other follow-up **[Go to *M0150*]**

   Transfer to an Inpatient Facility
   ☐   6 – Transferred to an inpatient facility—patient not discharged from agency **[Go to *M0830*]**
   ☐   7 – Transferred to an inpatient facility—patient discharged from agency **[Go to *M0830*]**

   Discharge from Agency — Not to an Inpatient Facility
   ☐   8 – Death at home **[Go to *M0906*]**
   ☐   9 – Discharge from agency **[Go to *M0150*]**
   ☐ 10 – Discharge from agency—no visits completed after start/resumption of care assessment
              [Go to *M0906*]

DEMOGRAPHICS AND PATIENT HISTORY

(M0140) **Race/Ethnicity** (as identified by patient): **(Mark all that apply.)**

   ☐   1 - American Indian or Alaska Native
   ☐   2 - Asian
   ☐   3 - Black or African-American
   ☐   4 - Hispanic or Latino
   ☐   5 - Native Hawaiian or Pacific Islander
   ☐   6 - White
   ☐ UK - Unknown

(M0150) **Current Payment Sources for Home Care:** **(Mark all that apply.)**

- ☐ 0 - None; no charge for current services
- ☐ 1 - Medicare (traditional fee-for-service)
- ☐ 2 - Medicare (HMO/managed care)
- ☐ 3 - Medicaid (traditional fee-for-service)
- ☐ 4 - Medicaid (HMO/managed care)
- ☐ 5 - Workers' compensation
- ☐ 6 - Title programs (e.g., Title III, V, or XX)
- ☐ 7 - Other government (e.g., CHAMPUS, VA, etc.)
- ☐ 8 - Private insurance
- ☐ 9 - Private HMO/managed care
- ☐ 10 - Self-pay
- ☐ 11 - Other (specify) _____
- ☐ UK - Unknown

(M0160) **Financial Factors** limiting the ability of the patient/family to meet basic health needs: **(Mark all that apply.)**

- ☐ 0 - None
- ☐ 1 - Unable to afford medicine or medical supplies
- ☐ 2 - Unable to afford medical expenses that are not covered by insurance/Medicare (e.g., copayments)
- ☐ 3 - Unable to afford rent/utility bills
- ☐ 4 - Unable to afford food
- ☐ 5 - Other (specify) _____

(M0170) From which of the following **Inpatient Facilities** was the patient discharged <u>during the past 14 days</u>? **(Mark all that apply.)**

- ☐ 1 - Hospital
- ☐ 2 - Rehabilitation facility
- ☐ 3 - Nursing home
- ☐ 4 - Other (specify) _____
- ☐ NA - Patient was not discharged from an inpatient facility **[If NA, go to *M0200*]**

(M0180) **Inpatient Discharge Date** (most recent):

__ __ / __ __ / __ __ __ __
month day   year

- ☐ UK - Unknown

(M0190) **Inpatient Diagnoses** and ICD code categories (three digits required; five digits optional) <u>for only those conditions treated during an inpatient facility stay within the last 14 days</u> (no surgical or V-codes):

Inpatient Facility Diagnosis	ICD
a. _____	(__ __ __ . __ __)
b. _____	(__ __ __ . __ __)

(M0200) **Medical or Treatment Regimen Change Within Past 14 Days:** Has this patient experienced a change in medical or treatment regimen (e.g., medication, treatment, or service change due to new or additional diagnosis, etc.) within the last 14 days?

- ☐ 0 - No **[If No, go to *M0220*]**
- ☐ 1 - Yes

(M0210) List the patient's **Medical Diagnoses** and ICD code categories (three digits required; five digits optional) <u>for those conditions requiring changed medical or treatment regimen</u> (no surgical or V-codes):

Changed Medical Regimen Diagnosis	ICD
a. _____	(__ __ __ . __ __)
b. _____	(__ __ __ . __ __)
c. _____	(__ __ __ . __ __)
d. _____	(__ __ __ . __ __)

(M0220) **Conditions Prior to Medical or Treatment Regimen Change or Inpatient Stay Within Past 14 Days**: If this patient experienced an inpatient facility discharge or change in medical or treatment regimen within the past 14 days, indicate any conditions which existed <u>prior to</u> the inpatient stay or change in medical or treatment regimen. **(Mark all that apply.)**

- ☐ 1 - Urinary incontinence
- ☐ 2 - Indwelling/suprapubic catheter
- ☐ 3 - Intractable pain
- ☐ 4 - Impaired decision-making
- ☐ 5 - Disruptive or socially inappropriate behavior
- ☐ 6 - Memory loss to the extent that supervision required
- ☐ 7 - None of the above
- ☐ NA - No inpatient facility discharge <u>and</u> no change in medical or treatment regimen in past 14 days
- ☐ UK - Unknown

(M0230/M0240) **Diagnoses and Severity Index**: List each medical diagnosis or problem for which the patient is receiving home care and ICD code category (three digits required; five digits optional – no surgical or V-codes) and rate them using the following severity index. (Choose one value that represents the most severe rating appropriate for each diagnosis.)

- 0 - Asymptomatic, no treatment needed at this time
- 1 - Symptoms well controlled with current therapy
- 2 - Symptoms controlled with difficulty, affecting daily functioning; patient needs ongoing monitoring
- 3 - Symptoms poorly controlled, patient needs frequent adjustment in treatment and dose monitoring
- 4 - Symptoms poorly controlled, history of rehospitalizations

(M0230) Primary Diagnosis	ICD	Severity Rating
a. _____	(__ __ __ . __ __)	☐ 0 ☐ 1 ☐ 2 ☐ 3 ☐ 4

(M0240) Other Diagnoses	ICD	Severity Rating
b. _____	(__ __ __ . __ __)	☐ 0 ☐ 1 ☐ 2 ☐ 3 ☐ 4
c. _____	(__ __ __ . __ __)	☐ 0 ☐ 1 ☐ 2 ☐ 3 ☐ 4
d. _____	(__ __ __ . __ __)	☐ 0 ☐ 1 ☐ 2 ☐ 3 ☐ 4
e. _____	(__ __ __ . __ __)	☐ 0 ☐ 1 ☐ 2 ☐ 3 ☐ 4
f. _____	(__ __ __ . __ __)	☐ 0 ☐ 1 ☐ 2 ☐ 3 ☐ 4

(M0250) **Therapies** the patient receives <u>at home</u>: **(Mark all that apply.)**

- ☐ 1 - Intravenous or infusion therapy (excludes TPN)
- ☐ 2 - Parenteral nutrition (TPN or lipids)
- ☐ 3 - Enteral nutrition (nasogastric, gastrostomy, jejunostomy, or any other artificial entry into the alimentary canal)
- ☐ 4 - None of the above

(M0260) Overall Prognosis: BEST description of patient's overall prognosis for <u>recovery from this episode of illness</u>.

☐   0 -   Poor: little or no recovery is expected and/or further decline is imminent
☐   1 -   Good/Fair: partial to full recovery is expected
☐ UK -   Unknown

(M0270) Rehabilitative Prognosis: BEST description of patient's prognosis for <u>functional status</u>.

☐   0 -   Guarded: minimal improvement in functional status is expected; decline is possible
☐   1 -   Good: marked improvement in functional status is expected
☐ UK -   Unknown

(M0280) Life Expectancy: (Physician documentation is not required.)

☐   0 -   Life expectancy is greater than 6 months
☐   1 -   Life expectancy is 6 months or fewer

(M0290) High Risk Factors characterizing this patient: **(Mark all that apply.)**

☐   1 -   Heavy smoking
☐   2 -   Obesity
☐   3 -   Alcohol dependency
☐   4 -   Drug dependency
☐   5 -   None of the above
☐ UK -   Unknown

LIVING ARRANGEMENTS

(M0300) Current Residence:

☐   1 -   Patient's owned or rented residence (house, apartment, or mobile home owned or rented by patient/couple/significant other)
☐   2 -   Family member's residence
☐   3 -   Boarding home or rented room
☐   4 -   Board and care or assisted living facility
☐   5 -   Other (specify) _____

(M0310) Structural Barriers in the patient's environment limiting independent mobility: **(Mark all that apply.)**

☐   0 -   None
☐   1 -   Stairs inside home which <u>must</u> be used by the patient (e.g., to get to toileting, sleeping, eating areas)
☐   2 -   Stairs inside home which are used optionally (e.g., to get to laundry facilities)
☐   3 -   Stairs leading from inside house to outside
☐   4 -   Narrow or obstructed doorways

(M0320) Safety Hazards found in the patient's current place of residence: **(Mark all that apply.)**

- ☐ 0 - None
- ☐ 1 - Inadequate floor, roof, or windows
- ☐ 2 - Inadequate lighting
- ☐ 3 - Unsafe gas/electric appliance
- ☐ 4 - Inadequate heating
- ☐ 5 - Inadequate cooling
- ☐ 6 - Lack of fire safety devices
- ☐ 7 - Unsafe floor coverings
- ☐ 8 - Inadequate stair railings
- ☐ 9 - Improperly stored hazardous materials
- ☐ 10 - Lead-based paint
- ☐ 11 - Other (specify) _____

(M0330) Sanitation Hazards found in the patient's current place of residence: **(Mark all that apply.)**

- ☐ 0 - None
- ☐ 1 - No running water
- ☐ 2 - Contaminated water
- ☐ 3 - No toileting facilities
- ☐ 4 - Outdoor toileting facilities only
- ☐ 5 - Inadequate sewage disposal
- ☐ 6 - Inadequate/improper food storage
- ☐ 7 - No food refrigeration
- ☐ 8 - No cooking facilities
- ☐ 9 - Insects/rodents present
- ☐ 10 - No scheduled trash pickup
- ☐ 11 - Cluttered/soiled living area
- ☐ 12 - Other (specify) _____

(M0340) Patient Lives With: (Mark all that apply.)

- ☐ 1 - Lives alone
- ☐ 2 - With spouse or significant other
- ☐ 3 - With other family member
- ☐ 4 - With a friend
- ☐ 5 - With paid help (other than home care agency staff)
- ☐ 6 - With other than above

SUPPORTIVE ASSISTANCE

(M0350) Assisting Person(s) Other than Home Care Agency Staff: (Mark all that apply.)

- ☐ 1 - Relatives, friends, or neighbors living outside the home
- ☐ 2 - Person residing in the home (EXCLUDING paid help)
- ☐ 3 - Paid help
- ☐ 4 - None of the above **[If None of the above, go to *M0390*]**
- ☐ UK - Unknown **[If Unknown, go to *M0390*]**

(M0360) Primary Caregiver taking <u>lead</u> responsibility for providing or managing the patient's care, providing the most frequent assistance, etc. (other than home care agency staff):

☐   0 -   No one person   **[If No one person, go to _M0390_]**
☐   1 -   Spouse or significant other
☐   2 -   Daughter or son
☐   3 -   Other family member
☐   4 -   Friend or neighbor or community or church member
☐   5 -   Paid help
☐ UK -   Unknown   **[If Unknown, go to _M0390_]**

(M0370) How Often does the patient receive assistance from the primary caregiver?

☐   1 -   Several times during day and night
☐   2 -   Several times during day
☐   3 -   Once daily
☐   4 -   Three or more times per week
☐   5 -   One to two times per week
☐   6 -   Less often than weekly
☐ UK -   Unknown

(M0380) Type of Primary Caregiver Assistance: (Mark all that apply.)

☐   1 -   ADL assistance (e.g., bathing, dressing, toileting, bowel/bladder, eating/feeding)
☐   2 -   IADL assistance (e.g., meds, meals, housekeeping, laundry, telephone, shopping, finances)
☐   3 -   Environmental support (housing, home maintenance)
☐   4 -   Psychosocial support (socialization, companionship, recreation)
☐   5 -   Advocates or facilitates patient's participation in appropriate medical care
☐   6 -   Financial agent, power of attorney, or conservator of finance
☐   7 -   Health care agent, conservator of person, or medical power of attorney
☐ UK -   Unknown

SENSORY STATUS

(M0390) Vision with corrective lenses if the patient usually wears them:

☐   0 -   Normal vision: sees adequately in most situations; can see medication labels, newsprint.
☐   1 -   Partially impaired: cannot see medication labels or newsprint, but <u>can</u> see obstacles in path, and the surrounding layout; can count fingers at arm's length.
☐   2 -   Severely impaired: cannot locate objects without hearing or touching them <u>or</u> patient nonresponsive.

(M0400) Hearing and Ability to Understand Spoken Language in patient's own language (with hearing aids if the patient usually uses them):

☐   0 -   No observable impairment. Able to hear and understand complex or detailed instructions and extended or abstract conversation.
☐   1 -   With minimal difficulty, able to hear and understand most multi-step instructions and ordinary conversation. May need occasional repetition, extra time, or louder voice.
☐   2 -   Has moderate difficulty hearing and understanding simple, one-step instructions and brief conversation; needs frequent prompting or assistance.
☐   3 -   Has severe difficulty hearing and understanding simple greetings and short comments. Requires multiple repetitions, restatements, demonstrations, additional time.
☐   4 -   <u>Unable</u> to hear and understand familiar words or common expressions consistently, <u>or</u> patient nonresponsive.

(M0410) Speech and Oral (Verbal) Expression of Language (in patient's own language):

- ☐ 0 - Expresses complex ideas, feelings, and needs clearly, completely, and easily in all situations with no observable impairment.
- ☐ 1 - Minimal difficulty in expressing ideas and needs (may take extra time; makes occasional errors in word choice, grammar or speech intelligibility; needs minimal prompting or assistance).
- ☐ 2 - Expresses simple ideas or needs with moderate difficulty (needs prompting or assistance, errors in word choice, organization or speech intelligibility). Speaks in phrases or short sentences.
- ☐ 3 - Has severe difficulty expressing basic ideas or needs and requires maximal assistance or guessing by listener. Speech limited to single words or short phrases.
- ☐ 4 - <u>Unable</u> to express basic needs even with maximal prompting or assistance but is not comatose or unresponsive (e.g., speech is nonsensical or unintelligible).
- ☐ 5 - Patient nonresponsive or unable to speak.

(M0420) Frequency of Pain interfering with patient's activity or movement:

- ☐ 0 - Patient has no pain or pain does not interfere with activity or movement
- ☐ 1 - Less often than daily
- ☐ 2 - Daily, but not constantly
- ☐ 3 - All of the time

(M0430) Intractable Pain: Is the patient experiencing pain that is <u>not easily relieved</u>, occurs at least daily, and affects the patient's sleep, appetite, physical or emotional energy, concentration, personal relationships, emotions, or ability or desire to perform physical activity?

- ☐ 0 - No
- ☐ 1 - Yes

INTEGUMENTARY STATUS

(M0440) Does this patient have a **Skin Lesion** or an **Open Wound**? This excludes "OSTOMIES."

- ☐ 0 - No **[If No, go to *M0490*]**
- ☐ 1 - Yes

(M0445) Does this patient have a **Pressure Ulcer**?

- ☐ 0 - No **[If No, go to *M0468*]**
- ☐ 1 - Yes

(M0450) Current Number of Pressure Ulcers at Each Stage: (Circle one response for each stage.)

	Pressure Ulcer Stages	Number of Pressure Ulcers				
a)	Stage 1: Nonblanchable erythema of intact skin; the heralding of skin ulceration. In darker-pigmented skin, warmth, edema, hardness, or discolored skin may be indicators.	0	1	2	3	4 or more
b)	Stage 2: Partial thickness skin loss involving epidermis and/or dermis. The ulcer is superficial and presents clinically as an abrasion, blister, or shallow crater.	0	1	2	3	4 or more
c)	Stage 3: Full-thickness skin loss involving damage or necrosis of subcutaneous tissue which may extend down to, but not through, underlying fascia. The ulcer presents clinically as a deep crater with or without undermining of adjacent tissue.	0	1	2	3	4 or more
d)	Stage 4: Full-thickness skin loss with extensive destruction, tissue necrosis, or damage to muscle, bone, or supporting structures (e.g., tendon, joint capsule, etc.)	0	1	2	3	4 or more
e)	In addition to the above, is there at least one pressure ulcer that cannot be observed due to the presence of eschar or a nonremovable dressing, including casts? ☐ 0 - No ☐ 1 - Yes					

(M0460) Stage of Most Problematic (Observable) Pressure Ulcer:

- ☐   1 -   Stage 1
- ☐   2 -   Stage 2
- ☐   3 -   Stage 3
- ☐   4 -   Stage 4
- ☐ NA -   No observable pressure ulcer

(M0464) Status of Most Problematic (Observable) Pressure Ulcer:

- ☐   1 -   Fully granulating
- ☐   2 -   Early/partial granulation
- ☐   3 -   Not healing
- ☐ NA -   No observable pressure ulcer

(M0468) Does this patient have a **Stasis Ulcer**?

- ☐   0 -   No **[If No, go to _M0482_]**
- ☐   1 -   Yes

(M0470) Current Number of Observable Stasis Ulcer(s):

- ☐   0 -   Zero
- ☐   1 -   One
- ☐   2 -   Two
- ☐   3 -   Three
- ☐   4 -   Four or more

(M0474) Does this patient have at least one **Stasis Ulcer that Cannot be Observed** due to the presence of a nonremovable dressing?

- ☐   0 -   No
- ☐   1 -   Yes

(M0476) Status of Most Problematic (Observable) Stasis Ulcer:

- ☐   1 -   Fully granulating
- ☐   2 -   Early/partial granulation
- ☐   3 -   Not healing
- ☐ NA -   No observable stasis ulcer

(M0482) Does this patient have a **Surgical Wound**?

- ☐   0 -   No **[If No, go to _M0490_]**
- ☐   1 -   Yes

(M0484) Current Number of (Observable) Surgical Wounds: (If a wound is partially closed but has <u>more</u> than one opening, consider each opening as a separate wound.)

- ☐   0 -   Zero
- ☐   1 -   One
- ☐   2 -   Two
- ☐   3 -   Three
- ☐   4 -   Four or more

(M0486) Does this patient have at least one **Surgical Wound that Cannot be Observed** due to the presence of a nonremovable dressing?

- ☐   0 -   No
- ☐   1 -   Yes

(M0488) Status of Most Problematic (Observable) Surgical Wound:

- ☐ 1 - Fully granulating
- ☐ 2 - Early/partial granulation
- ☐ 3 - Not healing
- ☐ NA - No observable surgical wound

RESPIRATORY STATUS

(M0490) When is the patient dyspneic or noticeably **Short of Breath**?

- ☐ 0 - Never, patient is not short of breath
- ☐ 1 - When walking more than 20 feet, climbing stairs
- ☐ 2 - With moderate exertion (e.g., while dressing, using commode or bedpan, walking distances less than 20 feet)
- ☐ 3 - With minimal exertion (e.g., while eating, talking, or performing other ADLs) or with agitation
- ☐ 4 - At rest (during day or night)

(M0500) Respiratory Treatments utilized at home: **(Mark all that apply.)**

- ☐ 1 - Oxygen (intermittent or continuous)
- ☐ 2 - Ventilator (continually or at night)
- ☐ 3 - Continuous positive airway pressure
- ☐ 4 - None of the above

ELIMINATION STATUS

(M0510) Has this patient been treated for a **Urinary Tract Infection** in the past 14 days?

- ☐ 0 - No
- ☐ 1 - Yes
- ☐ NA - Patient on prophylactic treatment
- ☐ UK - Unknown

(M0520) Urinary Incontinence or Urinary Catheter Presence:

- ☐ 0 - No incontinence or catheter (includes anuria or ostomy for urinary drainage) **[If No, go to *M0540*]**
- ☐ 1 - Patient is incontinent
- ☐ 2 - Patient requires a urinary catheter (i.e., external, indwelling, intermittent, suprapubic) **[Go to *M0540*]**

(M0530) When does **Urinary Incontinence** occur?

- ☐ 0 - Timed-voiding defers incontinence
- ☐ 1 - During the night only
- ☐ 2 - During the day and night

(M0540) Bowel Incontinence Frequency:

- ☐ 0 - Very rarely or never has bowel incontinence
- ☐ 1 - Less than once weekly
- ☐ 2 - One to three times weekly
- ☐ 3 - Four to six times weekly
- ☐ 4 - On a daily basis
- ☐ 5 - More often than once daily
- ☐ NA - Patient has ostomy for bowel elimination
- ☐ UK - Unknown

(M0550) Ostomy for Bowel Elimination: Does this patient have an ostomy for bowel elimination that (within the last 14 days): a) was related to an inpatient facility stay, <u>or</u> b) necessitated a change in medical or treatment regimen?

- ☐ 0 - Patient does <u>not</u> have an ostomy for bowel elimination.
- ☐ 1 - Patient's ostomy was <u>not</u> related to an inpatient stay and did <u>not</u> necessitate change in medical or treatment regimen.
- ☐ 2 - The ostomy <u>was</u> related to an inpatient stay or <u>did</u> necessitate change in medical or treatment regimen.

NEURO/EMOTIONAL/BEHAVIORAL STATUS

(M0560) Cognitive Functioning: (Patient's current level of alertness, orientation, comprehension, concentration, and immediate memory for simple commands.)

- ☐ 0 - Alert/oriented, able to focus and shift attention, comprehends and recalls task directions independently.
- ☐ 1 - Requires prompting (cuing, repetition, reminders) only under stressful or unfamiliar conditions.
- ☐ 2 - Requires assistance and some direction in specific situations (e.g., on all tasks involving shifting of attention), or consistently requires low stimulus environment due to distractibility.
- ☐ 3 - Requires considerable assistance in routine situations. Is not alert and oriented or is unable to shift attention and recall directions more than half the time.
- ☐ 4 - Totally dependent due to disturbances such as constant disorientation, coma, persistent vegetative state, or delirium.

(M0570) When Confused (Reported or Observed):

- ☐ 0 - Never
- ☐ 1 - In new or complex situations only
- ☐ 2 - On awakening or at night only
- ☐ 3 - During the day and evening, but not constantly
- ☐ 4 - Constantly
- ☐ NA - Patient nonresponsive

(M0580) When Anxious (Reported or Observed):

- ☐ 0 - None of the time
- ☐ 1 - Less often than daily
- ☐ 2 - Daily, but not constantly
- ☐ 3 - All of the time
- ☐ NA - Patient nonresponsive

(M0590) Depressive Feelings Reported or Observed in Patient: (Mark all that apply.)

- ☐ 1 - Depressed mood (e.g., feeling sad, tearful)
- ☐ 2 - Sense of failure or self reproach
- ☐ 3 - Hopelessness
- ☐ 4 - Recurrent thoughts of death
- ☐ 5 - Thoughts of suicide
- ☐ 6 - None of the above feelings observed or reported

(M0600) Patient Behaviors (Reported or Observed): (Mark all that apply.)

- ☐ 1 - Indecisiveness, lack of concentration
- ☐ 2 - Diminished interest in most activities
- ☐ 3 - Sleep disturbances
- ☐ 4 - Recent change in appetite or weight
- ☐ 5 - Agitation
- ☐ 6 - A suicide attempt
- ☐ 7 - None of the above behaviors observed or reported

(M0610) Behaviors Demonstrated <u>at Least Once a Week</u> (Reported or Observed): (Mark all that apply.)

- ☐ 1 - Memory deficit: failure to recognize familiar persons/places, inability to recall events of past 24 hours, significant memory loss so that supervision is required
- ☐ 2 - Impaired decision-making: failure to perform usual ADLs or IADLs, inability to appropriately stop activities, jeopardizes safety through actions
- ☐ 3 - Verbal disruption: yelling, threatening, excessive profanity, sexual references, etc.
- ☐ 4 - Physical aggression: aggressive or combative to self and others (e.g., hits self, throws objects, punches, dangerous maneuvers with wheelchair or other objects)
- ☐ 5 - Disruptive, infantile, or socially inappropriate behavior (**excludes** verbal actions)
- ☐ 6 - Delusional, hallucinatory, or paranoid behavior
- ☐ 7 - None of the above behaviors demonstrated

(M0620) Frequency of Behavior Problems (Reported or Observed) (e.g., wandering episodes, self abuse, verbal disruption, physical aggression, etc.):

- ☐ 0 - Never
- ☐ 1 - Less than once a month
- ☐ 2 - Once a month
- ☐ 3 - Several times each month
- ☐ 4 - Several times a week
- ☐ 5 - At least daily

(M0630) Is this patient receiving Psychiatric Nursing Services at home provided by a qualified psychiatric nurse?

- ☐ 0 - No
- ☐ 1 - Yes

<u>ADL/IADLs</u>

> For M0640-M0800, complete the "Current" column for all patients. For these same items, complete the "Prior" column only at start of care and at resumption of care; mark the level that corresponds to the patient's condition 14 days prior to start of care date (M0030) or resumption of care date (M0032). In all cases, record what the patient is *able to do.*

(M0640) Grooming: Ability to tend to personal hygiene needs (i.e., washing face and hands, hair care, shaving or make up, teeth or denture care, fingernail care).

Prior   Current
- ☐ ☐ 0 - Able to groom self unaided, with or without the use of assistive devices or adapted methods.
- ☐ ☐ 1 - Grooming utensils must be placed within reach before able to complete grooming activities.
- ☐ ☐ 2 - Someone must assist the patient to groom self.
- ☐ ☐ 3 - Patient depends entirely upon someone else for grooming needs.
- ☐   UK - Unknown

(M0650) Ability to Dress Upper Body (with or without dressing aids) including undergarments, pullovers, front-opening shirts and blouses, managing zippers, buttons, and snaps:

Prior	Current		
☐	☐	0 -	Able to get clothes out of closets and drawers, put them on and remove them from the upper body without assistance.
☐	☐	1 -	Able to dress upper body without assistance if clothing is laid out or handed to the patient.
☐	☐	2 -	Someone must help the patient put on upper body clothing.
☐	☐	3 -	Patient depends entirely upon another person to dress the upper body.
☐		UK -	Unknown

(M0660) Ability to Dress Lower Body (with or without dressing aids) including undergarments, slacks, socks or nylons, shoes:

Prior	Current		
☐	☐	0 -	Able to obtain, put on, and remove clothing and shoes without assistance.
☐	☐	1 -	Able to dress lower body without assistance if clothing and shoes are laid out or handed to the patient.
☐	☐	2 -	Someone must help the patient put on undergarments, slacks, socks or nylons, and shoes.
☐	☐	3 -	Patient depends entirely upon another person to dress lower body.
☐		UK -	Unknown

(M0670) Bathing: Ability to wash entire body. **Excludes grooming (washing face and hands only).**

Prior	Current		
☐	☐	0 -	Able to bathe self in shower or tub independently.
☐	☐	1 -	With the use of devices, is able to bathe self in shower or tub independently.
☐	☐	2 -	Able to bathe in shower or tub with the assistance of another person:
			(a) for intermittent supervision or encouragement or reminders, OR
			(b) to get in and out of the shower or tub, OR
			(c) for washing difficult to reach areas.
☐	☐	3 -	Participates in bathing self in shower or tub, but requires presence of another person throughout the bath for assistance or supervision.
☐	☐	4 -	Unable to use the shower or tub and is bathed in bed or bedside chair.
☐	☐	5 -	Unable to effectively participate in bathing and is totally bathed by another person.
☐		UK -	Unknown

(M0680) Toileting: Ability to get to and from the toilet or bedside commode.

Prior	Current		
☐	☐	0 -	Able to get to and from the toilet independently with or without a device.
☐	☐	1 -	When reminded, assisted, or supervised by another person, able to get to and from the toilet.
☐	☐	2 -	Unable to get to and from the toilet but is able to use a bedside commode (with or without assistance).
☐	☐	3 -	Unable to get to and from the toilet or bedside commode but is able to use a bedpan/urinal independently.
☐	☐	4 -	Is totally dependent in toileting.
☐		UK -	Unknown

(M0690) Transferring: Ability to move from bed to chair, on and off toilet or commode, into and out of tub or shower, and ability to turn and position self in bed if patient is bedfast.

Prior	Current		
☐	☐	0 -	Able to independently transfer.
☐	☐	1 -	Transfers with minimal human assistance or with use of an assistive device.
☐	☐	2 -	Unable to transfer self but is able to bear weight and pivot during the transfer process.
☐	☐	3 -	Unable to transfer self and is unable to bear weight or pivot when transferred by another person.
☐	☐	4 -	Bedfast, unable to transfer but is able to turn and position self in bed.
☐	☐	5 -	Bedfast, unable to transfer and is unable to turn and position self.
☐		UK -	Unknown

(M0700) Ambulation/Locomotion: Ability to <u>SAFELY</u> walk, once in a standing position, or use a wheelchair, once in a seated position, on a variety of surfaces.

Prior Current

☐ ☐ 0 - Able to independently walk on even and uneven surfaces and climb stairs with or without railings (i.e., needs no human assistance or assistive device).

☐ ☐ 1 - Requires use of a device (e.g., cane, walker) to walk alone <u>or</u> requires human supervision or assistance to negotiate stairs or steps or uneven surfaces.

☐ ☐ 2 - Able to walk only with the supervision or assistance of another person at all times.

☐ ☐ 3 - Chairfast, <u>unable</u> to ambulate but is able to wheel self independently.

☐ ☐ 4 - Chairfast, unable to ambulate and is <u>unable</u> to wheel self.

☐ ☐ 5 - Bedfast, unable to ambulate or be up in a chair.

☐   UK - Unknown

(M0710) Feeding or Eating: Ability to feed self meals and snacks. **Note: This refers only to the process of <u>eating</u>, <u>chewing</u>, and <u>swallowing</u>, <u>not preparing</u> the food to be eaten.**

Prior Current

☐ ☐ 0 - Able to independently feed self.

☐ ☐ 1 - Able to feed self independently but requires:
(a) meal set-up; <u>OR</u>
(b) intermittent assistance or supervision from another person; <u>OR</u>
(c) a liquid, pureed or ground meat diet.

☐ ☐ 2 - <u>Unable</u> to feed self and must be assisted or supervised throughout the meal/snack.

☐ ☐ 3 - Able to take in nutrients orally <u>and</u> receives supplemental nutrients through a nasogastric tube or gastrostomy.

☐ ☐ 4 - <u>Unable</u> to take in nutrients orally and is fed nutrients through a nasogastric tube or gastrostomy.

☐ ☐ 5 - Unable to take in nutrients orally or by tube feeding.

☐   UK - Unknown

(M0720) Planning and Preparing Light Meals (e.g., cereal, sandwich) or reheat delivered meals:

Prior Current

☐ ☐ 0 - (a) Able to independently plan and prepare all light meals for self or reheat delivered meals; <u>OR</u>
(b) Is physically, cognitively, and mentally able to prepare light meals on a regular basis but has not routinely performed light meal preparation in the past (i.e., prior to this home care admission).

☐ ☐ 1 - <u>Unable</u> to prepare light meals on a regular basis due to physical, cognitive, or mental limitations.

☐ ☐ 2 - Unable to prepare any light meals or reheat any delivered meals.

☐   UK - Unknown

(M0730) Transportation: Physical and mental ability to <u>safely</u> use a car, taxi, or public transportation (bus, train, subway).

Prior Current

☐ ☐ 0 - Able to independently drive a regular or adapted car; <u>OR</u> uses a regular or handicap-accessible public bus.

☐ ☐ 1 - Able to ride in a car only when driven by another person; <u>OR</u> able to use a bus or handicap van only when assisted or accompanied by another person.

☐ ☐ 2 - <u>Unable</u> to ride in a car, taxi, bus, or van, and requires transportation by ambulance.

☐   UK - Unknown

(M0740) Laundry: Ability to do own laundry -- to carry laundry to and from washing machine, to use washer and dryer, to wash small items by hand.

Prior	Current		
☐	☐	0 -	(a) Able to independently take care of all laundry tasks; <u>OR</u> (b) Physically, cognitively, and mentally able to do laundry and access facilities, <u>but</u> has not routinely performed laundry tasks in the past (i.e., prior to this home care admission).
☐	☐	1 -	Able to do only light laundry, such as minor hand wash or light washer loads. Due to physical, cognitive, or mental limitations, needs assistance with heavy laundry such as carrying large loads of laundry.
☐	☐	2 -	<u>Unable</u> to do any laundry due to physical limitation or needs continual supervision and assistance due to cognitive or mental limitation.
☐	UK -		Unknown

(M0750) Housekeeping: Ability to safely and effectively perform light housekeeping and heavier cleaning tasks.

Prior	Current		
☐	☐	0 -	(a) Able to independently perform all housekeeping tasks; <u>OR</u> (b) Physically, cognitively, and mentally able to perform <u>all</u> housekeeping tasks but has not routinely participated in housekeeping tasks in the past (i.e., prior to this home care admission).
☐	☐	1 -	Able to perform only <u>light</u> housekeeping (e.g., dusting, wiping kitchen counters) tasks independently.
☐	☐	2 -	Able to perform housekeeping tasks with intermittent assistance or supervision from another person.
☐	☐	3 -	<u>Unable</u> to consistently perform any housekeeping tasks unless assisted by another person throughout the process.
☐	☐	4 -	Unable to effectively participate in any housekeeping tasks.
☐	UK -		Unknown

(M0760) Shopping: Ability to plan for, select, and purchase items in a store and to carry them home or arrange delivery.

Prior	Current		
☐	☐	0 -	(a) Able to plan for shopping needs and independently perform shopping tasks, including carrying packages; <u>OR</u> (b) Physically, cognitively, and mentally able to take care of shopping, but has not done shopping in the past (i.e., prior to this home care admission).
☐	☐	1 -	Able to go shopping, but needs some assistance: (a) By self is able to do only light shopping and carry small packages, but needs someone to do occasional major shopping; <u>OR</u> (b) <u>Unable</u> to go shopping alone, but can go with someone to assist.
☐	☐	2 -	<u>Unable</u> to go shopping, but is able to identify items needed, place orders, and arrange home delivery.
☐	☐	3 -	Needs someone to do all shopping and errands.
☐	UK -		Unknown

(M0770) Ability to Use Telephone: Ability to answer the phone, dial numbers, and <u>effectively</u> use the telephone to communicate.

Prior Current

☐   ☐   0 -   Able to dial numbers and answer calls appropriately and as desired.

☐   ☐   1 -   Able to use a specially adapted telephone (i.e., large numbers on the dial, teletype phone for the deaf) and call essential numbers.

☐   ☐   2 -   Able to answer the telephone and carry on a normal conversation but has difficulty with placing calls.

☐   ☐   3 -   Able to answer the telephone only some of the time or is able to carry on only a limited conversation.

☐   ☐   4 -   <u>Unable</u> to answer the telephone at all but can listen if assisted with equipment.

☐   ☐   5 -   Totally unable to use the telephone.

☐   ☐   NA -   Patient does not have a telephone.

☐   UK -   Unknown

MEDICATIONS

(M0780) Management of Oral Medications: <u>Patient's ability</u> to prepare and take <u>all</u> prescribed oral medications reliably and safely, including administration of the correct dosage at the appropriate times/intervals. <u>**Excludes**</u> **injectable and IV medications. (NOTE: This refers to ability, not compliance or willingness.)**

Prior Current

☐   ☐   0 -   Able to independently take the correct oral medication(s) and proper dosage(s) at the correct times.

☐   ☐   1 -   Able to take medication(s) at the correct times if:
(a) individual dosages are prepared in advance by another person; <u>OR</u>
(b) given daily reminders; <u>OR</u>
(c) someone develops a drug diary or chart.

☐   ☐   2 -   <u>Unable</u> to take medication unless administered by someone else.

☐   ☐   NA -   No oral medications prescribed.

☐   UK -   Unknown

(M0790) Management of Inhalant/Mist Medications: <u>Patient's ability</u> to prepare and take <u>all</u> prescribed inhalant/mist medications (nebulizers, metered dose devices) reliably and safely, including administration of the correct dosage at the appropriate times/intervals. <u>**Excludes**</u> **all other forms of medication (oral tablets, injectable and IV medications).**

Prior Current

☐   ☐   0 -   Able to independently take the correct medication and proper dosage at the correct times.

☐   ☐   1 -   Able to take medication at the correct times if:
(a) individual dosages are prepared in advance by another person, <u>OR</u>
(b) given daily reminders.

☐   ☐   2 -   <u>Unable</u> to take medication unless administered by someone else.

☐   ☐   NA -   No inhalant/mist medications prescribed.

☐   UK -   Unknown

(M0800) **Management of Injectable Medications:** Patient's ability to prepare and take all prescribed injectable medications reliably and safely, including administration of correct dosage at the appropriate times/intervals. **Excludes IV medications.**

Prior Current

☐ ☐ 0 - Able to independently take the correct medication and proper dosage at the correct times.
☐ ☐ 1 - Able to take injectable medication at correct times if:
            (a) individual syringes are prepared in advance by another person, OR
            (b) given daily reminders.
☐ ☐ 2 - Unable to take injectable medications unless administered by someone else.
☐ ☐ NA - No injectable medications prescribed.
☐   UK - Unknown

EQUIPMENT MANAGEMENT

(M0810) **Patient Management of Equipment (includes ONLY oxygen, IV/infusion therapy, enteral/parenteral nutrition equipment or supplies):** Patient's ability to set up, monitor and change equipment reliably and safely, add appropriate fluids or medication, clean/store/dispose of equipment or supplies using proper technique. **(NOTE: This refers to ability, not compliance or willingness.)**

☐ 0 - Patient manages all tasks related to equipment completely independently.
☐ 1 - If someone else sets up equipment (i.e., fills portable oxygen tank, provides patient with prepared solutions), patient is able to manage all other aspects of equipment.
☐ 2 - Patient requires considerable assistance from another person to manage equipment, but independently completes portions of the task.
☐ 3 - Patient is only able to monitor equipment (e.g., liter flow, fluid in bag) and must call someone else to manage the equipment.
☐ 4 - Patient is completely dependent on someone else to manage all equipment.
☐ NA - No equipment of this type used in care **[If NA, go to *M0830*]**

(M0820) **Caregiver Management of Equipment (includes ONLY oxygen, IV/infusion equipment, enteral/parenteral nutrition, ventilator therapy equipment or supplies):** Caregiver's ability to set up, monitor, and change equipment reliably and safely, add appropriate fluids or medication, clean/store/dispose of equipment or supplies using proper technique. **(NOTE: This refers to ability, not compliance or willingness.)**

☐ 0 - Caregiver manages all tasks related to equipment completely independently.
☐ 1 - If someone else sets up equipment, caregiver is able to manage all other aspects.
☐ 2 - Caregiver requires considerable assistance from another person to manage equipment, but independently completes significant portions of task.
☐ 3 - Caregiver is only able to complete small portions of task (e.g., administer nebulizer treatment, clean/store/dispose of equipment or supplies).
☐ 4 - Caregiver is completely dependent on someone else to manage all equipment.
☐ NA - No caregiver
☐ UK - Unknown

EMERGENT CARE

(M0830) **Emergent Care:** Since the last time OASIS data were collected, has the patient utilized any of the following services for emergent care (other than home care agency services)? **(Mark all that apply.)**

☐ 0 - No emergent care services **[If no emergent care, go to *M0855*]**
☐ 1 - Hospital emergency room (includes 23-hour holding)
☐ 2 - Doctor's office emergency visit/house call
☐ 3 - Outpatient department/clinic emergency (includes urgicenter sites)
☐ UK - Unknown **[If UK, go to *M0855*]**

(M0840) Emergent Care Reason: For what reason(s) did the patient/family seek emergent care? **(Mark all that apply.)**

☐ 1 - Improper medication administration, medication side effects, toxicity, anaphylaxis
☐ 2 - Nausea, dehydration, malnutrition, constipation, impaction
☐ 3 - Injury caused by fall or accident at home
☐ 4 - Respiratory problems (e.g., shortness of breath, respiratory infection, tracheobronchial obstruction)
☐ 5 - Wound infection, deteriorating wound status, new lesion/ulcer
☐ 6 - Cardiac problems (e.g., fluid overload, exacerbation of CHF, chest pain)
☐ 7 - Hypo/Hyperglycemia, diabetes out of control
☐ 8 - GI bleeding, obstruction
☐ 9 - Other than above reasons
☐ UK - Reason unknown

DATA ITEMS COLLECTED AT INPATIENT FACILITY ADMISSION OR AGENCY DISCHARGE ONLY

(M0855) To which **Inpatient Facility** has the patient been admitted?

☐ 1 - Hospital **[Go to *M0890*]**
☐ 2 - Rehabilitation facility **[Go to *M0903*]**
☐ 3 - Nursing home **[Go to *M0900*]**
☐ 4 - Hospice **[Go to *M0903*]**
☐ NA - No inpatient facility admission

(M0870) Discharge Disposition: Where is the patient after discharge from your agency? **(Choose only one answer.)**

☐ 1 - Patient remained in the community (not in hospital, nursing home, or rehab facility)
☐ 2 - Patient transferred to a noninstitutional hospice **[Go to *M0903*]**
☐ 3 - Unknown because patient moved to a geographic location not served by this agency **[Go to *M0903*]**
☐ UK - Other unknown **[Go to *M0903*]**

(M0880) After discharge, does the patient receive health, personal, or support **Services or Assistance**? **(Mark all that apply.)**

☐ 1 - No assistance or services received
☐ 2 - Yes, assistance or services provided by family or friends
☐ 3 - Yes, assistance or services provided by other community resources (e.g., meals-on-wheels, home health services, homemaker assistance, transportation assistance, assisted living, board and care)

Go to *M0903*

(M0890) If the patient was admitted to an acute care **Hospital**, for what **Reason** was he/she admitted?

☐ 1 - Hospitalization for emergent (unscheduled) care
☐ 2 - Hospitalization for urgent (scheduled within 24 hours of admission) care
☐ 3 - Hospitalization for elective (scheduled more than 24 hours before admission) care
☐ UK - Unknown

(M0895) Reason for Hospitalization: (Mark all that apply.)

- ☐ 1 - Improper medication administration, medication side effects, toxicity, anaphylaxis
- ☐ 2 - Injury caused by fall or accident at home
- ☐ 3 - Respiratory problems (SOB, infection, obstruction)
- ☐ 4 - Wound or tube site infection, deteriorating wound status, new lesion/ulcer
- ☐ 5 - Hypo/Hyperglycemia, diabetes out of control
- ☐ 6 - GI bleeding, obstruction
- ☐ 7 - Exacerbation of CHF, fluid overload, heart failure
- ☐ 8 - Myocardial infarction, stroke
- ☐ 9 - Chemotherapy
- ☐ 10 - Scheduled surgical procedure
- ☐ 11 - Urinary tract infection
- ☐ 12 - IV catheter-related infection
- ☐ 13 - Deep vein thrombosis, pulmonary embolus
- ☐ 14 - Uncontrolled pain
- ☐ 15 - Psychotic episode
- ☐ 16 - Other than above reasons

  | Go to *M0903* |

(M0900) For what **Reason(s)** was the patient **Admitted** to a **Nursing Home**? **(Mark all that apply.)**

- ☐ 1 - Therapy services
- ☐ 2 - Respite care
- ☐ 3 - Hospice care
- ☐ 4 - Permanent placement
- ☐ 5 - Unsafe for care at home
- ☐ 6 - Other
- ☐ UK - Unknown

(M0903) Date of Last (Most Recent) Home Visit:

__ __ / __ __ / __ __ __ __
month day   year

(M0906) Discharge/Transfer/Death Date: Enter the date of the discharge, transfer, or death (at home) of the patient.

__ __ / __ __ / __ __ __ __
month day   year

Reprinted with permission from the Center for Health Services and Policy Research, Denver, 1998.

APPENDIX B: *FEDERAL REGISTER*

DEPARTMENT OF HEALTH AND HUMAN SERVICES

Health Care Financing Administration

[HCFA–3020–N]

RIN 0938–AJ54

Medicare and Medicaid Programs; Mandatory Use, Collection, Encoding, and Transmission of Outcome and Assessment Information Set (OASIS) for Home Health Agencies

AGENCY: Health Care Financing Administration (HCFA), HHS.

ACTION: Notice.

SUMMARY: This notice announces to home health agencies (HHAs), State survey agencies, Medicare and Medicaid beneficiaries, software vendors, and the general public changes to and effective dates for OASIS implementation. This notice announces the effective dates for the mandatory use, collection, encoding, and transmission of OASIS data for all Medicare/Medicaid patients receiving skilled services. For non-Medicare/non-Medicaid patients receiving skilled services, there will be no encoding and transmission until further notice, but HHAs must conduct comprehensive assessments and updates at the required time points. For patients receiving personal care only services, regardless of payor source, we are delaying the requirements regarding OASIS use, collection, encoding, and transmission

until further notice. We expect to begin implementation of OASIS for non-Medicare/non-Medicaid patients receiving skilled care and for patients receiving personal care only services in the Spring of 2000. A separate **Federal Register** notice will be published with instructions at that time. In addition, software changes described at the end of this notice are of interest to software vendors and HHAs. Also, a companion notice concerning the OASIS System of Records (SOR) is published elsewhere in this **Federal Register** and is available via the HCFA Internet site (http://www.hcfa.gov).

EFFECTIVE DATES: This notice is effective on July 19, 1999.

FOR FURTHER INFORMATION CONTACT: Tracey Mummert, (410) 786–3398, Mary Weakland, (410) 786–6835.

SUPPLEMENTARY INFORMATION:

I. Background

On January 25, we published a final regulation concerning the collection of OASIS data as part of the comprehensive assessment (64 FR 3764), and an interim final regulation concerning transmission of OASIS data (64 FR 3748). On April 7, 1999, we notified home health agencies (HHAs), State survey agencies, Medicare and Medicaid beneficiaries, software vendors, and the general public through the OASIS website that we delayed the effective date of the OASIS data transmission requirement. On April 27,

1999, we notified HHAs, State survey agencies, Medicare and Medicaid beneficiaries, software vendors, and the general public through the OASIS website, that the mandatory use, collection, and encoding of OASIS were also delayed, due to lack of Paperwork Reduction Act (PRA) clearances. A notice to this effect was published in the **Federal Register** on May 4, 1999 (64 FR 23846).

The appropriate PRA clearances have now been obtained and privacy procedures followed. Specifically, the PRA clearances for the final rule establishing OASIS collection and use, and the interim final rule for encoding and transmission have been obtained from the Office of Management and Budget (OMB) and approval numbers assigned. The respective OMB control numbers for these collections are 0938–0760 and 0938–0761 and the expiration dates are December 31, 1999. The Privacy Act System of Records (SOR) Notice has been carefully drafted in consultation with OMB and is published elsewhere in this **Federal Register**.

II. OASIS Effective Dates

Effective July 19, 1999, all HHAs participating in the Medicare/Medicaid programs are required to initiate the use of the standardized assessment data set, OASIS, as summarized in the following chart:

SUMMARY OF MANDATORY COLLECTION, ENCODING, AND TRANSMISSION DATES FOR OASIS

Patient classification	Collection effective date	Encoding effective date	Transmission effective date
Medicare [1]/Medicaid [2]—Skilled	July 19, 1999	July 19, 1999	August 24, 1999.
Non-Medicare/Non-Medicaid [3]—Skilled	July 19, 1999	Spring 2000	Spring 2000 [4].
Medicaid [5]—Personal Care Only	Spring 2000	Spring 2000	Spring 2000.
Non-Medicaid [3]—Personal Care Only	Spring 2000	Spring 2000	Spring 2000 [4].
• Patients under age 18; • Patients receiving pre & post partum maternity services; • Patients receiving only chore and housekeeping services.	Excluded	Excluded	Excluded.

[1] OASIS item (M0150) Current Payment Sources for Home Care: response 1 or 2.
[2] OASIS item (M0150) Current Payment Sources for Home Care: response 3 or 4.
[3] OASIS item (M0150) Current Payment Sources for Home Care: response 0, 5, 6, 7, 8, 9, 10, 11, or UK.
[4] Data transmitted with masked identifiers
[5] OASIS item (M0150) Current Payment Sources for Home Care: response 3.

III. Major Changes to OASIS

We are initiating OASIS activities as outlined in this notice which include the following changes:
• Administration of a standard notification to patients of their privacy rights on admission to the HHA.
• The addition of language in the SOR explaining limitations on "routine uses" of data under the Privacy Act, so that personally identifiable data will only be used where statistical

information is not sufficient. While this is usual practice, this language has not traditionally been included in SOR notices. Among other changes, personally identifiable data will no longer go to accrediting organizations such as the Joint Commission on Accreditation of Healthcare Organizations.
• Limiting the "routine uses" of data to other Federal and State agencies. Only those Federal and State agencies

that (1) contribute to the accuracy of HCFA's health insurance operations including payment, treatment, and coverage, and/or (2) support State agencies in the evaluations and monitoring of care provided by HHAs will have access to OASIS data.

• Major changes to the application of OASIS to private-pay patients under OASIS. We have decided that information on non-Medicare and non-Medicaid patients will not be transmitted to the States or HCFA in personally identifiable form.

• After careful attention to each question in OASIS, all questions but one were retained on the grounds of assuring quality of care and appropriate reimbursement. We did identify a sensitive question on patient financial factors that we consider less critical to achieving program goals, and this information will not be reported to HCFA or the States.

• Acceleration of efforts to encrypt data during transmission, to provide yet another level of protection. We expect to complete these efforts within a year.

• Delay and phase-in the requirement to collect, encode, and transmit OASIS data on patients receiving personal care only services until further notice. This allows States and associations to adjust to this requirement and allows us to evaluate issues pertaining to the content and frequency of OASIS data collection relative to other reporting requirements.

IV. OASIS Effective Dates in Detail

A. Medicare/Medicaid—Skilled

Effective July 19, 1999, for Medicare/ Medicaid patients receiving skilled services, HHAs must collect OASIS data as described in the final regulation published on January 25, 1999 (64 FR 3764) concerning use of the OASIS as part of the comprehensive assessment. This means that for all Medicare/ Medicaid patients receiving skilled services, currently under the care of the agency or admitted to the agency on or after July 19, 1999, HHAs must conduct comprehensive assessments and updates at the required time points, and incorporate the OASIS data set. The exception to this requirement are those patients receiving prepartum and postpartum services, patients under age 18, and patients receiving only housekeeping/chore services. OASIS data collection for patients receiving only personal care services is delayed. HHAs must collect start of care OASIS data and updates at the required time points on new admissions to the HHA on or after July 19, 1999. In addition, HHAs must collect OASIS data on patients already in service. At the next appropriate time point, that is, resumption of care, follow-up (that is, every 2 calendar months), transfer to an inpatient facility (with or without agency discharge) and death at home, on or after July 19, 1999, HHAs must collect OASIS data on all Medicare/ Medicaid patients receiving skilled services.

Effective July 19, 1999, for Medicare/ Medicaid patients receiving skilled services, HHAs must encode and lock

their OASIS data (that is, enter it into a computer), according to the requirements outlined in the interim final rule published January 25, 1999 (64 FR 3748) concerning transmission of OASIS data. This means that HHAs will encode and lock start of care OASIS data and updates at the required time points on new admissions to the HHA on or after July 19, 1999. In addition, HHAs must encode and lock OASIS data on patients already in service. At the next appropriate time point, that is, resumption of care, follow-up (i.e., every 2 calendar months), transfer to an inpatient facility (with or without agency discharge) and death at home, on or after July 19, 1999, HHAs must encode and lock OASIS data on all Medicare/Medicaid patients receiving skilled services. If the HHA patient's services are to be paid for by Medicare or Medicaid, the OASIS must be reported. There are no exceptions.

Effective August 18, 1999, HHAs must have completed a successful transmission of test OASIS data. HHAs must successfully transmit test OASIS data to the State agency for the purpose of determining connectivity with the State OASIS system and receive a feedback report on the test data. On August 19, 1999, States will begin to purge all data on the State OASIS systems to allow for acceptance of production data. Beginning August 24, 1999, HHAs must begin the transmission of production OASIS data, that is, OASIS assessments completed, encoded and locked the previous month.

EXAMPLE:

June 18, 1999—Publication of **Federal Register** Notice

July 19—August 18, 1999—Collection, encoding, and test transmission begins

August 19–24, 1999—States purge test data

August 25, 1999—Production transmission begins

At least monthly thereafter, HHA transmissions must include all OASIS data collected, encoded, and locked in the previous month.

B. Non-Medicare/Non-Medicaid— Skilled

Effective July 19, 1999, for non-Medicare/non-Medicaid patients receiving skilled services, HHAs must conduct comprehensive assessments and updates at the required time points as described in the final regulation concerning use of the OASIS as part of the comprehensive assessment published on January 25, 1999 (64 FR 3764), incorporating the OASIS data set.

HHAs must collect start of care OASIS data and updates at the required time points on new admissions to the HHA on or after July 19, 1999. In addition, HHAs must collect OASIS data on patients already in service. At the next appropriate time point, that is, resumption of care, follow-up (that is, every 2 calendar months), transfer to an inpatient facility (with or without agency discharge) and death at home, on or after July 19, 1999, HHAs must collect OASIS data on all non-Medicare/ non-Medicaid patients receiving skilled services. However, we are not requiring encoding and transmission of OASIS data at this time. These assessments must be retained as part of the patient's clinical record in the HHA.

We expect the effective date for encoding and transmission of OASIS data to begin in the Spring of 2000 for these patients. We will publish a notice in the **Federal Register** with instructions at that time. In the Spring of 2000, we will not expect HHAs to retroactively encode and transmit OASIS data collected between July 19, 1999 and the Spring of 2000. If a HHA mistakenly transmits identifiable non-Medicare/non-Medicaid data, we will reject this data at the State level. Rejection at this point ensures that the data will not get into the Federal data base until masking can be accomplished.

When the requirement to encode and transmit non-Medicare/non-Medicaid patient data begins, HHAs must submit non-identifiable OASIS data on these patients to the State agency. In this way, care provided by the HHA can be evaluated for all patients of the agency, and not just Medicare/Medicaid patients. However, these data will be not be individually identifiable, but will be masked, as discussed below.

C. Medicaid/Non-Medicaid—Personal Care Only

For patients receiving *only* personal care services, regardless of payor source, the effective date for OASIS implementation will be in the Spring of 2000. We will publish a notice in the **Federal Register** with instructions at that time. This is a delay in the implementation of OASIS for these patients, which we originally outlined in the preamble language to the January 25, 1999, regulation concerning use of the OASIS as part of the comprehensive assessment.

At this time, HHAs are not required to collect, encode and transmit OASIS data on patients receiving personal care or chore services unless skilled care is also provided. HHAs are required to collect, encode and transmit OASIS data on patients who receive personal care and/or chore services only if they also receive skilled care as described above, in addition to the personal care services.

We are delaying the requirement to allow States and associations to adjust to this requirement and allow us to evaluate issues pertaining to the content and frequency of OASIS reporting relative to other reporting requirements. In addition, this phase-in will allow HHAs more time to prepare, upgrade their systems and integrate the OASIS data set into their HHA and State specific instrument(s).

D. Masking

Masking refers to the concealing of individual data elements by the provider. Patient identifiable information is not known to HCFA or the OASIS State system. In OASIS terms, the data elements to be masked are patient's name, social security number, Medicare number, and Medicaid number. HHAs will keep the masked identifiers and the original data in their records. For non-Medicare/non-Medicaid patients, HCFA and other users will only be able to access data that does not contain any unique identifiers, including, no name, social security number, Medicare number and Medicaid number. With a consistent set of masked identifiers, we are still able to do the longitudinal data linking across patient care settings that is necessary for outcome measurement and targeting patients for sampling during the State survey agency certification review. At a minimum, we will follow the Federal Government FIPS 46–2 Data Encryption Standard (DES).

Implementation of a masking system for non-Medicare/non-Medicaid OASIS data is expected to occur in the Spring of 2000. The steps required to accomplish this task include acquiring and evaluating tools that follow the FIPS 46–2 DES, developing system specifications required to incorporate the data masking tool, making the necessary program changes to the HCFA-provided HAVEN data entry software, as well as making other necessary changes to the OASIS State system and HCFA data specifications. For HHAs not using HAVEN, we are providing the opportunity for software vendors to make the required changes and properly test their software by posting these data specifications on the OASIS website in the near future. In addition, Year 2000 testing must take place after all program changes have been incorporated, to ensure that all systems are millennium compliant.

Until such time as a system of masking patient identifiers is

implemented, HHAs must assess and collect OASIS information from all patients as required by the regulation but only encode and transmit assessments with a Medicare/Medicaid payment source. To ensure only assessments with a Medicare/Medicaid payment source are received by the OASIS State system, the OASIS State system will reject all assessments with a non-Medicare/non-Medicaid payment source.

E. Encryption

HHAs are required to send OASIS assessment data for patients who have a Medicare or Medicaid payor source. Currently, these data are sent to the respective State via a private telephone line that connects directly into the OASIS State system. Although this is a relatively secure method, additional protection may be provided by using encryption. The use of 128-bit server certificates will provide strong encryption for all users who use either the domestic or export version of the latest leading browsers. HCFA plans to require this method in the near future. Several Federal agencies such as the U.S. Department of Commerce and the United States Postal Services have an expanded license to issue 128-bit serve digital certificates.

A 128-bit encryption is standard for Netscape and Microsoft Internet Explorer, the two major web browsers. Both products are available free off the Internet or by mail for a nominal fee (less than $20.00). There are some system requirements to run these browsers. This includes a 32-bit operating system, that is, a computer that runs Windows 95, 98, or NT. HCFA's Y2K compliance requirements also require computers to have a 32-bit operating system. HHAs using the recommended computer system requirements described in the interim final regulations published on January 25, 1999 (64 FR 3738), concerning transmission of OASIS data will not require additional changes. The projected date for full 128-bit encryption transmission by HHAs is July 2000.

V. More Background on Changes to OASIS

A. Patient Rights

Existing regulations at 42 CFR 484.10, Conditions of Participation: Home Health Agencies, specify that the patient has the right to be informed of his or her rights with respect to care provided by the HHA. Under the terms of this condition, HHA patients whose data will be collected and used by the

Federal government must receive a notice of their privacy rights. These rights include: (1) the right to be informed that OASIS information will be collected and the purpose of collection; (2) the right to have the information kept confidential and secure; (3) the right to be informed that OASIS information will not be disclosed except for legitimate purposes allowed by the Federal Privacy Act; (4) the right to refuse to answer questions; and (5) the right to see, review, and request changes on their assessment. The statements of patient privacy rights with regard to the OASIS collection (one for Medicare/Medicaid patients, one for all other patients served by the HHA) are included in this notice. They will also be available via the HCFA Internet site (http://www.hcfa.gov). These statements may be revised in accordance with the OMB Paperwork Reduction Act reapproval process. Future revisions to these statements will be available via the HCFA Internet site (http://www.hcfa.gov) and in other instructional materials issued by HCFA.

Consumer testing was undertaken to determine whether Medicare beneficiaries understood the overall message of the proposed Medicare notice. The findings indicated that beneficiaries understood that the notice was informing them about their rights relating to their personal health care information and that these protections were good. In addition, the majority of the beneficiaries found the notice's language to be clear and easy to understand. For Medicare/Medicaid patients, transmission of the assessment data to HCFA will be a condition for payment and an essential tool in ensuring that both programs are paying for quality health care services. As such, we are providing HHAs with a copy of the notice that HHAs must incorporate into their admission process.

● *Notice to Medicare/Medicaid Patients*

HHAs must incorporate into their admission process for Medicare/Medicaid patients Attachments A and B. Please refer to Attachment A—Statement of Patient Privacy Rights (front), and Attachment B—Privacy Act Statement—Health Care Records (back) of this notice for this document.

● *Notice to Non-Medicare/Non-Medicaid Patients*

Attachment C—Notice About Privacy for Patients Who Do Not Have Medicare or Medicaid Coverage. This is the notice that HHAs must incorporate into their admission process for non-Medicare/non-Medicaid patients.

B. Administering the Assessment

The OASIS items should be answered as a result of the clinician's total assessment process, not completed as a checklist during an interview. Conducting a patient assessment involves both interview and observation. Many times the two processes complement each other. Information gained through interview is verified through observation. Many clinicians begin the assessment process with an interview, sequencing the questions to build rapport and gain trust and then proceed with observation. Others choose to start the assessment process with a familiar procedure such as taking vital signs to demonstrate clinical competence to the patient before proceeding to the interview. Very few OASIS data items rely solely on patient interview. In the rare instance that an assessment cannot be made due to lack of patient information, agencies must report the most appropriate response, based on their professional judgement. Patients should not be forced to cooperate with the assessment process.

If patients refuse to answer some questions that are part of the OASIS assessment, the HHA may still deliver care to the patient as long as it completes and submits the OASIS assessment to the best of its ability.

Some changes have been made to the OASIS User's manual with regard to the conventions involved in collecting and recording OASIS data in the context of the comprehensive assessment process, particularly for mental health assessments. These changes are available via the HCFA Internet site (http://www.hcfa.gov). Alternately, these changes can be accessed directly at www.hcfa.gov/medicare/hsqb/oasis/hhedtrng.htm which is where the entire OASIS User's manual is available for downloading free of charge. The purpose of these changes is to clarify the definitions, instructions, and assessment strategies for selected OASIS items, as follows:

• Pages 8.2 and 8.3 of the OASIS User's Manual have been modified to clarify the means of administering the OASIS items in the context of the comprehensive assessment.

• An introductory page (8.82) has been inserted into the Item-by-Item Tips section regarding the assessment of mental and emotional status, to provide further clarification concerning observational and interview techniques that are effective in eliciting the needed information while minimizing burden and intrusion on the patient.

• Item-by-item tips have been changed for item M0540 and items M0560 through M0620. The purpose of these changes is to emphasize observational techniques and to provide further guidance for clinicians in assessing these characteristics especially in situations where patients refuse to answer direct questions.

C. Financial Factors Limiting the Ability of the Patient/Family to Meet Basic Health Needs (M0160)

HCFA is not requiring the transmission of OASIS data item M0160 to the OASIS State system at this time. Because this data item assesses the patient's ability to meet basic health needs, the HHA may need this information to provide appropriate care. Therefore, HCFA requires the collection, assessment and encoding of this item. HCFA's data entry software (HAVEN Version 2.0) will blank out this encoded item as it is prepared for transmission to the OASIS State system. Additionally, the State system will reject this data item if it is inadvertently transmitted to the OASIS State system from software that does not meet HCFA specifications. Vendor software must be changed to accommodate this and other changes. This is discussed elsewhere in this notice.

VI. Technical Information for HHAs and Vendors

A. Medicare/Medicaid Patients

At this time, HCFA requires the encoding and transmission of OASIS information on patients who are receiving Medicare/Medicaid benefits. This means that for patients who have selected a payor source of (1) Medicare (traditional fee-for-service), (2) Medicare (HMO/managed care), (3) Medicaid (traditional fee-for-service), or (4) Medicaid (HMO/managed care) on OASIS item M0150, the HHA must collect, encode and transmit all required OASIS information to the State agency. The payor source for services provided as part of a Medicaid waiver or home and community-based waiver (HCBW) program by a Medicare-approved HHA are coded as (3) Medicaid (traditional fee-for-service) at item M0150.

B. Non-Medicare/Non-Medicaid Patients

For non-Medicare/non-Medicaid patients, the HHA will only assess and collect OASIS as part of the comprehensive assessment and agency medical record. Until such time as we develop and implement a system to mask individual-level identifying data, encoding and transmission of OASIS

data items is not required for patients with payor sources other than Medicare/Medicaid. Non-Medicare/non-Medicaid payor sources include private insurance, private HMO/managed care, self pay programs funded under the Social Security Act: for example, Title III, V, XX or other Government programs.

C. Automation Information

Software Changes Made

The following section is of interest to software vendors and includes the changes that *have been made* to accommodate requirement changes for the OASIS:

1. *HAVEN Software:* HAVEN has changed the export function to allow the user to select Medicare/Medicaid only assessments, non-Medicare/non-Medicaid assessments only, or all assessments. The HAVEN export function produces an ASCII text file from the HAVEN database. This file meets the OASIS data specifications that must be transmitted to the State agency. If a user selects Medicare/Medicaid only, as defined earlier, all assessments with a reason for assessment (M0100) value of 1, 2, 3, 4, 5, and 9 *and* a payment source (M0150) value of 1, 2, 3, or 4, as well as, all assessments with a reason for assessment (M0100) with a value of 6, 7, 8, and 10 will be selected for export. If a user selects non-Medicare/non-Medicaid only, as previously defined, all assessments with a reason for assessment (M0100) value of 1, 2, 3, 4, 5, and 9 *and* a payment source (M0150) value other than 1, 2, 3, or 4 will be selected for export. Therefore, the HHA controls assessments to be sent to the State agency. As stated previously in this notice, these procedures ensure that only assessments with a Medicare/Medicaid payment source are received by the OASIS State system as the OASIS State system will reject all assessments with a non-Medicare/non-Medicaid payment source.

In addition to this change, HAVEN will blank out responses and move spaces to the Financial Factors data item (M0160) on *all* assessments prior to creating the export file. This data will remain in the original format in the HHA database but will exist as spaces at the State database. No data is collected at the State system on this item.

2. *OASIS State System:* The OASIS State system has been changed to reject any assessment with a reason for assessment (M0100) value of 1, 2, 3, 4, 5, and 9 *and* a payment source (M0150) value other than 1, 2, 3, or 4. The validation report will reflect that an

assessment meeting the above criteria has been rejected.

In addition to this change, the OASIS State system will blank out and move spaces to the Financial Factors data (M0160) on *all* assessments prior to editing a file submitted by a HHA. This data will remain in the original format in the HHA database but as spaces at the State database. These changes in the HAVEN software are available via the HCFA Internet site (http://www.hcfa.gov) in our revised HAVEN software, version 2.0. Registered HAVEN users will be mailed a copy of the revised HAVEN software, version 2.0 by July.

The following changes *still need to be made* to accommodate requirement changes for the OASIS data base:

Software Changes Pending

1. HAVEN Software: The HAVEN software will need to incorporate all requirements to mask designated identifiers for any assessment with a reason for assessment (M0100) value of 1, 2, 3, 4, 5, and 9 *and* a payment source (M0150) value other than 1, 2, 3, or 4. Specifications for this are scheduled to be available via the HCFA Internet site (http://www.hcfa.gov) by July 1, 1999, and scheduled to become effective in April 2000.

2. OASIS State System: The OASIS State system will make the necessary edits to reject any assessment with a reason for assessment (M0100) value of 1, 2, 3, 4, 5, *and* 9 *and* a payment source (M0150) value other than 1, 2, 3, or 4 that does not have the designated identifiers masked. This edit is scheduled to be effective in April 2000.

HCFA Websites

Revisions and updates to OASIS implementation will be available via the HCFA Internet site (http://www.hcfa.gov). Alternatively, the OASIS Internet site is accessible directly at the following address: www.hcfa.gov/medicare/hsqb/oasis/oasishmp.htm. This is the OASIS home page. A summary of OASIS website content is available at this site.

OMB Review

In accordance with the provisions of Executive Order 12866 this document was reviewed by the Office of Management and Budget.

(Catalog of Federal Domestic Assistance Program No. 93.778, Medical Assistance Program; No. 93.773 Medicare—Hospital Insurance Program)

Dated: June 11, 1999.

Nancy-Ann Min DeParle,
Administrator, Health Care Financing Administration.

BILLING CODE 4120-03-P

Attachment A

Home Health Agency
Outcome and Assessment Information Set (OASIS)
STATEMENT OF PATIENT PRIVACY RIGHTS

As a home health patient, you have the privacy rights listed below.

● **You have the right to know why we need to ask you questions.**
We are required by law to collect health information to make sure:
  1) you get quality health care, and
  2) payment for Medicare and Medicaid patients is correct.

● **You have the right to have your personal health care information kept confidential.**
You may be asked to tell us information about yourself so that
we will know which home health services will be best for you.
We keep anything we learn about you confidential.
This means, only those who are legally authorized to know, or who
have a medical need to know, will see your personal health information.

● **You have the right to refuse to answer questions.**
We may need your help in collecting your health information.
If you choose not to answer, we will fill in the information as best we can.
You do not have to answer every question to get services.

● **You have the right to look at your personal health information.**
  ■ We know how important it is that the information we collect about you is
  correct. If you think we made a mistake, ask us to correct it.
  ■ If you are not satisfied with our response, you can ask the Health Care
  Financing Administration, the federal Medicare and Medicaid agency, to
  correct your information.

You can ask the Health Care Financing Administration
to see, review, copy, or correct
your personal health information which that Federal agency maintains in its
HHA OASIS System of Records. See the back of this Notice for CONTACT INFORMATION.
If you want a more detailed description of your privacy rights, see the back of this Notice:
PRIVACY ACT STATEMENT - HEALTH CARE RECORDS.

This is a Medicare & Medicaid
Approved Notice.

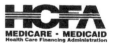

32990   Federal Register / Vol. 64, No. 117 / Friday, June 18, 1999 / Notices

Attachment B

PRIVACY ACT STATEMENT - HEALTH CARE RECORDS

THIS STATEMENT GIVES YOU ADVICE REQUIRED BY LAW (the Privacy Act of 1974).
THIS STATEMENT IS NOT A CONSENT FORM. IT WILL NOT BE USED TO RELEASE OR TO USE YOUR HEALTH CARE INFORMATION.

I. AUTHORITY FOR COLLECTION OF YOUR INFORMATION, INCLUDING YOUR SOCIAL SECURITY NUMBER, AND WHETHER OR NOT YOU ARE REQUIRED TO PROVIDE INFORMATION FOR THIS ASSESSMENT.
Sections 1102(a), 1154, 1861(o), 1861(z), 1863, 1864, 1865, 1866, 1871, 1891(b) of the Social Security Act.

Medicare and Medicaid participating home health agencies must do a complete assessment that accurately reflects your current health and includes information that can be used to show your progress toward your health goals. The home health agency must use the "Outcome and Assessment Information Set" (OASIS) when evaluating your health. To do this, the agency must get information from every patient. This information is used by the Health Care Financing Administration (HCFA, the federal Medicare & Medicaid agency) to be sure that the home health agency meets quality standards and gives appropriate health care to its patients. You have the right to refuse to provide information for the assessment to the home health agency. If your information is included in an assessment, it is protected under the federal Privacy Act of 1974 and the "Home Health Agency Outcome and Assessment Information Set" (HHA OASIS) System of Records. You have the right to see, copy, review, and request correction of your information in the HHA OASIS System of Records.

II. PRINCIPAL PURPOSES FOR WHICH YOUR INFORMATION IS INTENDED TO BE USED

The information collected will be entered into the Home Health Agency Outcome and Assessment Information Set (HHA OASIS) System No. 09-70-9002. Your health care information in the HHA OASIS System of Records will be used for the following purposes:
* support litigation involving the Health Care Financing Administration;
* support regulatory, reimbursement, and policy functions performed within the Health Care Financing Administration or by a contractor or consultant;
* study the effectiveness and quality of care provided by those home health agencies;
* survey and certification of Medicare and Medicaid home health agencies;
* provide for development, validation, and refinement of a Medicare prospective payment system;
* enable regulators to provide home health agencies with data for their internal quality improvement activities;
* support research, evaluation, or epidemiological projects related to the prevention of disease or disability, or the restoration or maintenance of health,
   and for health care payment related projects; and
* support constituent requests made to a Congressional representative.

III. ROUTINE USES

These "routine uses" specify the circumstances when the Health Care Financing Administration may release your information from the HHA OASIS System of Records without your consent. Each prospective recipient must agree in writing to ensure the continuing confidentiality and security of your information. Disclosures of the information may be to:
1. the federal Department of Justice for litigation involving the Health Care Financing Administration;
2. contractors or consultants working for the Health Care Financing Administration to assist in the performance of a service related to this system of records and who need to access these records to perform the activity;
3. an agency of a State government for purposes of determining, evaluating, and/or assessing cost, effectiveness, and/or quality of health care services provided in the State; for developing and operating Medicaid reimbursement systems; or for the administration of Federal/State home health agency programs within the State;
4. another Federal or State agency to contribute to the accuracy of the Health Care Financing Administration's health insurance operations (payment, treatment and coverage) and/or to support State agencies in the evaluations and monitoring of care provided by HHAs;
5. Peer Review Organizations, to perform Title XI or Title XVIII functions relating to assessing and improving home health agency quality of care;
6. an individual or organization for a research, evaluation, or epidemiological project related to the prevention of disease or disability, the restoration or maintenance of health, or payment related projects;
7. a congressional office in response to a constituent inquiry made at the written request of the constituent about whom the record is maintained.

IV. EFFECT ON YOU, IF YOU DO NOT PROVIDE INFORMATION

The home health agency needs the information contained in the Outcome and Assessment Information Set in order to give you quality care. It is important that the information be correct. Incorrect information could result in payment errors. Incorrect information also could make it hard to be sure that the agency is giving you quality services. If you choose not to provide information, there is no federal requirement for the home health agency to refuse you services.

NOTE: This statement may be included in the admission packet for all new home health agency admissions. Home health agencies may **request** you or your representative to sign this statement to document that this statement was given to you. **Your signature is NOT required.** If you or your representative sign the statement, the signature merely indicates that you received this statement. You or your representative must be supplied with a copy of this statement.

CONTACT INFORMATION

If you want to ask the Health Care Financing Administration to see, review, copy, or correct your personal health information which that Federal agency maintains in its HHA OASIS System of Records:

Call 1-800-638-6833, toll free, for assistance in contacting the HHA OASIS System Manager.
TTY for the hearing and speech impaired: 1-800-820-1202.

Federal Register / Vol. 64, No. 117 / Friday, June 18, 1999 / Notices   32991

Attachment C

Home Health Agency
Outcome and Assessment Information Set (OASIS)

NOTICE ABOUT PRIVACY
For Patients Who Do Not Have Medicare or Medicaid Coverage

- As a home health patient, there are a few things that you need to know about our collection of your personal health care information.

    - Federal and State governments oversee home health care to be sure that we furnish quality home health care services, and that you, in particular, get quality home health care services.

    - We need to ask you questions because we are required by law to collect health information to make sure that you get quality health care services.

    - We will make your information anonymous. That way, the Health Care Financing Administration, the federal agency that oversees this home health agency, cannot know that the information is about you.

- We keep anything we learn about you confidential.

This is a Medicare & Medicaid
Approved Notice.

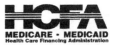

MEDICARE · MEDICAID
Health Care Financing Administration

Community Health Accreditation
    Program, 25
Community integration
    testing of, *99*, 117
    training in, by physical therapists,
        108, 218
Community services, OT assessment of,
    138
Competency assessment, 26-27, 32,
        294-304
    for OASIS, 206, *207-14*
    in pediatrics, 83
Compliance. *See also* Documentation
    hospice, 92
    Medicare, 13-14
Conditions of Participation
    changes in, 170, 172
    comprehensive assessment, 174-78
    Medicare Part A and, 9, 11
    OASIS and, 7
Consultation, SLP and, 125, 134
Continuing education, 27
Coordination, of care. *See* Care
        coordination
COPs. *See* Conditions of Participation
Cost-based reimbursement, 6-7
Costs, escalation of, 25
COTAs. *See* Certified occupational
        therapy assistants
Counseling, by SLP, 125
Cranial nerve integrity, testing of, *99*, 117
Cross training, 27, 32
Crutches. See Assistive devices
Cultural factors, in SLP, 128
Customer service, 33-36
    in hospice, 92
Customers. **See also** Caregivers; Patients
    defining, 35-36
CWF. *See* Common working file

D

DDST. *See* Denver Developmental
    Screening Test

Deductions, Medicare Part A and, 9
Denver Developmental Screening Test, 77
Diabetes education
    home care bag contents for, *31*
    Medicare and, 8
    referral requirements for, *63*
Diagnosis
    PT and, *97*, 104, 111
    for SLP referrals, *127*
    tracking visits by, 32
Diathermy therapy, coverage of, 46
Dietitians
    coverage of, 50
    home care bag contents for, *29*
    referral requirements for, *61*
    SLP and, 50
Disabled persons
    Medicare coverage of, 5
    resources on, 395
Discontinuation of services, by OT, 141,
        152-53
Disease management. *See* Health
        maintenance
DME. *See* Durable medical equipment
DMERCs, *12*
Doctor orders. *See* Physician orders
Documentation, 13, 14, 18-24. *See also*
        Form 485; OASIS
    of care coordination, 69-70
    of competency, 26-27, 32
    corrections on, 19
    on homebound status, 18
    for hospice, 92-93, *94*, 95
    of patient communication, 35-36
    in pediatrics, 77, *80-82*
    problems in, 22-24
    in PT, *106*, 113, 115, 119, 218
    in SLP, 128
    to support covered care, 14-15
Domains
    of home care, *3*, 3-4
    standardization of (*See* OASIS)

Pages in italics indicate figures or boxes

Pages in italics indicate figures or boxes

Pages in italics indicate figures or boxes

NOTES